Synopsis of Systemic
Pathology for Surgeons

Synopsis of Systemic Pathology for Surgeons

R.A.J. Spence MA, MD, FRCS(Ed), FRCS(I)
Consultant Surgeon, Belfast City Hospital, Belfast

J.M. Sloan MD, FRC(Path)
Consultant Pathologist, Royal Victoria Hospital, Belfast

G. McCluggage MB, MRC(Path)
Consultant Pathologist, Royal Victoria Hospital, Belfast

A member of the Hodder Headline Group
LONDON
Co-published in the USA by
Oxford University Press Inc., New York

First published in Great Britain in 2001 by
Arnold, a member of the Hodder Headline Group,
338 Euston Road, London NW1 3BH

http://www.arnoldpublishers.com

Co-published in the USA by
Oxford University Press Inc.,
198 Madison Avenue, New York, NY10016
Oxford is a registered trademark of Oxford University Press

Whilst the advice and information in this book are believed to be true and
accurate at the date of going to press, neither the authors nor the publisher
can accept any legal responsibility or liability for any errors or omissions
that may be made. In particular (but without limiting the generality of the
preceding disclaimer) every effort has been made to check drug dosages;
however, it is still possible that errors have been missed. Furthermore,
dosage schedules are constantly being revised and new side-effects
recognized. For these reasons the reader is strongly urged to consult the
drug companies' printed instructions before administering any of the drugs
recommended in this book.

British Library Cataloguing in Publication Data
A catalogue record for this book is available from the British Library

Library of Congress Cataloging-in-Publication Data
A catalog record for this book is available from the Library of Congress

ISBN 0 340 76378 7

1 2 3 4 5 6 7 8 9 10

Publisher: Geoffrey Smaldon
Production Editor: James Rabson
Production Controller: Bryan Eccleshall
Cover Design: Terry Griffiths

Typeset in 8/9 pt Palatino by Genesis Typesetting, Rochester, Kent
Printed and bound in Great Britain by MPG Books Ltd, Bodmin, Cornwall

What do you think about this book? Or any other Arnold title?
Please send your comments to feedback.arnold@hodder.co.uk

To Carol

JMS

To Ursula and Erin

GMcC

To Di, Robert, Andrew and Katherine

RAJS

Contents

Preface

This text has been written following the publication of two editions of our textbook *Pathology for Surgeons*. With the change in the examinations in postgraduate surgery, and with the advent of the MRCS and the Inter-Collegiate Fellowship, a rapid reference revision text was felt to be of benefit by our trainees and colleagues who examine in surgery.

The text is written by two consultant pathologists and a general surgeon with an interest in surgical pathology. One of us (RAJS) is an examiner on the Board of Examiners of the Royal Colleges of Surgeons of Ireland and of Edinburgh and is also an examiner in the Inter-Collegiate Fellowship Examination in General Surgery. The text, written in a synopsis format, has been revised where appropriate following the publication of the second edition of *Pathology for Surgeons*.

The text is written in an easy to understand systematic fashion which should allow easy and rapid revision. The text has been written to provide either the trainee surgeon, or indeed the established surgeon, who wants an easy and rapid referral to a particular condition, with access for information either for personal use or for teaching purposes. While the text is written primarily for surgeons in training, it will be of interest also to established surgeons in practice, and undergraduate students in medicine will find it to be useful for revision purposes.

We acknowledge the help and advice given by Dr Geoffrey Smaldon, of Butterworth-Heinemann, in the preparation and publication of this text.

RAJS
JMS
GMcC

Sources

Tables and figures in this book have been reproduced or adapted from the following sources.

Azzopardi, J.G. (1979) *Problems in Breast Pathology.* W.B. Saunders, London.

Davis, N.C. (1982) Malignant melanoma: clinical presentation and differential diagnosis. In: Emmett, A.J. and O'Rourke, M.G.E. (eds) *Malignant Skin Tumours.* Churchill Livingstone, Edinburgh.

Goligher, J.C. (1984) *Surgery of the Anus, Rectum and Colon.* Baillière Tindall, London.

Katzenstein, A.L. and Askin, F.B. (1982) *Surgical Pathology of Non-neoplastic Lung Disease.* W.B. Saunders, Philadelphia.

Medical Research Council's Working Party on Embryonal Tumours in Childhood (1978) Management of nephroblastoma in childhood. Clinical study of two forms of maintenance chemotherapy. *Arch. Dis. Child.* **53**, 112–119.

Olbourne, N.A. (1975) Choledochal Cysts. A review of the cystic anomalies of the biliary tree. *Ann. R. Coll. Surg. Engl.* **56**, 26–32.

Peckham, M.J. (1981) *The Management of Testicular Tumours.* Edward Arnold, London.

Pugh, R.C.B. (1976) *Pathology of the Testis.* Blackwell Science Publications, Oxford.

Robbins, S.L., Cotran, R.S. and Kumar, V. (1984) *Pathologic Basis of Disease,* 3rd edn. W.B. Saunders, Philadelphia.

Seifert, G., Miehlke, A., Haubrich, J. *et al.* (1986) *Diseases of the Salivary Glands: Pathology – Diagnosis – Treatment – Facial Nerve Surgery.* p. 171. Georg Thieme Verlag, Stuttgart.

Sufrin, G. (1982) The challenges of renal adenocarcinoma. In: Far, W.R. (ed.) *The Surgical Clinics of North America: Urological Surgery,* vol. 2, no. 6, pp 1101–1118. W.B. Saunders, Philadelphia.

Tompkins, R.K., Thomas, D., Wile, A. *et al.* (1981) Prognostic factors in bile duct carcinoma. Analysis of 96 cases. *Ann. Surg.* **194**, 447–457.

The oral cavity, salivary glands and neck ■ 1

Normal structure

- lined by squamous epithelium – keratinised on hard palate, lips and gingiva

TONGUE PAPILLAE

- filiform – small – keratinised
- fungiform – large – non-keratinised
- circumvallate – divides anterior two-thirds from posterior one-third
- accessory (minor) salivary glands are distributed throughout the oral mucosa
- anterior two-thirds of tongue arises from 1st and 2nd branchial arch
- posterior one-third of tongue arises from 3rd branchial arch

Traumatic lesions

TRAUMATIC ULCERS

- caused by sharp teeth
- linear
- heal in a few weeks

FIBROUS HYPERPLASIA

- tumour-like nodules of fibrous tissue
- common in cheek, lip, tongue, palate, gingiva
- may be denture induced

Infectious lesions – viral

ACUTE HERPETIC STOMATITIS

- cause: usually type I herpes simplex virus, rarely type II
- more common in children, adolescents
- grossly vesicles and/or ulcers
- microscopy shows viral inclusion bodies
- self-limiting
- 30% susceptible to recurrent infections

RECURRENT HERPES SIMPLEX

- presents as clear vesicle with red base
- virus persists in trigeminal nerve ganglia
- on lips – cold sores
- reactivated by variety of stimuli, e.g. febrile illness, sunlight
- self-limiting

COXSACKIE TYPE A

- acute infection (herpangina/acute oropharyngitis)
- self-limiting

INFECTIOUS MONONUCLEOSIS

- caused by Epstein-Barr virus
- small petechiae on palate
- pharyngitis common

Infectious lesions – bacterial

May be associated with immunodeficiency and malnutrition

ACUTE NECROTISING ULCERATIVE GINGIVITIS (VINCENT'S DISEASE)

- symbiotic organisms: *Borrelia vincentii* and *Fusiformis fusiformis*
- spread to cheeks in malnourished children

SYPHILIS

- primary, secondary or tertiary

TUBERCULOSIS

- ulcers on dorsum of tongue or lip
- microscopy shows caseating granulomas with Langhan's type giant cells

CERVICOFACIAL ACTINOMYCOSIS

- *Actinomyces israelii* is usual cause
- infection often follows surgical trauma or fractures
- sinuses are common
- pus contains sulphur granules

LUDWIG'S ANGINA

- spreading infection of submandibular space
- infection of lower molars
- oedema in floor of mouth, tongue

Infectious lesions – fungal

CANDIDOSIS

- due to *Candida albicans*
- acute candidosis (thrush, angular stomatitis)
- chronic candidosis (denture stomatitis, candidal leukoplakia, chronic mucocutaneous candidosis, angular stomatitis)
- may be associated with debility, antibiotics, AIDS

White lesions

WHITE SPONGE NAEVUS

- inherited
- any part of oral mucosa
- harmless lesion
- microscopically there is parakeratosis and acanthosis

SMOKERS' KERATOSIS

- usually lips
- microscopy shows epithelial atrophy and hyperkeratosis
- may get associated dysplasia

LICHEN PLANUS

- white lacy striae on buccal mucosa and tongue
- microscopy shows degeneration of basal layer of epidermis, 'saw-tooth' rete ridge pattern, lymphocyte infiltration in dermis
- occurs in 1% of population

LEUKOPLAKIA

'white patch or plaque which cannot be classified clinically or pathologically as another disease entity – WHO'

- essentially a clinical diagnosis with no specific histological implications
- microscopically ranges from simple hyperkeratosis and hyperplasia to severe dysplasia
- may develop squamous carcinoma
- higher risk of malignancy with females, iron deficiency, excess alcohol or smoking

TUMOURS OF ORAL CAVITY

Tumours of covering epithelium

SQUAMOUS PAPILLOMA

- benign, common
- sessile or pedunculated
- microscopy shows fronds of squamous epithelium with connective tissue core
- human papilloma virus may be a cause

EPITHELIAL DYSPLASIA AND CARCINOMA *IN SITU*

- may regress, remain static or progress
- microscopy shows nuclear pleomorphism, hyperchromatism and increased mitoses

SQUAMOUS CARCINOMA

Epidemiology and aetiology

- commonest malignant tumour of oral cavity
- 5% of all cancers in West, 50% of all cancers in India
- more common in males
- usually middle-aged or elderly
- steady decline in United Kingdom
- cigarette smoking, pipe and cigar smoking, tobacco chewing, (reversed smoking India), chewing betel nut
- alcohol excess
- Plummer-Vinson syndrome
- sunlight predisposes to lip cancer

Gross appearance

- change in colour of mucous membrane
- erythroplakia (red patch)
- ulceration
- exophytic lesions
- distribution – lip (25%), floor of mouth (15%), gingiva (10%), tongue (30%), buccal mucosa (10%), palate (10%)

Microscopically

- typical squamous carcinoma with epithelial nests and keratin pearls

Table 1.1 TNM Classification of oral cavity cancer

T1	<2 cm
T2	2–4 cm
T3	>4 cm
T4	Extension to bone or muscle
N1	Ipsilateral movable nodes
N2	Contralateral or bilateral movable nodes
N3	Fixed nodes
M0	No distant metastases
M1	Presence of distant metastases

Lip

- usually well differentiated
- more favourable prognosis than other types of oral cancer
- 5-year survival is 85%
- spread first to submental and submandibular nodes

Floor of mouth

- anterior floor usually
- usually well differentiated
- 5-year survival is 50%
- spread first to submandibular nodes

Tongue

- malignant ulcer with raised edges
- lateral border of middle third is commonest site followed by posterior third
- tumours of anterior two-thirds spreads to submental and submandibular nodes unilaterally
- tumours of posterior one-third spread to upper deep cervical nodes bilaterally
- tumours of tongue have least favourable prognosis of all intraoral squamous carcinomas
- 5-year survival is approximately 30%

Buccal mucosa

- usually adjacent to lower third molar teeth
- older patients
- aggressive
- spread to submandibular, deep cervical nodes

Gingiva

- well differentiated
- molar, premolar area
- lower jaw more often than upper
- spread to submandibular and deep cervical nodes
- 5-year survival is 40%

Palate

- more common in soft than hard palate, occasionally arises in uvula
- well differentiated
- direct invasion occurs
- spread to submandibular and deep cervical nodes

VARIANTS OF SQUAMOUS CARCINOMA OF THE ORAL MUCOSA

Verrucous carcinoma

- elderly men
- appears grossly as warty growth
- well differentiated microscopically
- good prognosis
- invades adjacent structures including bone
- absent or very late appearance of metastases
- radiotherapy contraindicated as risk of anaplastic transformation

Spindle cell carcinoma

- fleshy, polypoid tumour
- occurs after radiation
- microscopically may be mistaken for sarcoma

MALIGNANT MELANOMA

- 1% of oral tumours
- may originate in benign naevus or more commonly *de novo*
- occurs on hard palate
- may or may not be pigmented
- poor prognosis

BASAL CELL CARCINOMA

- usually upper lip
- arises from skin but may extend to mucocutaneous junction

Cysts and tumours of odontogenic epithelium

DENTAL CYST (RADICULAR CYST, PERIAPICAL CYST)

- commonest of odontogenic cysts
- apex of root of dead tooth

DENTIGEROUS CYST

- developmental in origin
- surrounds crown of unerupted tooth

ODONTOGENIC KERATOCYST

- lined by squamous epithelium
- may recur following operative removal
- associated with Gorlin Goltz syndrome – basal cell carcinoma of skin, skeletal anomalies, intracranial calcification, ocular defects

AMELOBLASTOMA (ADAMANTINOMA)

- tumour of intermediate malignancy
- most commonly arises in mandible (80%)
- slow growing but locally invasive
- microscopy shows palisading of cells (similar to basal cell carcinoma)
- molar region is most frequent location
- rarely metastasises

Connective tissue tumours

NERVE SHEATH TUMOURS

- neurofibromas and schwannomas
- if multiple may be associated with neurofibromatosis

HAEMANGIOMA

- occurs on lips and buccal mucosa
- on tongue may enlarge and obstruct airway
- if multiple –associated with Rendu-Weber-Osler disease

KAPOSI'S SARCOMA

- associated with AIDS

LYMPHANGIOMA

- most commonly occurs on tongue
- difficult to excise because of ramifying nature

MISCELLANEOUS CONDITIONS

Aphthous ulcers

- common on oral mucosa
- often multiple and recurrent
- cause unknown but may be trauma, stress, hormonal factors
- minor and major forms

MINOR

- common, shallow ulcers
- 10–40 year age group
- lasts for 4–10 days
- heals with no scar

MAJOR

- large painful ulcers
- lasts for 10–40 days
- heals with scar

Behcet's syndrome

- oral and genital ulcers
- uveitis, neurological disease
- predominantly young men

Crohn's disease

- may get aphthous ulcer, swelling of lips
- microscopically there may be granulomas

Median rhomboid glossitis

- dark red, rhomboidal area in midline of tongue
- may be painful
- candidal infection implicated in aetiology

Geographic tongue

- common condition (1–2% of population)
- smooth red tongue
- atrophy of filiform papillae
- cause unknown

Dermoid cyst

- 2% of dermoids occur in floor of mouth
- young adults
- squamous epithelial lining
- benign

Giant cell epulis

- red or maroon swelling of gingiva
- microscopically composed of spindle cells and giant cells
- benign

Congenital epulis

- occurs in newborn
- usually in maxillary region
- more common in females
- microscopy shows granular cells
- benign

Fibrous epulis

- common
- sessile or pedunculated swelling of gingiva
- microscopically there is fibroblastic proliferation and inflammation
- benign

Pregnancy epulis

- identical to pyogenic granuloma
- occurs in second and third trimesters of pregnancy
- microscopy shows inflamed vascular tissue
- benign

Granular cell tumour

- tongue is most common site
- presents as painless nodule
- occurs at any age

- Schwann cell origin
- usually benign, rarely malignant
- microscopy shows cells with abundant granular cytoplasm
- hyperplasia of overlying squamous epithelium may simulate carcinoma

Thyroglossal cyst

- arises at foramen caecum in posterior part of tongue and in floor of mouth

SALIVARY GLANDS

MAJOR

- parotid
- submandibular
- sublingual

MINOR

- accessory

Normal structure

PAROTID

- parotid sheath derived from deep cervical fascia
- facial nerve – 5 branches from anterior border
- Stensen's duct enters mouth opposite second upper molar tooth
- lymphatic drainage is to anterior-superior deep cervical nodes via intraparotid node
- microscopically composed mainly of serous acini

SUBMANDIBULAR

- superficial and deep lobes
- mylohyoid divides lobes
- Wharton's duct is long and narrow and prone to stone formation
- lymphatic drainage is to submandibular nodes
- microscopically is composed of serous and mucous acini

SUBLINGUAL

- smallest of major salivary glands
- lies above mylohyoid muscle in lingual sulcus of floor of mouth
- several ducts connect to oral cavity (largest is Bartholin duct)
- microscopically composed of serous and mucous acini

ACCESSORY

- dispersed within mucosa of oral cavity
- microscopically composed of serous or mucous acini

Salivary gland biopsy

- avoid incisional biopsy as risk of local recurrence of tumour
- care, as with parapharyngeal mass, chemodectoma is differential diagnosis
- fine needle aspiration (FNA) biopsy is accurate with no risk of tumour seedling
- trucut biopsy – avoid due to risk of tumour seedling
- frozen section – interpretation difficult

Non-neoplastic lesions of salivary glands

MUCOCOELE

- commonest lesion of accessory salivary glands
- occurs in submucosa of lips, floor of mouth
- either retention or extravasation cysts due to obstruction of duct
- recurrence common

CALCULI

- 90% in submandibular gland as Wharton's duct is long and narrow
- most common in middle-aged males
- pain and swelling after eating
- plasma calcium normal

Viral infections

- mumps is commonest cause of parotiditis
- children of school age

Bacterial infections

ACUTE SIALADENITIS

- most common in parotid
- may occur postoperatively
- systemic illness with pain and swelling
- retrograde infection from mouth is the main cause
- microscopy shows acute inflammatory infiltrate with abscesses

MYOEPITHELIAL SIALADENITIS (MESA)

- usually middle-aged females
- diffuse lymphocytic infiltration with lymphoepithelial lesions
- destruction of acini
- usually bilateral
- may predispose to lymphoma development

SICCA SYNDROME

- keratoconjunctivitis sicca and xerostomia (due to MESA in lacrimal glands and accessory salivary glands)

SJOGREN'S SYNDROME

- keratoconjunctivitis sicca, xerostomia and associated connective tissue disorder, usually rheumatoid arthritis

MIKULICZ'S SYNDROME

- clinical term
- bilateral lacrimal and salivary swellings due to a variety of causes, e.g. tuberculosis, sarcoidosis

SARCOIDOSIS

- parotid glands involved in 6% of cases
- microscopy shows non-caseating granulomas

Tumours of salivary glands

- incidence – approximately 1/100000 population
- 85% occur in parotid glands
- 10% occur in submandibular glands
- 5% occur in sublingual or minor glands
- 1/10 parotid tumours are malignant
- 1/3 submandibular tumours are malignant

CLASSIFICATION

Table 1.2 Classification of salivary gland neoplasms (Seifert *et al.* 1986)

ADENOMAS
Pleomorphic adenoma
Monomorphic adenoma
Cystadenolymphoma
Duct adenoma
Basal cell adenoma
Oncocytoma
Sebaceous adenoma
Clear cell adenoma
Other
MALIGNANT EPITHELIAL TUMOURS
Acinic cell tumour
Mucoepidermoid tumour
Carcinoma
Adenoid cystic carcinoma
Adenocarcinoma
Squamous cell carcinoma
Carcinoma ex-pleomorphic adenoma
Duct carcinoma
Undifferentiated carcinoma
Other
NON-EPITHELIAL TUMOURS
METASTATIC TUMOURS

Benign salivary gland tumours

PLEOMORPHIC ADENOMA

- commonest tumour
- occurs in any gland, but commonest in parotid
- painless mass with slow growth
- more common in males
- commonest in fourth and fifth decades
- preoperative diagnosis – FNA
- smooth and lobulated on gross appearance
- microscopically
  - epithelial and mesenchymal components
  - ducts lined by epithelial cells – chondromyxoid stroma
  - incomplete capsule
  - satellite nodules common
- treatment is superficial parotidectomy
- prone to recurrence due to satellite nodules and incomplete capsule
- small risk of malignant transformation, especially with repeated recurrences
- poor prognosis if malignant transformation occurs

MONOMORPHIC ADENOMAS

Adenolymphoma (Warthin's tumour)

- usually occur in sixth to seventh decades
- more common in males
- usually affect parotid
- 10% are bilateral
- preoperative diagnosis – FNA
- brown and cystic on gross appearance
- microscopically – cystic spaces lined by oncocytic epithelium, lymphocytic infiltration
- treatment is wide local excision
- benign

Oncocytoma (oxyphilic adenoma)

- rare
- elderly patients
- slightly more common in women
- usually encapsulated
- microscopically composed of large polygonal cells with eosinophilic cytoplasm
- benign

Other types of monomorphic adenoma

- rare
- parotid or minor salivary glands
- lip is commonest site
- basal cell adenoma, canalicular adenoma, tubular adenoma, trabecular adenoma, myoepithelioma

Malignant salivary gland tumours

MUCOEPIDERMOID CARCINOMA

- most common in parotid gland
- age – 20–60 years
- children and adults
- more common in females
- may have associated facial nerve palsy
- tan-yellow colour and cystic on gross appearance
- microscopy shows mucoid, squamoid (epidermoid) and intermediate cells in varying proportions
- classified as low, intermediate or high grade
- all have malignant potential
- local recurrence common
- prognosis dependent on stage, grade and adequacy of treatment
- low grade tumours rarely metastasise
- high grade tumours may metastasise to lung, brain and bone

ADENOID CYSTIC CARCINOMA

- most common in parotid
- more common in females
- usually fourth to sixth decades
- usually slow growing
- characteristically invades nerves
- tenderness, pain and facial nerve palsy common
- firm grey, white mass on gross appearance
- microscopy shows cribriform, tubular and solid patterns
- perineural invasion characteristic
- slowly growing but recurrences common
- late onset of metastases
- good 5-year survival but poor 10–20 year survival

ACINIC CELL CARCINOMA

- usually occurs in parotid
- more common in females
- occurs in children and adults
- usually slowly enlarging mass
- satellite lesions are common
- microscopy shows basophilic cells
- recurrence rate approximately 35%
- approximately 20% metastasise

ADENOCARCINOMA

- most common in parotid
- more common in women
- microscopy shows glandular formation
- prognosis depends on grade and stage

SQUAMOUS CARCINOMA

- most common in parotid
- more common in males
- rare
- aggressive with poor prognosis
- pain and nerve palsy are common
- may be associated with prior exposure to radiation

POLYMORPHOUS LOW GRADE ADENOCARCINOMA

- almost always affects minor salivary glands
- low grade tumour
- more common in females
- microscopically shows a polymorphous pattern
- characteristically shows perineural invasion
- prone to local recurrence

SALIVARY DUCT CARCINOMA

- high grade tumour
- rare
- most common in parotid
- more common in males
- microscopically resembles intraduct carcinoma of breast
- highly aggressive with tendency to lymphatic and vascular permeation
- poor prognosis

MISCELLANEOUS LESIONS IN THE NECK

Branchial cyst

- more common in males
- usually age 20–30 years
- fluctuant swelling – anterior to sternocleidomastoid muscle
- diagnosis – FNA
- straw-coloured fluid and cholesterol crystals on aspiration
- microscopy shows cystic spaces lined by squamous or columnar epithelium, lymphoid infiltration
- there may be superimposed infection
- carcinoma rarely develops

Branchial fistula and sinus

- arises from the second branchial cleft
- internal opening in posterior pillar of fauces
- mostly sinus; fistula is rare
- lined by ciliated columnar epithelium on histology

Thyroglossal duct cyst

- most cases clinically evident during childhood
- result of localised persistence of thyroglossal duct
- anywhere from foramen caecum of tongue to skin of suprasternal notch
- usually midline of neck in region of hyoid bone
- lined by squamous or columnar epithelium, may contain thyroid tissue

Carotid body tumours

- normal carotid body lies at bifurcation of carotid artery and has a chemoreceptor function
- hyperplasia occurs with chronic hypoxia, e.g. living at altitude
- alternative names for carotid body tumour are paraganglioma or chemodectoma
- painless lump in neck is presenting feature
- equal incidence in males and females
- age 30–60 years
- 10% have a positive family history
- 10% are bilateral
- macroscopically have a brown fleshy appearance
- microscopically contain polygonal cells with eosinophilic cytoplasm
- extremely vascular stroma
- usually benign but rarely malignant
- histology is not reliable means of predicting malignant behaviour
- risk of haemorrhage operatively

Cystic hygroma

- developmental anomaly with lymphatic origin
- multiloculated, cystic structure
- 50% present at birth
- microscopy shows multiple lymphatic spaces
- diagnosis is by CT or MRI
- may result in compressive symptoms

The oesophagus

2

NORMAL STRUCTURE

- oesophagus measures 25–30 cm in length and extends from the cricoid cartilage (C6) to the cardia (T11). The distal 2 cm is intra-abdominal
- the squamocolumnar junction at the lower end of the oesophagus is 40 cm from the incisor teeth and is recognised by an irregular line (Z line)
- oesophageal wall consists of mucosa (with a discontinuous muscularis mucosa), submucosa and a muscular layer (muscularis propria). The intra-abdominal part has a serosa
- epithelium is non-keratinising stratified squamous
- connective tissue papillae containing capillaries extend upward into the epithelium from the lamina propria. The submucosa contains oesophageal mucus glands
- muscle layer has inner circular and outer longitudinal coat. In the upper third the muscle is skeletal in type and merges with smooth muscle in the middle third. The lower third is composed of smooth muscle only
- oesophageal muscle is supplied by branches of vagus nerve. The oesophageal blood supply is from vessels arising directly from the aorta
- a lower oesophageal sphincter is present at the distal end of the oesophagus

CONGENITAL OESOPHAGEAL DISORDERS

Oesophageal atresia (OA) and tracheo-oesophageal fistula (TOF)

- oesophageal atresia (OA) occurs with or without tracheo-oesophageal fistula (TOF)
- incidence is 1 in 3000 births
- in some cases there are associated congenital heart problems, gastrointestinal anomalies, vertebral defects or renal anomalies
- chronic respiratory problems may persist into adult life as a result of aspiration secondary to a stricture following operative procedures
- the main types are shown in Figure 2.1

Duplications and cysts

- rare
- true duplication of a segment of oesophagus can occur
- oesophageal duplication cyst presents as a mediastinal mass (usually posterior)
- have a muscle coat and are lined by columnar or squamous epithelium
- may cause pressure on the oesophagus and trachea causing dysphagia and dyspnoea
- often associated with vertebral abnormalities

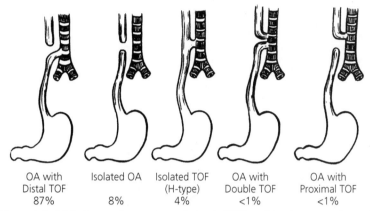

OA with	Isolated OA	Isolated TOF	OA with	OA with
Distal TOF		(H-type)	Double TOF	Proximal TOF
87%	8%	4%	<1%	<1%

Figure 2.1 Main types of oesophageal atresia (OA) and tracheo-oesophageal fistula (TOF)

Diverticula of the oesophagus

- defined as a pouch lined by epithelium
- due to either pressure from within (pulsion diverticulum) or traction from without (traction diverticulum)
- may cause dysphagia if a large diverticulum presses on the oesophageal wall

Congenital oesophageal web and stenosis

- occur usually in the upper oesophagus or at junction between the middle and lower thirds
- occur in combination with single or multiple oesophageal stenoses

Congenital diaphragmatic hernia

- due to maldevelopment of diaphragm
- abdominal contents herniate into thorax

MOTOR DISORDERS

Achalasia

- characterised by three abnormalities: absent oesophageal peristalsis, incomplete relaxation of lower oesophageal sphincter, and increased resting pressure of lower oesophageal sphincter
- affects males and females equally and usually presents between the ages of 35 and 45 years
- body of the oesophagus is grossly dilated with tapering of the lower end

- microscopically there is diminution of number or absence of ganglion cells and neurons particularly in the dilated segment
- superimposed inflammation is common
- overspill into the lungs results in aspiration pneumonia and lung abscess
- oesophageal squamous carcinoma is an uncommon but recognised complication

Chagas' disease

- caused by the protozoan *Trypanosoma cruzi*
- destroys the myenteric ganglia of oesophagus and other parts of the gut
- causes aperistalsis
- microscopically there is reduction in the number of ganglion cells
- may be associated with cardiomyopathy, megacolon and megaureter

Scleroderma and systemic sclerosis

- oesophageal involvement may be localised or part of a generalised systemic disorder
- 75% of patients with systemic sclerosis have oesophageal involvement
- smooth muscle of lower two-thirds of the oesophagus is involved. This becomes atrophied and fibrosed
- causes reduced peristalsis and decreased resting pressure of lower oesophageal sphincter
- produces incompetence with subsequent reflux
- Barrett's oesophagus and adenocarcinoma is a rare complication

REFLUX (PEPTIC) OESOPHAGITIS

- due to reflux of acid gastric contents into lower oesophagus
- symptoms of reflux oesophagitis are extremely common
- often obese females
- usually present with heartburn, worse after meals and associated with bending and smoking
- dysphagia is a later feature
- chest pain, indistinguishable from angina, occurs in 10% of patients
- main anti-reflux mechanisms are:
  - intrinsic physiological lower oesophageal sphincter (LOS) maintains resting pressure between 10 and 30 mmHg
  - intra-abdominal oesophagus acts as a flutter valve. The intra-abdominal pressure is higher than the intra-oesophageal pressure and causes closure of the intra-abdominal oesophagus
- failure of anti-reflux mechanisms may be due to an intrinsic defect in the LOS or increased intra-abdominal pressure
- other factors include the potency of the reflux material. A mixture of gastric acid and bile may be particularly harmful
- prolonged oesophageal clearance may also be a factor
- severe ulcerative oesophagitis appears at endoscopy as a red lower oesophagus with greyish/white areas of necrotic slough
- microscopically there is hyperplasia of the basal cell layer of the squamous epithelium

- microscopic criteria for a diagnosis of reflux oesophagitis are a basal zone thickness of greater than 15% of the total epithelial thickness and connective tissue papillae extending for more than two-thirds of the thickness of the epithelium. An acute inflammatory cell infiltrate consisting of eosinophils and neutrophils is also present
- poor correlation between symptoms and histology, especially with lesser degrees of oesophagitis

Complications

FIBROUS STRICTURE

- in some patients the inflammatory process heals by fibrosis with subsequent stricture formation

PEPTIC ULCERATION

- occurs in area of heterotopic gastric mucosa or in areas of columnar cell metaplasia
- may be associated with haemorrhage, stricture or perforation
- microscopically there is ulcerated mucosa, necrotic debris and granulation tissue

RESPIRATORY COMPLICATIONS

- reflux of gastric contents into the oesophagus causes bronchial hyperreactivity in patients with asthma

BARRETT'S OESOPHAGUS

- columnar cell lining epithelium of the lower oesophagus; also known as columnar epithelial-lined lower oesophagus (CELLO)
- caused by metaplastic replacement of normal squamous epithelium by columnar epithelium
- usually occurs as a continuous sheet but sometimes as scattered islands
- secondary to gastro-oesophageal reflux
- at endoscopy has a prominent red colour compared with normal pale oesophageal mucosa
- microscopically there are three types of epithelium:
  - specialised columnar epithelium resembling intestinal metaplasia of the stomach with goblet cells
  - junctional type epithelium similar to gastric cardia
  - gastric fundal/body type epithelium containing parietal cells
- specialised columnar epithelium with goblet cells is the commonest and some reserve the term Barrett's oesophagus for this type of epithelium
- many patients are asymptomatic but retrosternal pain, heartburn and dysphagia are common
- dysphagia is usually due to associated fibrous stricturing
- dysplasia occurs in the specialised columnar epithelium of Barrett's oesophagus in 25% of patients. Low grade dysplasia is most common but is of uncertain clinical significance. High grade dysplasia generally precedes or accompanies adenocarcinoma
- adenocarcinoma may arise in Barrett's oesophagus. The risk of developing adenocarcinoma in Barrett's oesophagus is 40 times that of the general population

HIATUS HERNIA

- in a sliding hiatus hernia the lower oesophageal sphincter is displaced into the thorax due to weakening of its diaphragmatic attachment. Contributory factors include an increase in intra-abdominal pressure, chronic coughing, kyphosis, obesity and pregnancy
- in a paraoesophageal hiatus hernia (rolling hernia) part of the stomach rotates anti-clockwise into the thorax
- a traumatic hiatus hernia is due to a breach in the diaphragm

Sliding hiatus hernia presenting in infancy (partial thoracic stomach)

- occurs in 1 in 400 births
- usually presents in the first week of life with persistent blood-stained vomiting
- the absence of an abdominal segment of oesophagus results in gastro-oesophageal incompetence and reflux oesophagitis

PATERSON-BROWN-KELLY SYNDROME (PLUMMER-VINSON SYNDROME)

- the association of post-cricoid oesophageal web, glossitis, koilonychia and iron-deficiency anaemia
- presents with dysphagia
- most common in women aged 40–50 years
- a post-cricoid web consists of a fold of squamous epithelium with a connective tissue core
- webs occlude most of lumen of oesophagus
- the syndrome is associated with a high incidence of post-cricoid squamous carcinoma

OESOPHAGEAL VARICES

- bleeding oesophageal varices account for 5% of admissions for haematemesis and melaena
- most are associated with liver cirrhosis. Some are associated with extrahepatic portal hypertension
- at endoscopy, oesophageal varices are seen as large blood vessels protruding longitudinally into the oesophageal lumen. If superficially placed, they appear blue or red, but if deeply placed they appear white in colour
- small red blebs (cherry-red spots or varices upon varices) may occur on the surface
- microscopically there are large venous channels in the oesophageal lamina propria and submucosa with small vascular channels within the squamous epithelium
- approximately 50% of patients admitted to hospital with bleeding varices will die during their first admission and most of the survivors will rebleed within 1 year
- only 25% survive for 2 years or more. Patients with extrahepatic portal hypertension have good liver function and a better prognosis. Patients with liver cirrhosis have poor liver function and a poor prognosis
- varices are difficult to detect at autopsy as they collapse after death

MALLORY-WEISS SYNDROME

- due to vomiting and severe retching
- there are partial oesophageal tears, usually just above cardia
- may be associated with severe haemorrhage

OESOPHAGEAL PERFORATION

- instrumental perforation is probably the commonest cause. This may occur during rigid oesophagoscopy, dilatation of strictures, attempted intubation and variceal tamponade
- spontaneous perforation occurs after alcohol excess or in association with severe vomiting
- ingestion of fish bones and other foreign objects may result in perforation
- perforation may follow the ingestion of corrosive compounds
- benign ulcers of the oesophagus may also perforate
- oesophageal carcinoma may rarely perforate
- mediastinitis, empyema and surgical emphysema are usual complications

INFECTIOUS LESIONS OF THE OESOPHAGUS

- multiple infections may occur in association with AIDS (see Chapter 22)

Candidal oesophagitis

- usual cause is *Candida albicans*, although other candidal species may be involved
- may occur with or without associated oral infection
- predisposing factors include broad spectrum antibiotics, steroids, immuno-suppression
- candidal organisms may colonise pre-existing ulcers
- presenting features are dysphagia and retrosternal pain
- in early stages white mucosal plaques are seen on endoscopy. Later the mucosa becomes necrotic and ulcerated

Herpes simplex oesophagitis

- most common visceral site of infection
- may be associated with immunosuppression
- usually type I herpes simplex virus
- virus may cause oesophageal infection either by direct spread from the mouth or by reactivation of the virus in the sensory ganglia of vagus nerve
- usually middle and distal thirds of oesophagus affected
- painful multiple ulcers occur on the oesophageal mucosa
- microscopy may show characteristic intranuclear inclusion bodies
- immunohistochemistry using specific antiviral antibody is useful in diagnosis

Chemical and drug-induced oesophagitis

- following ingestion of corrosive fluids, hot substances, drugs
- ulceration followed by healing with fibrous stricture formation

BENIGN TUMOURS OF THE OESOPHAGUS

Squamous papilloma

- rare
- sessile lesion composed of papillary projections of squamous epithelium
- may be multiple and associated with human papilloma virus (HPV) infection
- little or no malignant potential

Fibrous polyp

- relatively common
- occurs anywhere within the oesophagus as a fleshy pedunculated polyp
- may ulcerate and cause haemorrhage
- consists of a connective tissue core covered by squamous epithelium

Leiomyoma

- most common benign tumour of the oesophagus
- more common in males
- occurs most often in the lower oesophagus
- arises in the muscularis mucosa or more commonly in the muscularis propria
- may present as a polypoid intraluminal mass, as an intramural tumour or rarely projects to the external surface of the oesophagus
- microscopically composed of bundles of regular spindle-shaped cells
- may get malignant forms (leiomyosarcoma)
- behaviour difficult to predict from histology. The most reliable indicators of malignancy are cellularity, number of mitoses, tumour size, necrosis

Granular cell tumour

- rare
- usually presents as polyp
- benign
- microscopically composed of cells with abundant granular cytoplasm
- Schwann cell origin

Neurofibroma

- rare submucosal tumour
- may be sporadic or multiple in association with von Recklinghausen's disease

MALIGNANT TUMOURS OF THE OESOPHAGUS

Oesophageal carcinoma

- the most common type is squamous carcinoma
- in recent years there has been a marked increase in the incidence of adenocarcinoma involving the lower oesophagus. In some regions this is now more common than squamous carcinoma
- squamous carcinoma of the oesophagus has a high incidence in areas of Iran and China
- heavy intake of tobacco and/or alcohol are common predisposing factors
- dietary factors also important, e.g. consumption of hot beverages
- genetic influences are of minor importance with the exception of tylosis, a rare autosomal dominant condition associated with hyperkeratosis of palms and soles and high risk of oesophageal squamous carcinoma
- predisposing factors to development of squamous carcinoma include Paterson-Brown-Kelly syndrome, strictures and previous irradiation
- half of squamous carcinomas arise in the middle third of the oesophagus
- squamous carcinoma of the middle and lower thirds is more common in males
- post-cricoid carcinoma is more common in females and may be associated with Paterson-Brown-Kelly syndrome
- adenocarcinoma is most common in the lower oesophagus and usually arises within specialised columnar epithelium of Barrett's oesophagus. May also rarely arise from submucosal oesophageal glands
- microscopically squamous carcinomas of the oesophagus consist of nests of squamous cells with central keratin pearls. Adenocarcinomas are composed of glandular structures with varying degrees of mucus secretion
- lymphatic spread occurs early due to the rich submucosal lymphatic network
- lung and liver are common sites of distant blood-borne spread
- the TNM system of clinical staging is shown in Table 2.1.
- in Western series the prognosis is poor. Five-year survival is approximately 10% for squamous carcinoma
- lymph node metastases and venous invasion are important independent prognostic factors
- early oesophageal cancer indicates tumour confined to mucosa and submucosa. The prognosis is much better than that of advanced cancer

Carcinosarcoma

- a rare tumour in which both epithelial and connective tissue stromal elements are malignant
- often presents as polypoid mass
- better prognosis than other malignant tumours due to metastases occurring late
- normally the sarcomatous element metastasises

Leiomyosarcoma

- see section on leiomyoma (p. 22)
- rare and differs from leiomyoma in having areas of increased cellularity, high mitotic count and necrosis
- borderline lesions occur in which the behaviour cannot be predicted
- prognosis is better than carcinoma

Table 2.1   TNM pretreatment clinical classification

Tis   Preinvasive carcinoma (carcinoma-*in-situ*)

T0   No evidence of primary tumour

T1   Tumour involving 5 cm or less of the oesophageal length, producing no obstruction, does not involve the entire circumference of the oesophagus and shows no evidence of extra-oesophageal spread

T2   Tumour involving more than 5 cm of the oesophageal length and with no evidence of extra-oesophageal spread, or tumour of any size producing obstruction and/or involvement of the entire circumference of the oesophagus but with no extra-oesophageal spread

T3   Tumour with evidence of extra-oesophageal spread, such as recurrent laryngeal, phrenic or sympathetic nerve involvement, fistula formation, involvement of trachea or bronchial tree, vena cava or azygos vein obstruction or malignant effusion

Cervical oeseophagus
N0   No evidence of regional lymph node involvement
N1   Evidence of involvement of movable unilateral regional nodes
N2   Evidence of involvement of movable bilateral regional nodes
N3   Evidence of fixed regional nodes

Thoracic oesophagus
N0   No evidence of regional node involvement on exploration or mediastinoscopy
N1   Involved regional nodes

Distant metastases
M0   No evidence
M1   Presence of distal metastases

Malignant melanoma

- rare primary tumour of the oesophagus
- usually in the elderly
- may be black in colour
- usually occurs in the middle or lower third of the oesophagus
- need to exclude secondary spread from a primary elsewhere
- prognosis is poor

Small cell undifferentiated (oat cell) carcinoma

- rare
- highly aggressive tumour
- shows neuroendocrine differentiation with immunohistochemistry or electron microscopy
- prognosis poor, most patients die within a year
- secondary spread from a primary bronchial small cell carcinoma must be excluded
- treatment with chemotherapy and/or radiotherapy is more effective than surgery

Secondary tumours

- rare
- most commonly direct spread from gastric, bronchial or thyroid carcinoma
- lymphatic or vascular spread from other sites

Leukaemias and lymphomas

- rare
- usually secondary involvement of oesophagus

The stomach and duodenum

3

NORMAL STRUCTURE OF STOMACH

- the stomach is divided anatomically into four parts: the cardia surrounds the oesophagogastric junction; the fundus lies above a horizontal line drawn through the cardia; the body is between the fundus and the incisura; the antrum is between the body and the pylorus
- the fundus and body have thick mucosal folds. Beyond the incisura the antral mucosa is flat
- the stomach wall consists of mucosa, submucosa, muscularis propria and serosa (Figure 3.1)
- three types of mucosa are seen in the stomach:
  1. Cardiac mucosa containing mucus-secreting glands

  2. Body and fundal mucosa containing test-tube shaped glands incorporating large numbers of parietal cells (produce acid and intrinsic factor) and chief cells (produce pepsin)

  3. Antral or pyloric mucosa containing glands mainly lined by mucus-secreting cells. Gastrin-producing cells (G cells) and other neuroendocrine cells are found in this area. A tongue of antral mucosa extends proximally along the lesser curvature

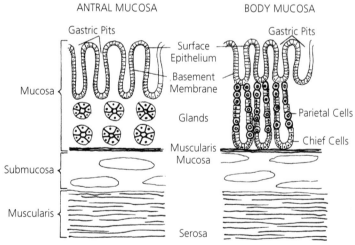

Figure 3.1 Schematic diagram to show the structure of antral and body gastric mucosa

- blood supply of stomach is from the coeliac axis. The main arteries are the left and right gastric arteries and left and right gastroepiploic arteries; short gastric arteries supply the fundus
- venous drainage is to the portal vein
- lymphatic drainage is to the left and right gastric nodes, subpyloric nodes, pancreatic nodes, splenic nodes and right gastroepiploic nodes

NORMAL STRUCTURE OF DUODENUM

- adult duodenum is 20–25 cm in length
- almost entirely retroperitoneal
- divided anatomically into four parts
- pancreatic and bile ducts open into second part
- duodenal wall consists of mucosa, submucosa, muscularis propria and serosa
- mucosa contains numerous villous processes
- blood supply of upper duodenum is from coeliac axis. The remainder of the duodenum receives blood supply from superior mesenteric artery
- venous drainage is to the superior mesenteric and portal veins

GASTRIC BIOPSY

- adequate numbers of biopsies (at least six) should be taken at endoscopy from any significant lesion to minimise sampling error
- biopsy from the edge of an ulcer is more informative than from the base which may be covered with necrotic slough

DUODENAL BIOPSY

- must be properly orientated to assess villous pattern

CONGENITAL CONDITIONS

Infantile hypertrophic pyloric stenosis

- see p. 3

Duodenal atresia

- atresia is complete loss of continuity
- duodenal atresias account for 40% of small bowel atresias and are associated with Down's syndrome
- may be due to vascular insufficiency during fetal development
- incompatible with survival unless promptly recognised and bypassed surgically

ULCERS AND EROSIONS

- an erosion is a mucosal defect which does not penetrate the muscularis mucosa
- an acute ulcer penetrates the muscularis mucosa but contains no fibrous tissue
- a chronic ulcer is one in which fibrous tissue is formed in the base of the ulcer

Acute erosions and ulcers

- causes of acute erosions and ulcers are given in Table 3.1
- usually occur in stomach
- Cushing's ulcers or erosions occur secondary to intracranial disease or surgery. These are prone to perforation
- acute erosions and ulcers appear 3–6 days following the stressful event
- present as haematemesis, melaena or perforation
- also known as acute haemorrhagic gastritis or acute stress ulcers
- the lesions are multiple, usually occur in the fundus and body and seldom exceed 0.5 cm in diameter
- often dark red due to altered blood
- surrounding mucosa is congested and contains petechial haemorrhages
- acute ulcers are larger than erosions and are associated with more severe bleeding

Table 3.1   Causes of acute erosions and ulcers

Drugs – aspirin, indomethacin, other NSAIDs, alcohol
Cushing's ulcers
Stress ulcers
Trauma
Surgery
Sepsis
Burns (Curling's ulcer)
Myocardial infarction
Respiratory failure

Chronic peptic ulcer

- occurs in stomach or duodenum
- the course of chronic peptic ulcer disease has been radically altered in recent years following the introduction of efficient therapeutic suppression of gastric acid secretion (H_2-receptor antagonists and proton pump inhibitors). The value of therapy to eradicate *Helicobacter pylori* is now apparent
- most patients do not now require surgical treatment
- chronic peptic ulceration is a multifactorial disease and occurs when there is a disturbance in the balance between secretion of acid/pepsin and mucosal resistance
- factors important in the pathogenesis of chronic peptic ulcer include:
  1. *Helicobacter pylori*
     - Gram-negative bacterium possessing urease activity
     - found in the mucus layer on the surface of gastric mucosa, especially antral mucosa

- causes chronic active gastritis
- microscopically associated with neutrophil infiltration of lamina propria
- found in 90% of patients with chronic duodenal and 70% with chronic gastric ulcer
- probably the major aetiological factor in chronic peptic ulcer
- Giemsa stain is useful for demonstration of organisms in histological sections
- eradication of the organism is usually associated with permanent ulcer healing

2. Acid secretion
   - peptic ulceration does not occur in achlorhydria
   - duodenal ulcer patients often have increased fasting and stimulated gastric acid levels, especially at night
   - Zollinger-Ellison syndrome is characterised by marked hyperacidity (due to gastrin secretion) and is a rare cause of severe and often multiple duodenal ulceration
   - in gastric ulcer patients acid secretion is normal or even low

3. Mucosal defence mechanisms
   - surface mucus layer traps bicarbonate secreted by surface epithelial cells and forms a protective coat
   - this layer is vulnerable to ischaemia, aspirin and related drugs

4. Prostaglandins
   - endogenous prostaglandin production in the gastric mucosa increases mucosal blood flow, bicarbonate secretion and mucus secretion

5. Drugs
   - aspirin and other non-steroidal anti-inflammatory drugs (NSAIDs) may cause acute gastric erosions
   - chronic use of such drugs is associated with peptic ulcer disease (especially in the elderly)

6. Miscellaneous
   - other aetiological factors include stress, bile reflux and smoking
   - duodenal ulceration is more common in blood group O

Pathology

- gastric ulcers usually occur in antral mucosa on the lesser curvature
- most gastric ulcers are less than 3 cm in diameter
- large gastric ulcers raise the possibility of malignancy
- the base of a chronic peptic ulcer is composed of fibrous tissue. This contracts and results in radiating mucosal folds adjacent to the ulcer
- 90% of chronic duodenal ulcers occur in the first part of the duodenum
- anterior wall is the commonest site of duodenal ulceration
- 10–15% of duodenal ulcers are multiple
- microscopically chronic peptic ulcers are composed of necrotic tissue with fibrinous exudate on the surface and granulation tissue with fibroblasts and immature blood vessels and mature dense fibrous tissue in the base of the ulcer
- blood vessels in the ulcer base show thickening of the vessel wall (endarteritis obliterans)

Complications

HAEMORRHAGE

- haemorrhage is the commonest complication with a mortality of 4–10%
- mortality is more likely with recurrent haemorrhage and in the elderly
- most bleeding peptic ulcers will heal spontaneously. In the remainder, endoscopy frequently shows a visible vessel in the ulcer base

PERFORATION

- perforation is much more common in duodenal than gastric ulcer
- the usual site of perforation is the anterior duodenal wall
- ingestion of NSAIDs contributes to perforation in elderly patients

STENOSIS

- peptic ulceration (especially in region of pylorus or first part of duodenum) may result in local fibrosis and stenosis with signs of obstruction

MALIGNANT TRANSFORMATION

- the term ulcer-cancer denotes a chronic peptic ulcer with carcinoma in its margins
- should be distinguished from ulcerating carcinoma
- rarely occurs in chronic gastric ulcer and almost never in chronic duodenal ulcer

PATHOLOGY OF THE POSTOPERATIVE STOMACH

- after surgery for benign ulcer disease, a range of abnormalities may occur in the stomach or duodenum. These include:

1. Lesser curve necrosis may occur after proximal gastric vagotomy. This presents with perforation

2. Afferent loop obstruction occurs after Polya gastrectomy or gastrojejunostomy. The acute variety may be caused by internal herniation of the afferent loop, oedema around the stoma or intussusception of jejunal mucosa into stomach. The chronic variety presents as bile vomiting after meals. Secretion of bile and pancreatic fluid is stimulated by a meal and accumulates under pressure in the afferent loop which is partially obstructed by adhesions, herniation or kinking

3. Postoperative bile gastritis
   - bile reflux is associated with burning epigastric pain and bilious vomiting
   - microscopically there is oedema, foveolar hyperplasia and presence of smooth muscle fibres in the lamina propria of the stomach

4. Recurrent ulcer
   - recurrence after duodenal ulcer surgery occurs at stoma or in the duodenum
   - occasionally recurrent ulceration occurs in the stomach due to stasis following inadequate drainage
   - after proximal gastric vagotomy and/or vagotomy and pyloroplasty recurrence is invariably in the duodenum
   - after vagotomy and gastroenterostomy or Polya gastrectomy it is more common at the stoma

5. Postoperative gastric carcinoma
   - the risk of gastric carcinoma increases significantly 15–20 years after gastric surgery
   - risk is higher after surgery for gastric ulcer than for duodenal ulcer
   - cancer most frequently occurs around the stoma and has a poor prognosis
   - postoperative patients with dysplastic mucosal changes on biopsy should be closely followed up

GASTRIC OUTLET OBSTRUCTION (PYLORIC STENOSIS)

Causes include:

Peptic ulcer

- occurs in 1% of peptic ulcer patients
- presents with vomiting and signs of destruction

Infantile hypertrophic pyloric stenosis

- occurs in 2.5 per 1000 live births in UK
- four times more common in males
- usually presents between second and fourth weeks of life
- polygenic pattern of inheritance with increased risk in siblings
- association with other congenital intestinal obstruction
- pylorus is increased in length and diameter, duodenum is not affected
- circular muscle layer is markedly thickened due to hyperplasia and hypertrophy of muscle cells. The stomach proximal to the obstruction is dilated
- operative procedure is pyloromyotomy (Ramstedt's procedure)

Adult hypertrophic pyloric stenosis

- aetiology unknown
- may be manifestation of less severe form of infantile disease
- pylorus is grossly thickened
- microscopy shows hyperplasia of circular muscle layers

Carcinoma and other gastric tumours

- a short history of pyloric stenosis in middle-aged or elderly patients raises the suspicion of gastric malignancy
- biopsy is essential
- other tumours such as malignant lymphoma may also result in pyloric stenosis

Other miscellaneous causes

- annular pancreas
- extrinsic adhesions
- Crohn's disease
- mucosal diaphragm

GASTRITIS, GASTRIC ATROPHY, INTESTINAL METAPLASIA AND DYSPLASIA

- gastritis is characterised by neutrophils (acute gastritis), mononuclear cells (chronic gastritis), or most commonly both types of cells (active chronic gastritis) in mucosa of stomach
- atrophy implies loss of the specialised cells of gastric glands, either the acid- and pepsin-producing cells of the body and fundus, or the mucus and endocrine cells of the antrum
- intestinal metaplasia is characterised by replacement of gastric epithelial cells by intestinal type cells
- dysplasia implies premalignant cellular atypia of epithelial cells confined to gastric glands

Acute gastritis

- acute gastritis is common and is usually transitory requiring no treatment
- in severe cases acute gastritis may be associated with multiple gastric erosions
- may be caused by alcohol or aspirin and related drugs
- acute phlegmonous or suppurative gastritis is rare. This implies acute suppurative inflammation of the full thickness of the stomach wall. The most common implicated organisms are haemolytic streptococci. If gas-forming organisms are responsible the condition is known as emphysematous gastritis

Chronic gastritis

TYPE A

- relatively uncommon
- principally affects the mucosa of the body of the stomach
- mucosa is atrophic, flat and thin
- microscopy shows loss of parietal and chief cells and a scanty chronic inflammatory cell infiltrate
- characterised by extensive intestinal metaplasia
- most frequently seen in association with pernicious anaemia (PA)
- PA patients have antibodies to parietal cells and often to intrinsic factor/vitamin B12 complex
- parietal cell loss results in hypochlorhydria or achlorhydria
- gastrin (G) cell hyperplasia occurs, occasionally resulting in the formation of small neuroendocrine tumours
- increased risk of gastric dysplasia and carcinoma

TYPE B

- relatively common and affects both antrum and body of stomach
- microscopy shows infiltration of the upper part of the lamina propria by neutrophils, lymphocytes and plasma cells. Lymphoid follicle formation may occur
- presence of neutrophils indicates activity
- may get atrophy of mucosal glands
- *Helicobacter pylori* infection in the gastric mucus layer and within gastric pits is the commonest cause of type B gastritis

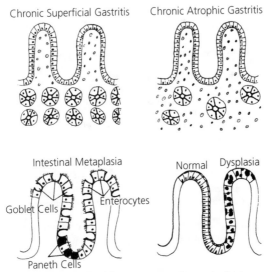

Figure 3.2   Schematic diagram to demonstrate the main features of chronic superficial gastritis, chronic atrophic gastritis, intestinal metaplasia and dysplasia

- organisms most commonly occur in the antrum of the stomach but may also be found within the body
- there is poor correlation between symptoms, endoscopic appearances and histological gastritis

TYPE C

- type C or reflux gastritis is associated with bile reflux
- most pronounced in the postoperative stomach
- microscopy shows oedema of the lamina propria, foveolar hyperplasia and paucity of inflammatory cells
- a similar histological picture may be seen with chronic NSAID ingestion
- a recent semiquantitative system for the histological classification of gastritis (the Sydney system) recognises acute, chronic and special forms. In this system the degree of inflammation, atrophy and intestinal metaplasia are evaluated

Intestinal metaplasia (IM)

(see Figure 3.2)

- there is focal replacement of gastric mucosa by intestinal epithelium
- common in the general population
- marked increase in incidence with advancing age
- commonly associated with mucosal atrophy
- may occur in type A or B gastritis
- intestinal-type gastric cancers may arise in areas of intestinal metaplasia

Dysplasia

(see Figure 3.2)
- dysplasia can only be diagnosed microscopically and cannot be recognised endoscopically
- microscopically there are large, irregular, hyperchromatic nuclei, loss of cellular polarity and glandular architectural abnormality
- low grade dysplasia may regress but high grade dysplasia may be associated with or may progress to carcinoma
- diagnosis of dysplasia in biopsy necessitates careful follow up

DUODENITIS

- duodenal ulcer symptoms
- endoscopy shows inflamed, friable duodenal mucosa, sometimes with superficial erosions
- gastric metaplasia is often present. This consists of islands of gastric mucosa which may be colonised by *Helicobacter pylori*

GASTRIC POLYPS

Epithelial polyps

- two main types are recognised:
  1. Hyperplastic or regenerative polyps
     - sessile, found in the presence of gastritis
     - single or multiple
     - commonest in gastric antrum
     - probably arise on the basis of excessive regeneration following mucosal change
     - microscopically show elongated gastric pits, cystic dilatation of glands, oedema and inflammation
     - have little or no malignant potential
  2. Adenomatous polyps
     - sessile or pedunculated
     - predominate in antrum
     - microscopically have tubulovillous pattern. Glands are lined by epithelial cells showing intestinal metaplasia and dysplasia
     - have considerable malignant potential, especially if over 2 cm diameter
     - patients with familial adenomatous polyposis (FAP) may have gastric adenomatous polyps
     - also associated with pernicious anaemia

Other polyps

These include:
1. Heterotopias (presence of tissue not normally found in the area)
   - commonest is pancreatic tissue, usually situated in the submucosa of the pylorus

2. Fundic gland polyps
   - often multiple
   - usually occur in the fundus and body
   - microscopically consist of cystic glands lined by parietal cells
   - do not possess malignant potential
   - may be associated with familial adenomatous polyposis (FAP)

3. Hamartomas (abnormal development of tissues which are normally found in the area)
   - Peutz-Jeghers' and juvenile polyps may occur in the stomach (see Chapter 4)

4. Inflammatory fibroid polyps
   - small polyps, usually occurring singly in the antrum
   - microscopically show vascular connective tissue and inflammatory cells, especially eosinophils
   - no malignant potential

5. Cronkhite-Canada syndrome
   - unknown aetiology, no familial tendency
   - gastrointestinal polyposis associated with alopecia, atrophy of nails and skin pigmentation
   - patients usually get watery diarrhoea
   - grossly polyps have a glistening appearance
   - microscopically there is oedema and cystic change in glands

GASTRIC CANCER

Epidemiology, aetiology and pathogenesis

- gastric cancer shows marked geographical variation in its incidence
- common in Japan, China, Columbia and Brazil, while Canada, USA and Australia have a low incidence
- incidence has declined in Western countries over the past 30 years
- while incidence of carcinoma of the distal stomach has declined, that of the proximal stomach has increased markedly
- maximum incidence is 55–65 year age group
- incidence is greater in males than females
- diet has been incriminated in various high risk areas. There is an increased risk with high consumption of salt, and preserved meat together with low consumption of fresh fruit and vegetables
- N-nitroso compounds are potent carcinogens in experimental animals
- bacteria in gastric juice reduce dietary nitrate to nitrite and then further reduce nitrite to N-nitroso compounds
- emigrants from Japan (high-risk area) to the USA (low-risk area) exhibit a fall in incidence supporting the influence of environmental factors
- *Helicobacter pylori* infection has been implicated in the pathogenesis of gastric cancer

Pre-malignant conditions

- atrophic gastritis and intestinal metaplasia are common and are associated with an increased risk of gastric cancer

- pernicious anaemia is associated with severe and widespread atrophic gastritis and intestinal metaplasia and an increased risk of gastric cancer

Pathology

- almost all are adenocarcinomas
- the antrum is the commonest site of gastric carcinoma
- most cancers are nodular or ulcerating
- 7% show diffuse infiltration of the wall of the stomach (linitis plastica)
- one of the most commonly used histological classifications is the Lauren classification which recognises intestinal and diffuse type adenocarcinomas
- microscopically intestinal adenocarcinomas show attempted glandular formation and the surrounding mucosa often shows intestinal metaplasia
- microscopically diffuse adenocarcinoma is composed of sheets or columns of tumour cells with little or no attempt at glandular formation. Signet ring cells containing mucin are characteristic

Spread

- direct spread through and within the gastric wall occurs early
- gastric mucosa is rich in lymphatics and lymphatic spread occurs early. The pattern of spread depends on the location of the tumour within the stomach. Pancreatic and splenic nodes are commonly affected
- blood spread to liver and lung
- transperitoneal spread may result in bilateral involvement of ovaries (Krukenberg tumours)
- peritoneal seedling by tumour may occur

Prognosis

- overall 5-year survival for advanced cancer after gastrectomy is 20–30%
- much better results for early gastric cancer (see below)
- approximately one-third of patients in whom tumour has infiltrated to the serosa of the stomach have metastatic spread to lymph nodes
- when tumour extends beyond the serosa the proportion with lymph node metastases rises to 80%

Early gastric cancer (EGC)

- defined as cancer confined to the mucosa or submucosa irrespective of lymph node involvement
- frequently multifocal. Lymph node metastases are present in 15–20%
- in Japan up to 30% of gastric cancers are resected at the EGC stage. This is because of screening programmes for gastric cancer
- in the West the proportion is much smaller
- prognosis is much better than in advanced gastric cancer
- 5-year survival is up to 90%
- when lymph nodes are involved the 5-year survival rate is around 75%

OTHER GASTRIC TUMOURS

Carcinoid tumours

- about 50% are associated with atrophic gastritis and in this setting are often multiple
- most commonly found in the antrum of stomach
- usually benign or of low grade malignancy
- those not associated with atrophic gastritis are usually solitary and are more likely to exhibit malignant behaviour
- tumours are typically yellow on cut surface
- microscopically show insular and trabecular arrangements of tumour cells

Stromal tumours

- spindle cell tumours arising in the submucosa or muscularis propria of the stomach and other parts of the intestine are now grouped under the term gastrointestinal stromal tumours (GIST)
- may show smooth muscle, neural or non-specific mesenchymal differentiation
- those showing smooth muscle differentiation are also known as leiomyomas, leiomyoblastomas or leiomyosarcomas
- stromal tumours can occur throughout the gastrointestinal tract but are most common in the stomach and small intestine
- they vary greatly in size. Large tumours may ulcerate the overlying mucosa causing haematemesis, melaena or anaemia
- microscopically they are composed of spindle shaped cells
- prognosis is unpredictable
- lesions greater than 5 cm in size should be regarded as at least potentially malignant
- mitotic activity, necrosis and cellular pleomorphism may also be related to prognosis
- small low grade tumours have a good prognosis but high grade tumours have a 5-year survival rate of 30–40%
- those showing neural differentiation may be associated with von Recklinghausen's disease (neurofibromatosis)

MALIGNANT LYMPHOMA

- the stomach is the commonest site for primary gut lymphoma but it is much less common than gastric carcinoma
- gastric lymphomas are the commonest of the mucosa-associated lymphoid tissue (MALT) lymphomas
- gastric lymphomas usually occur in the antrum
- may resemble carcinoma on endoscopy and clinical presentation
- microscopically the majority are non-Hodgkin's lymphomas of B-cell origin. Most are low grade
- gastric lymphoma is related to *Helicobacter pylori* infection
- eradication of *Helicobacter pylori* may result in regression of some cases of early low grade lymphoma
- prognosis is better than gastric carcinoma or nodal malignant lymphoma

- tend to remain localised to the stomach
- overall prognosis is good
- most lesions previously reported as gastric pseudolymphoma probably represent low grade lymphomas

OTHER GASTRIC NEOPLASMS

- other gastric neoplasms are rare and include lipoma, plasmacytoma, glomus tumour, granular cell tumour and Kaposi's sarcoma (usually in the setting of AIDS)

TUMOURS OF THE DUODENUM

- these are rare

Adenoma

- Brunner's gland adenomas are found in the duodenum and may present with melaena. They consist of collections of Brunner's glands and are benign
- tubular, tubulovillous and villous adenomas, similar to those found in the large intestine also occur
- these are found mainly in the region of the ampulla of Vater and most often have a villiform pattern
- dysplasia is common and malignant transformation may occur
- patients with familial adenomatous polyposis (FAP) and Gardner's syndrome may have duodenal adenomas

Carcinoma

- duodenal carcinoma is rare and usually involves the first or second part of the duodenum, especially around the ampulla of Vater
- some may arise on the basis of a pre-existing adenoma
- periampullary tumours frequently present with obstructive jaundice
- microscopically they are adenocarcinomas and vary from well differentiated papillary lesions to anaplastic or signet ring carcinomas
- may rarely be associated with coeliac or Crohn's disease
- prognosis depends on histological grade and tumour stage
- periampullary carcinomas tend to be well differentiated tumours with invasion limited to the wall of the common bile duct and have a 5-year survival rate of over 70%
- neoplasms elsewhere tend to be more advanced at operation and the overall 5-year survival is around 20%

Other duodenal neoplasms

- carcinoid tumours may arise in the duodenum, as in other parts of the small intestine

- gangliocytic paraganglioma is a rare neuroendocrine tumour, usually confined to the duodenum. It may occur in association with von Recklinghausen's disease. Histologically it is composed of neuroendocrine cells and ganglion cells

MISCELLANEOUS CONDITIONS

Acute dilatation of the stomach

- pathogenesis is unclear although reflex inhibition of intrinsic electrical pace-maker activity has been proposed
- may follow any surgery, especially splenectomy
- often occurs during prolonged immobilisation
- early symptoms include hiccup and vomiting. Later pain or collapse from hypovolaemia occurs

Ménétrier's disease

- affects the stomach
- usually presents with epigastric pain, weight loss, vomiting and diarrhoea
- characterised by giant rugal mucosal folds either along the greater curve or throughout the fundus and body of the stomach. The antrum is usually spared
- microscopy shows hypertrophy of mucosa with marked elongation of gastric pits, cyst formation and parietal cell loss
- gastric malignancy is a rare complication

Volvulus

- rarely occurs in stomach
- predisposing factors include abnormal bands or adhesions and tumours
- may be acute or chronic
- acute volvulus presents as an acute abdomen and has a high mortality
- chronic volvulus presents with pain, vomiting and bloating
- complications include ulceration, haemorrhage, obstruction, strangulation, gangrene and perforation

Diverticula

- gastric diverticula are rare and are mostly found near the cardia. Less often they occur in the pylorus
- duodenal diverticula are also rare and are often identified as an incidental finding on barium studies
- complications include haemorrhage due to mucosal ulceration, perforation, obstruction of the common bile or pancreatic duct and malabsorption due to bacterial overgrowth

Bezoars

- foreign bodies in the stomach
- may be composed of hair (trichobezoars) or vegetable material (phytobezoars)

- usually occur in young children or persons with chronic mental disorders
- present as epigastric mass or with obstruction
- complications include gastric ulceration, obstruction or perforation

Mallory-Weiss syndrome

(see also Chapter 2)
- upper gastrointestinal bleeding from a linear mucosal tear in the region of the cardia
- lacerations may be confined to the gastric mucosa or may extend across the gastro-oesophageal junction
- the linear tear is in the long axis of the stomach
- usually caused by violent vomiting, coughing or abdominal trauma
- most cases present with haematemesis and respond to conservative measures

Congestive gastropathy and gastric varices

- portal hypertensive gastropathy is now well recognised in patients with cirrhosis of the liver
- on endoscopy lesions range from mucosal mosaic pattern to multiple red mucosal spots which are most noticeable in the fundus
- gastric varices arise because of either generalised or segmental portal hypertension
- splenic vein thrombosis results in varices in the body and fundus of the stomach but not usually in the oesophagus
- gastric varices arising in patients with generalised portal hypertension are usually accompanied by oesophageal varices

Dieulafoy's lesion

- a gastric erosion consisting of a small mucosal defect up to 5 mm in diameter
- usually located high in the fundus on the lesser curvature of the stomach
- a solitary, usually large and tortuous artery is aneurysmally dilated and protrudes through the defect. This aneurysm can rupture and produce bleeding
- lesions occur at any age and are more common in men

The intestines

4

NORMAL STRUCTURE

- small intestine consists of the duodenum, jejunum and ileum. In the adult, the duodenum measures 20–25 cm in length. Of the remainder of the small intestine, the jejunum accounts for the proximal 40% and the ileum for the distal 60%
- wall of small intestine consists of mucosa, submucosa, muscularis propria and serosa
- mucosal villi are lined by absorptive cells (enterocytes) and goblet cells (secrete mucus). Between villi are crypts lined by Paneth cells, neuroendocrine cells, enterocytes and goblet cells
- jejunum and ileum are supplied by superior mesenteric artery and venous drainage is to the portal vein. Lymphatics drain to the superior mesenteric nodes
- large intestine consists of caecum (with attached appendix), ascending colon, hepatic flexure, transverse colon, splenic flexure, descending colon, sigmoid colon and rectum
- caecum is that part adjacent to the ileocaecal valve
- sigmoid colon extends from brim of pelvis to rectum
- rectum starts opposite the sacral promontory
- large intestinal wall consists of mucosa, submucosa, muscularis propria and serosa
- mucosa contains non-branching tubular glands
- surface cells are mainly absorptive. The crypts are lined mainly by goblet cells with occasional neuroendocrine cells
- muscularis propria has inner circular and outer longitudinal layer
- longitudinal coat of muscle is condensed into three bands (taeniae coli)
- the colon from the caecum to the splenic flexure is supplied by the superior mesenteric artery. The remainder of the colon is supplied by the inferior mesenteric artery. The rectum is supplied by the superior rectal artery (a branch of the inferior mesenteric), middle rectal artery (a branch of the internal iliac) and inferior rectal arteries (from the internal pudendal). Lymphatic drainage is to paracolic or pararectal nodes

DEVELOPMENTAL ABNORMALITIES

Rotational abnormalities

- during sixth week of fetal life the gut herniates into the umbilical cord. When it returns it undergoes complex rotation, failure of which leads to anatomical abnormalities
- abnormalities include the small bowel lying entirely to the right of midline with the caecum in the left iliac fossa
- the midgut tends to have a long narrow mesentery and is subsequently prone to torsion

Atresia and stenosis

- atresia is complete discontinuity of the intestinal lumen for a variable distance. Stenosis is narrowing of the lumen
- these are most common in the ileum (60%) but may also occur in the jejunum and duodenum (40%)
- these conditions may be associated with Down's syndrome

Duplications and cysts

- duplications may be complete or partial and communication with the main gastrointestinal tract is variable
- enterogenous cysts may occur in the wall of the bowel, in the mesentery or completely separate from the bowel
- duplications or cysts occasionally cause obstruction, haemorrhage or intussusception

Meckel's diverticulum

- commonest congenital abnormality of gastrointestinal tract, present in 2% of population
- commoner in males
- the vitello-intestinal duct connects the midgut to the umbilicus
- proximal portion may persist and form a Meckel's diverticulum
- lies on the antimesenteric border of the ileum, approximately 90 cm above the ileocaecal valve
- microscopically is usually lined by small intestinal mucosa
- gastric mucosa or ectopic pancreatic tissue are occasionally present
- complications include peptic ulceration, haemorrhage, obstruction, perforation and herniation (Littré's hernia)

Hirschsprung's disease

- due to congenital absence of ganglion cells in segment of large bowel, usually the rectum
- usually starts at the anus and extends proximally for a variable distance
- incidence is 1 in 20 000 births and the condition is five times more common in males than females
- familial tendency
- may present in the neonatal period, in infancy or occasionally in later life (adult Hirschsprung's disease)
- neonates present with failure to pass meconium. In older children constipation, abdominal distension and vomiting are usual
- classified as ultra-short, short and long segment disease according to the length of the aganglionic segment. The aganglionic segment is narrow and the proximal bowel grossly dilated
- diagnosis is made by full thickness rectal biopsy or by partial thickness suction biopsy consisting of mucosa and some submucosa. Biopsies should be taken at 1-cm intervals proximal to the dentate line until normal intestine is reached

- microscopically there is absence of ganglion cells and increase in number and size of cholinergic nerve fibres in all layers of the bowel wall
- histochemistry to demonstrate acetylcholinesterase is required
- complications include obstruction, ischaemic necrosis, perforation and enterocolitis

CONDITIONS OCCURRING IN CHILDHOOD

Neonatal necrotising enterocolitis

- unknown aetiology
- affects premature infants in first week of life
- infants present with abdominal distension, vomiting and bloody diarrhoea
- terminal ileum and right colon are most often affected and exhibit mucosal haemorrhage, necrosis and ulceration. Gas bubbles appear as cyst-like spaces in submucosa
- surgical resection of the affected area may be necessary

Intussusception

- invagination of one part of the small or large intestine into the immediately distal part
- commonest cause of intestinal obstruction in young children
- in children often not possible to detect a cause. However, 10% of children have anatomical causes such as Meckel's diverticulum or a polyp. Hypertrophy of lymphoid tissue in Peyer's patches may also be a cause
- most common site is ileocolic but ileum, jejunum or colon may be affected

CHRONIC INFLAMMATORY BOWEL DISEASE (CIBD)

- comprises ulcerative colitis (UC) and Crohn's disease (CD)
- in some cases distinction between UC and CD is impossible (colitis indeterminate)

Epidemiology, aetiology and pathogenesis

- both UC and CD have an annual incidence in Western populations of approximately 5 per 100 000. The incidence of Crohn's disease is rising. Both conditions are more common in USA and Northern Europe than in Africa and Asia
- peak incidence for CIBD is early adult life. A second peak occurs in patients over 55 years
- infectious agents have long been suspected to be implicated in the causation of CIBD, but evidence for a transmissible agent is unproven
- there is a genetic predisposition to the development of both UC and CD with an increased prevalence of CIBD amongst first degree relatives of affected patients

- there is an association of CIBD with HLA-B27 in patients with ankylosing spondylitis
- it has been suggested that CD is a granulomatous vasculitis causing multiple ischaemic infarcts in bowel wall. This is not universally accepted

Ulcerative colitis

- commonly a chronic intermittent disease in which symptoms are episodic
- during exacerbations may get many bowel movements per day and in severe cases there may be marked constitutional symptoms. Severe attacks may be complicated by acute dilatation of the colon (toxic megacolon)
- in endoscopically active disease diffuse small ulcers on a red granular mucosa are seen. The mucosa is friable and bleeds on contact
- inflammatory polyps may be seen
- in quiescent disease mucosa may appear normal or may be smooth and atrophic with loss of folds
- disease tends to be most severe in the rectum
- colectomy may be necessary for failed medical treatment, in severe attacks or for complications such as toxic megacolon, perforation or haemorrhage
- microscopically there is inflammation usually confined to the mucosa and submucosa with polymorphs invading glandular crypts and forming crypt abscesses. Granulomas are not seen
- mucosal ulceration and depletion of goblet cells occur
- in quiescent cases the ulcerated mucosa becomes re-epithelialised and inflammation subsides but mucosal glands are distorted and shortened

Crohn's disease

- chronic intermittent disease
- may affect any part of the gastrointestinal tract
- propensity to occur in small bowel, especially terminal ileum
- commonest clinical presentation is diarrhoea and abdominal pain
- 30% of patients require surgical intervention in the first year following diagnosis. The remainder require surgery at 5% per year
- grossly affected areas show thickening of bowel wall due to fibrosis and oedema
- mucosa shows deep fissuring ulcers and often has a cobblestone appearance
- the mucosa between the discontinuous affected areas appears normal, resulting in so-called skip lesions
- loops of adjacent gut may be matted together, with concomitant abscess and fistula formation
- perianal lesions such as fistulae, fissures and abscesses are more common in CD than UC
- microscopically there is deep fissure ulceration of the mucosa with oedema and fibrosis. The inflammatory infiltrate affects all layers of the bowel wall (transmural inflammation). Granuloma formation occurs in 50–70% of cases

Course of CIBD

- 5–10% of patients have long-term remission after the first attack; 10% experience continuous symptoms and the remainder have remissions and exacerbations
- recurrence is common in CD after surgical resection. Around 50% of patients suffer recurrence over 10 years

Complications of CIBD

- external fistulae occur in 25% of patients with CD
- toxic megacolon affects 2–4% of patients with UC. It may also occur occasionally in CD. In toxic megacolon there is intense transmural inflammation with extensive mucosal ulceration, dilatation of the colon and thinning of the bowel wall
- patients with extensive UC for more than 10 years have an increased risk of developing colorectal cancer
- 15–20% of patients with UC will develop cancer after 30 years. Dysplasia is frequently found on biopsy in patients who have UC complicated by colorectal cancer and patients with long-standing disease should have colonoscopy and biopsy
- cancer developing in UC may be difficult to detect endoscopically and multiple lesions may occur
- there is an increased risk of colorectal cancer in CD, although this is not as high as in UC
- there is an increased risk of small intestinal adenocarcinoma in CD
- there appears to be a slightly increased risk of colorectal lymphoma in patients with CIBD
- following construction of an ileal pouch approximately 10% of patients will develop pouchitis. This is characterised by increased frequency and urgency of bowel movement sometimes accompanied by blood staining. In some cases there may be abdominal discomfort, fever or arthritis. Endoscopy shows mucosal congestion, bleeding and ulceration. Microscopically there is villous atrophy, acute and chronic inflammation, mucosal ulceration and occasionally granuloma formation

Extra-intestinal manifestations of CIBD

LIVER

- fatty change and pericholangitis occur in association with UC. Many patients with primary sclerosing cholangitis have underlying UC. These conditions are also rarely associated with CD

SKIN

- erythema nodosum and pyoderma gangrenosum occur occasionally in patients with UC and less often with CD

EYES

- episcleritis and uveitis may occur

JOINTS

- arthritis occurs in 6% of patients. Both UC and CD may be associated with ankylosing spondylitis

URINARY TRACT

- renal amyloid is a rare complication
- increased frequency of urinary calculi in CIBD, especially in patients with ileostomy

Idiopathic proctitis

- in this condition macroscopic and microscopic findings identical to UC are found restricted to the rectum. Many authorities consider that this differs from UC only in the extent of bowel involvement

OTHER INFLAMMATORY CONDITIONS OF THE INTESTINES

Infective colitis

- presents as an acute illness with bloody diarrhoea. Can be difficult to distinguish from UC and CD
- organisms responsible include *Shigella, Salmonella,* certain strains of *Escherichia coli* and *Campylobacter.* Chlamydial infection may cause proctitis
- microscopic findings are oedema of the lamina propria with a predominantly polymorphonuclear infiltrate. This is unlike UC and CD which have both acute and chronic inflammatory cells
- distortion of mucosal glands which occurs in both UC and CD is usually not a feature of infective colitis
- usually self-limiting

Yersinia enterocolitis

- *Yersinia pseudotuberculosis* and *Yersinia entercolitica* may cause acute enteritis with fever and diarrhoea
- terminal ileum and caecum are usually affected. Mucosa appears congested and oedematous with superficial ulceration
- microscopically there is inflammation with granuloma formation. Typically there are characteristic micro-abscesses in bowel wall and in enlarged draining lymph nodes
- diagnosis is usually by isolation of the organism from blood or by demonstration of specific antibodies in rising titres

Amoebic dysentery

- caused by the protozoan parasite *Entamoeba histolytica*
- occurs in the large bowel and may be confused with both UC and CD
- small yellow mucosal lesions are seen which break down to form flask-shaped mucosal ulcers with surface necrotic debris
- diagnosis is by identification of the organism in the stool or in rectal biopsy
- rarely the colon perforates or an amoeboma forms. This is a chronic form of the disease with much associated fibrosis and which may present as a tumorous mass
- amoebae may invade vessels in the bowel wall and spread to the liver with the development of a hepatic amoebic abscess

Pseudomembranous colitis

- may rarely develop after major abdominal surgery but is most commonly seen as a complication of antibiotic administration

- especially associated with lincomycin and clindamycin therapy, although it has been reported with a wide range of antibiotics
- *Clostridium difficile* and its toxin can be isolated from the stool in 90% of cases
- macroscopically mucosal surface contains yellow friable plaques which may become confluent
- microscopically there are disrupted epithelial crypts with a surface 'cap' of debris, mucin, fibrin and polymorphs. Later there is complete mucosal necrosis with overlying necrotic membrane
- *Clostridium difficile* is sensitive to vancomycin which is the treatment of choice
- occasionally toxic megacolon may supervene

Tuberculosis

- most frequently involves the terminal ileum and caecum
- may be primary, due to infection with the bovine bacillus or secondary, due to swallowed sputum in patients with open pulmonary tuberculosis
- infection with atypical mycobacteria is common in patients with AIDS
- macroscopically there is ulceration of the mucosa. The ulcers lie transverse to the long axis of the bowel. Fibrosis occurs later leading to single or multiple strictures
- microscopically there are caseating granulomas especially in draining lymph nodes
- bacilli can be demonstrated with Ziehl-Neelsen stain
- distinction from Crohn's disease or ischaemic stricture may be difficult

Cryptosporidiosis

- small intestine is usual site of involvement
- usually occurs in immunodeficiency, including AIDS

Diversion colitis

- occurs in segments of bowel which have been excluded from the faecal stream by surgical diversion via a colostomy
- symptoms include mucoid and bloody discharge and rectal discomfort
- endoscopy shows inflamed friable mucosa with ulceration
- microscopically there is non-specific mucosal inflammation with prominent lymphoid follicles
- occasionally granulomas are present

DIVERTICULAR DISEASE OF THE LARGE INTESTINE

- often asymptomatic, but if diverticula become inflamed, local and/or systemic symptoms such as pain, intestinal obstruction and rectal bleeding may occur
- incidence increases with age. In the UK at least one in three people over 60 years have colonic diverticula
- more common in Western countries than in Africa, India, South America or Japan. This may be due to a high dietary fibre intake in the latter areas
- colonic diverticula are pulsion in type
- their development depends on the intraluminal pressure and the strength of the colonic wall

- the sigmoid colon is predominantly affected but the proximal colon may also be involved. The rectum is not involved due to its complete investing layers of both muscle coats
- diverticula consist of pouches of mucosa which herniate through the circular muscle coat. They often contain a faecolith
- they appear in rows between the taeniae coli at points of weakness where blood vessels enter. Inflammation within diverticula and adjacent mucosa is common
- the circular muscle layer is markedly thickened and the affected segment of bowel is shortened
- there may be redundant folds of mucosa which, in combination with muscle thickening and fibrosis, may cause stenosis

Complications of diverticular disease

INFLAMMATION (DIVERTICULITIS)

- may arise due to ulceration of the mucosal lining of a diverticulum by a faecolith or due to obstruction of the mouth of a diverticulum
- inflammation may spread through the diverticular wall and along the external surface of the bowel to affect other diverticula
- may result in abscess formation with a localised peritonitis and subsequent fibrosis
- may present as a hard mass which may mimic a carcinoma

PERFORATION

- necrosis and perforation of the wall of a diverticulum may occur
- perforation may be contained forming an abscess or may give rise to generalised peritonitis

OBSTRUCTION

- diverticulitis heals by fibrosis. The fibrous tissue contracts leading to stenosis of the bowel. This may be compounded by contraction of taeniae coli and thickening of the circular muscle coat. This may result in acute or chronic intestinal obstruction

HAEMORRHAGE

- haemorrhage may occur without preceding symptoms
- diverticula protrude through the colonic wall where blood vessels enter. Erosion or ulceration of the wall may lead to haemorrhage

FISTULA

- a pericolic abscess may perforate into the bladder, uterus, vagina, ureter, small intestine or the skin with formation of a fistula. Colovesical fistula is the commonest and usually presents with pneumaturia and cystitis

ISCHAEMIC DISORDERS OF THE INTESTINE

- ischaemic disorders of the intestine are due to a reduction or absence of intestinal blood flow. This may be caused by arterial disease, venous disease, systemic hypotension or a combination of these factors

Arterial obstruction

- most commonly involves the superior mesenteric artery
- the most common cause of arterial obstruction is atheroma. Atheroma typically affects the ostium and the first few centimetres of the superior mesenteric artery, sparing the more peripheral branches
- predisposing factors include hypertension, diabetes mellitus, hypercholesterolaemia and smoking
- may rarely be caused by an arteritis (e.g. collagen vascular diseases), radiation, dissecting aneurysm or tumours which compress or invade arteries

Venous occlusion

- may result from local causes such as compression within a hernial sac or by an abdominal or pelvic mass
- may be a result of generalised disease which precipitates intravascular thrombosis such as polycythaemia. Cases have been reported with the oral contraceptive pill

Systemic hypotension

- may occur secondary to severe blood loss or left ventricular heart failure. Both result in massive splanchnic vasoconstriction

CLASSIFICATION OF ISCHAEMIC DISORDERS OF INTESTINE

Acute intestinal failure

- sudden complete occlusion of the superior mesenteric artery rapidly leads to necrosis and gangrene of the small intestine and ascending colon. This may also be due to sudden venous occlusion or severe hypotension
- presents as an abdominal emergency with severe pain and circulatory collapse
- serosal surface of the bowel is deep red in colour and later becomes black
- peristalsis ceases and, in arterial occlusion, mesenteric pulsation is absent
- vascular congestion and necrosis of the intestinal wall occur
- mortality from acute superior mesenteric artery occlusion is 80%. Venous infarction has a mortality of 40%

Ischaemic colitis

- acute ischaemia of the colon usually affects the splenic flexure as this has a poor blood supply. If this is severe there is full thickness necrosis of the intestinal wall. This usually presents with severe left-sided abdominal pain
- in less severe cases there is partial-thickness necrosis and presentation is with colicky pain and bloody diarrhoea. The mucosal surface becomes congested and ulcerated. Microscopy reveals necrosis of the superficial mucosa
- in the reparative phase the mucosa re-epithelialises and fibrosis of the gut wall may result in stricture formation

Chronic intestinal ischaemia

- causes symptoms of abdominal angina, characterised by colicky abdominal pain occurring 30 minutes after eating
- usually caused by atheroma of superior mesenteric artery

OTHER VASCULAR ABNORMALITIES

Haemangiomas

- may be single or multiple and occur in both small and large bowel. Some cases are associated with multiple haemangiomas outside the gastrointestinal tract, e.g. hereditary haemorrhagic telangiectasia (Rendu-Weber-Osler disease)
- may present with gastrointestinal haemorrhage, anaemia, obstruction or intussusception

Angiodysplasia

- small vascular lesions consisting of dilated mucosal and submucosal blood vessels
- most commonly found in caecum and ascending colon of elderly patients
- an important cause of lower gastrointestinal bleeding in the elderly
- diagnosis is by angiography. Tortuous arteries, vascular lakes and early filling veins are seen
- at colonoscopy lesions appear as cherry-red areas 2–5 mm in diameter
- microscopic confirmation of the diagnosis is difficult as blood vessels collapse. Prominent dilated thin walled vascular channels are seen within the mucosa and submucosa of the intestine

SOLITARY RECTAL ULCER

- term is misleading as lesion is not necessarily solitary nor ulcerated
- aetiology is not fully understood, but trauma secondary to partial rectal prolapse is implicated in most cases
- condition often affects patients under 40 years. They usually present with rectal bleeding and the passage of mucus. Difficulty in initiation of defaecation is common
- on sigmoidoscopy the lesion occurs 7–10 cm from the anal verge on the anterior wall of the rectum. There is ulceration or localised erythema of the mucosa
- microscopy shows smooth muscle fibres extending upwards into the lamina propria from a thickened muscularis mucosa. Ulceration may or may not be present

SMALL BOWEL TUMOURS

- primary tumours of the small bowel are rare. The commonest benign tumours are adenoma, leiomyoma (stromal tumour) and lipoma. Malignant tumours include adenocarcinoma, lymphoma, carcinoid tumour and leiomyosarcoma

Benign tumours of the small intestine

ADENOMAS

- have the same gross and histological features as large bowel adenomas but are much less common
- they occur with decreasing frequency from the duodenum to the ileum. The most common site is in the duodenum around the ampulla of Vater
- patients with familial adenomatous polyposis (FAP) and Gardner's syndrome may develop multiple small bowel adenomas and carcinomas
- small bowel adenomas may develop into adenocarcinoma

LEIOMYOMAS

- these are discussed under the heading Intestinal stromal tumours (see p. 53)

PEUTZ-JEGHERS' POLYPS

- occur as part of the Peutz-Jeghers' syndrome
- autosomal dominant syndrome
- hamartomatous leisons and not truly neoplastic
- syndrome consists of pigmented spots in mucus membrane of oral cavity and skin with multiple polyps of gastrointestinal tract
- polyps occur mainly in jejunum and ileum but less commonly in stomach, duodenum and large intestine
- polyps are lobulated and sessile or pedunculated
- microscopically show proliferation and branching of muscularis mucosa. The covering epithelium is normal and non-dysplastic
- malignant transformation within Peutz-Jeghers' polyps is rare but recognised. There is an increased tendency to intestinal and extra-intestinal tumour formation
- syndrome may include a characteristic ovarian sex cord tumour (sex cord stromal tumour with annular tubules) and carcinoma of breast, pancreas, endocervix, stomach and colon

Carcinoma of the small bowel

- much less common than carcinoma of large intestine
- the vast majority of adenocarcinomas may arise in adenomas
- most common site is around ampulla of Vater
- many have metastasised to mesenteric lymph nodes or distant sites at diagnosis
- macroscopically common type is annular and the rest are polypoid
- microscopically similar to other adenocarcinomas of gastrointestinal tract
- may be associated with Crohn's disease, coeliac disease or ileostomy stoma

Carcinoid tumours (neuroendocrine tumours)

- the appendix is the commonest site for carcinoid tumours within the gastro-intestinal tract. In this site the vast majority are benign
- outside the appendix the terminal ileum is the commonest site followed by the rectum and stomach. Such tumours show variable degrees of malignancy and may be multiple

- local complications include intussusception, haemorrhage and small bowel obstruction
- many are functional and secrete several amines including 5-hydroxytrypt-amine(5HT), 5-hydroxy-tryptaphan, histamine and bradykinin. 5HT is degraded in the urine to 5-hydroindoleacetic acid (5HIAA). This may be used for diagnosis
- carcinoid syndrome occurs when liver metastases are present and amines are secreted into systemic circulation bypassing the liver. The syndrome is characterised by paroxysms of flushing, wheezing and diarrhoea. Pulmonary stenosis and tricuspid insufficiency may develop
- carcinoid tumours are nodular and located within the submucosa. On cut section they are yellow in colour
- microscopically they are composed of uniform tumour cells growing in a variety of patterns, the commonest being 'insular' and 'trabecular'
- may metastasise to mesenteric lymph nodes, liver and lungs
- immunohistochemistry for neuroendocrine markers and electron microscopy to demonstrate characteristic dense core granules are useful for pathological diagnosis

Lymphomas of small intestine

- benign hyperplasia of lymphoid tissue occurs in terminal ileum in region of ileocaecal valve in infants and children. This may cause bowel obstruction, intussusception or haemorrhage
- many primary malignant lymphomas of small intestine are part of spectrum of mucosa-associated lymphoid tissue (MALT) lymphoma
- in the West most small bowel lymphomas arise in the terminal ileum, whereas in the Middle East the jejunum and ileum are equally affected
- malignant lymphomas of the small intestine are usually B cell in type
- most patients with malignant lymphoma present with obstruction, bleeding or perforation
- adjacent mesenteric lymph nodes may be involved
- the prognosis is not as good as for gastric lymphoma. Low grade lymphomas have a better outlook than high grade
- malignant lymphomatous polyposis is a rare malignant lymphoma which may affect the terminal ileum, but more often involves the colon and rectum. The condition presents with multiple lymphomatous polyps
- in malignant lymphomatous polyposis spread to lymph nodes and bone marrow occurs early and the prognosis is poor
- Burkitt-type lymphoma, a high-grade tumour of B-cell origin, occurs in the ileocaecal region
- Burkitt-type lymphoma mainly affects young children and is relatively rare in Western countries
- primary Hodgkin's disease involving the gut is very rare
- coeliac disease may predispose to pleomorphic T-cell lymphoma of small bowel (especially jejunum)
- this lymphoma type is aggressive with early involvement of mesenteric nodes, spleen, liver and bone marrow
- alpha-chain disease, otherwise known as immunoproliferative small intestinal disease (IPSID) or Mediterranean lymphoma, occurs mainly in the Middle East or in immigrants from that region
- this lymphoma frequently affects young adults and presents with malabsorption, bleeding, obstruction or perforation

- microscopically this lymphoma is characterised by massive infiltration of the bowel wall by lymphoplasmacytoid cells and plasma cells
- in the early stages IPSID responds to antibiotic therapy (tetracyclines)
- malignant lymphoma complicating AIDS is discussed in Chapter 22. The small intestine and anorectal region are the most frequently affected sites

Intestinal stromal tumours syn. gastrointestinal stromal tumours (GIST)

- most were previously classified as leiomyoma or leiomyosarcoma but immuno-histochemical studies indicate that many show no evidence of smooth muscle differentiation and thus the term intestinal stromal tumour was introduced
- the stomach is the commonest site for such tumours (see Chapter 3) but they may also occur in the small intestine
- occasionally occur in colon and rectum
- often are asymptomatic but may cause obstruction, intussusception and bleeding
- tumours arise from muscularis propria or muscularis mucosa and project internally into the gut lumen or externally from the serosal surface
- cut surface is whorled
- microscopy shows spindle-shaped cells
- prognosis is unpredictable
- tumour size is an important prognostic factor. Tumours exceeding 5 cm in diameter should be considered as potentially malignant. Small tumours have a good prognosis
- other adverse prognostic factors, apart from large size, include increased mitotic activity, nuclear pleomorphism and vascular invasion by tumour cells

Inflammatory fibroid polyps

(see Chapter 3)
- may occur in the small intestine and are benign
- usually arise in submucosa
- may cause mucosal ulceration and obstruction
- microscopically composed of fibroblasts and loose connective tissue which is characteristically infiltrated by inflammatory cells, notably eosinophils

COLONIC POLYPS

- colonic polyps may be hamartomatous, metaplastic, inflammatory or neoplastic

Hamartomatous polyps

- hamartomas are disorders of growth and consist of an abnormal mixture of those tissues normally found in the organ concerned
- colonic hamartomas include Peutz-Jeghers' polyps (see p. 51) and juvenile polyps
- juvenile polyps most commonly occur in children, less often in adolescents and occasionally in adults

- they have a nodular smooth surface and occur mainly in the rectosigmoid region
- microscopy shows cystically dilated glands in an excess of inflamed lamina propria
- single juvenile polyps have no malignant potential
- juvenile polyposis is a syndrome usually presenting in infancy and characterised by juvenile polyps in the colon, stomach and small intestine
- haemorrhage or intussusception may occur
- juvenile polyposis is associated with an increased incidence of gastrointestinal malignancy, especially colorectal carcinoma
- regular colonoscopic surveillance is recommended

Metaplastic polyps (hyperplastic polyps)

- seldom exceed 1 cm
- found throughout colon but mainly in the sigmoid and rectum
- often multiple and very common in patients over 40 years
- metaplastic polyps are not neoplastic but are frequently associated with synchronous adenomatous polyps

Inflammatory polyps

- may be secondary to various insults to the colorectal mucosa
- most frequent cause is ulcerative colitis
- other causes include Crohn's disease and ischaemic bowel disease

Neoplastic polyps (adenomas)

- large intestinal adenomas are classified as tubular, villous or tubulo-villous
- may or may not have a stalk
- large colorectal adenomas tend to be commonest in countries with a high incidence of colorectal cancer
- adenomas occur throughout the large intestine but are commonest in sigmoid and descending colon
- incidence increases with age and they are very common in elderly patients
- 50% of colonic adenomas exceed 1 cm in diameter
- microscopically the epithelial lining shows some degree of dysplasia which is generally more severe in larger lesions

Malignancy arising in colorectal adenomas

- majority of colonic carcinomas arise in a pre-existing adenoma
- adenomas are more common in surgically resected colorectal specimens with cancer than in resected specimens without cancer
- focal carcinoma may be seen microscopically arising within an adenoma
- adenomas are found more frequently in geographical areas with a high incidence of colorectal cancer. The distribution of adenomas within the colon matches that of colonic cancer
- in untreated colonic adenomas, the risk of malignancy developing at the site of the polyp is 24% after 20 years

- most important risk factors for development of carcinoma in a colonic adenoma are the size of the adenoma and its configuration. Villous adenomas have a higher likelihood of malignancy developing than other types
- the incidence of severe dysplasia and the risk of carcinoma increase in proportion to the size of the polyp and in association with a predominantly villous architecture

MANAGEMENT OF COLONIC ADENOMAS

- colonoscopy should be performed in all patients with colonic adenomas and lesions greater than 5 mm diameter should be removed
- patients with a large adenoma or multiple adenomas should probably undergo colonoscopy every 3–5 years, but cost implications are considerable

Familial adenomatous polyposis (FAP) (familial polyposis coli)

- an inherited autosomal dominant disease in which multiple polyps (by definition over 100) arise in colon in early adult life (second or third decade)
- most cases are hereditary but 25% arise due to new mutations and have no family history
- the genetic abnormality is on the long arm of chromosome 5 and causes hyperproliferative mucosa throughout the gastrointestinal tract
- gastric lesions comprising fundic gland polyps and adenomas may coexist
- duodenal adenomas, usually affecting the second part of the duodenum, may occur
- periampullary carcinoma arising in the region of the ampulla of Vater in the duodenum may occur
- congenital hypertrophy of retinal pigment epithelium (CHRPE lesion) may be useful as a preliminary screening investigation
- female patients with FAP have an increased incidence of papillary thyroid carcinoma
- multiple adenomatous polyps develop throughout the large intestine from the age of 10 years
- adenomas tend to be more common in the distal colon and rectum
- microscopically polyps are tubular, tubulovillous or villous adenomas
- untreated the development of cancer is invariable

OTHER POLYPOSIS SYNDROMES

Gardner's syndrome

- FAP coexisting with extra-intestinal disease such as osteomas, desmoid tumours of abdominal wall and mesentery, lipomas, fibromas and epidermoid cysts
- autosomal dominant

Turcot's syndrome

- rare
- autosomal recessive inheritance

- colonic polyps are associated with central nervous system malignancy, usually medulloblastoma
- adenomas are fewer in number than in FAP

COLORECTAL CANCER

- the essential criterion for a diagnosis of colorectal cancer is the presence of malignant glands or cells which have infiltrated across the muscularis mucosa into the submucosa
- when limited to the colonic mucosa only, carcinoma has very little potential to metastasise. In this scenario, the term intramucosal carcinoma may be used

Epidemiology, aetiology and pathogenesis

- second to carcinoma of the bronchus as the commonest cause of death from malignant disease in the UK
- three times more common in first degree relatives of affected patients than in general population
- common in Western countries and much less common in Africa and Asia
- in recent years in countries with a high incidence there has been a relative reduction in the number of cancers of the rectum and left side of the colon and a corresponding increase in cancers of the right colon
- dietary factors are thought to be implicated in the development of colorectal carcinoma. Suggested dietary factors contributing to colorectal cancer include low dietary fibre, low intake of fresh vegetables and a high dietary content of animal fat
- colorectal cancer is much more common in first degree relatives
- there is an association between colorectal cancer and familial adenomatous polyposis (see above)
- hereditary non-polyposis colorectal cancer (HNPCC) is associated with an early onset of colorectal cancer, an increased incidence of proximal bowel cancer and a slightly improved prognosis. This condition is characterised by mutations in DNA mismatch repair genes and probably accounts for less than 10% of cases of colorectal cancer
- a sequence of genetic mutations occurs in the progression from hyperplastic colonic epithelium through early and late adenomas to invasive carcinoma
- these genetic mutations mainly affect chromosomes 5q, 18q and 17p
- a large proportion of colorectal cancers arise from pre-existing adenomatous polyps
- there is an increased risk of carcinoma in long-standing cases of chronic inflammatory bowel disease (CIBD), especially ulcerative colitis (see p. 44)
- there is an increased risk of colorectal cancer with schistosomiasis

Pathology

- in recent years there has been a relative shift from distal to proximal colonic tumours
- most are ulcerated. Many involve the whole circumference of the bowel resulting in constricting annular tumours which may present with obstruction

- majority are adenocarcinomas
- mucinous adenocarcinoma is a rare variant characterised by the production of large amounts of mucus

Spread of colorectal cancer

- direct spread through colonic wall, especially at points where blood vessels enter
- longitudinal spread is not usually prominent
- lymphatic spread is common. This takes place in a contiguous fashion, first involving nodes adjacent to the tumour and then involving distant nodes
- vascular spread usually results in hepatic metastases

Staging of colorectal cancer

- prognosis depends to a large extent on staging. Staging of colorectal cancer is based on Dukes' classification (Figure 4.1)
- Dukes' A – tumour is confined to the wall of the bowel but has not spread outside the muscularis propria
- Dukes' B – tumour has spread through the bowel wall to the serosal surface
- Dukes' C – there is lymph node involvement. This is divided into Dukes' C1 (only local lymph nodes are involved) and C2 (mesenteric nodes involved at the level of ligation of the vascular pedicle, i.e. apical lymph node is involved)
- Dukes' D – distant metastases are present
- other staging systems include the Astler Coller system (see Figure 4.1)

Prognosis of colorectal cancer

DIRECT SPREAD
- local extramural spread is of major prognostic importance especially in the rectum. Involvement of the lateral limits of resection by tumour carries a high risk of local recurrence

HISTOLOGICAL GRADE
- this is based on the degree of gland or tubule formation within the tumour
- poorly differentiated tumours have a worse prognosis than moderately or well differentiated

TUMOUR TYPE
- mucinous adenocarcinomas frequently have a poor prognosis and are more common in the right side of the colon

LYMPH NODE STATUS
- this is the most important single prognostic factor
- if more than four lymph nodes are involved by secondary carcinoma, the prognosis is poor

DUKES (Original Classification)

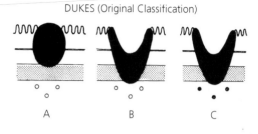

ASTLER/COLLER MODIFICATION

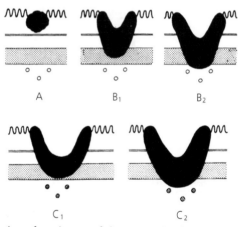

Figure 4.1 Staging of carcinoma of the rectum by the Dukes' original classification and by the Astler/Coller modification. Unshaded circles represent uninvolved lymph nodes and shaded circles represent involved lymph nodes

VASCULAR INVASION

- tumour invasion of large extramural veins is associated with a poor prognosis

OTHER FACTORS

- diploid tumours on flow cytometry have a better prognosis than aneuploid tumours
- tumours showing p53 gene mutation have a worse prognosis than those in which this is absent
- rectal carcinoma in younger patients often presents at an advanced stage and is associated with a poor prognosis

Complications of colorectal cancer

INTESTINAL OBSTRUCTION

- often a presenting feature with annular carcinomas

PERFORATION

- may occur at the tumour site or proximal to this
- may result in a malignant fistula

OTHER TUMOURS OF THE LARGE BOWEL

Neuroendocrine (carcinoid) tumours

- neuroendocrine cells secreting 5HT and polypeptide hormones occur throughout the large intestine
- occasionally give rise to carcinoid tumours
- carcinoid tumours are much less common than in the small intestine or appendix
- the caecum and rectum are the commonest sites
- prognosis is related to tumour size, nuclear pleomorphism, high mitotic activity and tumour necrosis

Tumours of lymphoid tissue

BENIGN

- small benign lymphoid polyps are a common finding in lower rectum
- these may be sessile or pedunculated
- they are probably inflammatory in nature and consist of reactive lymphoid tissue with lymphoid follicles

MALIGNANT

- large intestine may be involved as part of a generalised lymphoma
- primary malignant lymphomas of the colon and rectum are rare
- the caecum is the commonest site followed by the rectum
- most colonic lymphomas are non-Hodgkins B cell in type and present as a tumorous mass
- the incidence of malignant lymphoma of the rectum is increased in AIDS (see Chapter 22)
- multiple lymphomatous polyposis is a rare multicentric malignant lymphoma which presents as multiple polypoid deposits in the mucosa and submucosa, usually of the colon and rectum. The prognosis is poor
- malignant B-cell lymphomas occasionally develop in association with long-standing chronic inflammatory bowel disease
- in children, Burkitt's type lymphomas may involve the ileocaecal region

Stromal tumours

- occur occasionally in the colon and rectum (see p. 53)

Lipomas

- benign tumours which occur mainly in the right colon, most frequently in the region of the ileocaecal valve
- submucosal in location and often asymptomatic
- may result in intussusception or may ulcerate and bleed

MISCELLANEOUS CONDITIONS

Volvulus

- the sigmoid colon is the commonest part of the intestine to undergo volvulus
- sigmoid volvulus usually occurs in elderly patients
- may be associated with a large redundant sigmoid loop and peritoneal adhesions
- clinical presentation is with abdominal distension due to acute large bowel obstruction
- twisting of bowel initially causes venous obstruction and then arterial insufficiency with resulting ischaemia, necrosis, perforation and peritonitis. Without elective operation recurrence is common
- caecal volvulus also occurs. The terminal ileum and ascending colon are usually involved with the caecum

Pneumatosis cystoides intestinalis

- gaseous cysts may occur in the bowel, usually in the submucosa or subserosa
- contain oxygen and nitrogen under pressure
- more common in small than in large bowel
- aetiology is unknown, but may be associated with chronic obstructive airways disease, peptic ulceration and connective tissue diseases
- usually presents in middle-aged males but may occur in infants
- may cause change in bowel habit, rectal bleeding and pneumoperitoneum
- cysts cause gross irregularity of mucosal surface and may project from the serosa
- microscopically cysts are lined by macrophages and multinucleate giant cells

Pseudo-obstruction

- symptoms and signs of intestinal obstruction without presence of a lesion causing mechanical obstruction
- cause is probably abnormal motility in the small bowel, colon or both
- lesion may be primary without a known cause or may be secondary to conditions such as scleroderma, amyloid or diabetes mellitus

Radiation enteropathy

- radiation, often for gynaecological malignancy (especially carcinoma of the cervix), may result in damage to the small and large intestine
- acute effect in the small intestine results in shortening of villi. Ulceration and perforation may occur in the small or large intestine

- microscopically recovery usually occurs in 6 months
- symptoms of acute radiation effects include pain, diarrhoea, bleeding and mucoid discharge
- chronic radiation effects may have similar symptoms but presentation is often with subacute obstruction
- affected segments of gut are thickened with telangiectasia and mucosal ulceration. There may be perforation or fistula formation with adhesions between adjacent loops of bowel
- in the late stages there may be stricture formation
- microscopy shows hyalinised endarteritis, submucosal fibrosis and oedema, lymphatic ectasia and abnormally shaped fibroblasts

Isolated small bowel ulceration

- a proportion of small bowel ulcers do not fit into recognised inflammatory, vascular or neoplastic categories and are termed non-specific
- some are due to ingestion of enteric-coated potassium compounds or non-steroidal anti-inflammatory drugs (NSAIDs)
- a few remain of unknown aetiology
- clinical presentation includes intermittent intestinal obstruction, bleeding and perforation

Solitary non-specific colonic ulcer

- may occur in any part of the colon but most common in caecum, ascending and sigmoid colon
- aetiology is unclear
- some cases are associated with drugs (especially NSAIDs), ischaemia, diverticular disease or colonic stenosis at a more distal site

THE APPENDIX

Normal structure

- the normal adult appendix is, on average, 7 cm in length. In children it normally arises from the distal end of the caecum and in adults it normally arises from the medial wall of the caecum below the ileocaecal valve. However, it may be variable in position
- blood supply is from a branch of caecal artery. The lymphatic drainage is to the ileocaecal and right paracolic nodes
- histology is similar to the rest of large bowel
- many lymphoid follicles occur in the lamina propria. These are especially prominent in children but tend to diminish with increasing age

Appendicitis

- acute appendicitis is the commonest abdominal surgical emergency
- the highest incidence is in the second and third decades at a time when the amount of lymphoid tissue in the appendix is maximal

EPIDEMIOLOGY, AETIOLOGY AND PATHOGENESIS

- incidence is greatest in developed countries
- a combination of bacterial infection and obstruction of the appendiceal lumen is a common cause of acute appendicitis. Obstruction may be caused by a faecolith, food debris, hypertrophy of lymphoid tissue, tumour or kinking

PATHOLOGY

- initially get hyperaemia of serosal surface with a fibrinopurulent exudate
- when gangrene occurs the wall becomes green or black and perforation is common
- microscopically there is ulceration of the mucosa and transmural infiltration by polymorphs

COMPLICATIONS

- although some cases undergo resolution and fibrosis, many perforate if not treated
- perforation occurs at an earlier stage in young children and usually results in generalised peritonitis. In adults perforation may result in a palpable mass of inflamed omentum, an appendix mass or abscess
- pus may track forming either a pelvic or subphrenic abscess
- obliteration of the lumen by fibrosis may result in formation of a mucocoele

Mucocoele of the appendix

- the appendix becomes distended by the accumulation of luminal mucus
- a simple mucocoele may develop following appendicitis if the lumen becomes obstructed by fibrosis
- a mucocoele may also be secondary to a mucus-secreting adenoma (cystadenoma) or carcinoma (cystadenocarcinoma) of the appendix
- rupture of a mucocoele may result in pseudomyxoma peritoneii (see p. 63)

Miscellaneous conditions

- the appendix may be involved in ileocolic Crohn's disease
- chronic appendiceal abscess formation may be associated with actinomycosis infection
- *Yersinia* infection of the terminal ileum may involve the appendix
- endometriosis occasionally involves the serosal surface or wall of the appendix
- diverticula may be present in 1% of appendicectomy specimens. They are often multiple

Tumours of the appendix

- carcinoid tumour is the most common primary tumour of the appendix. Cystadenomas and cystadenocarcinomas are rare. Metaplastic polyps and Peutz-Jegher polyps may also occur

ADENOMAS

- these are mucinous cystadenomas. They may produce excess mucus resulting in a mucocoele
- microscopically there are papillary formations of mucus-secreting epithelium
- adenomas show dysplastic features and are pre-malignant
- appendiceal adenomas may be associated with adenomas or carcinomas elsewhere in colon and rectum

ADENOCARCINOMAS

- most are mucinous cystadenocarcinomas and arise from pre-existing adenomas
- need to see histological infiltration of submucosa for a definitive diagnosis
- prognosis depends on depth of invasion and histological grade
- spread occurs to mesoappendiceal and ileocolic lymph nodes

PSEUDOMYXOMA PERITONEII

- mucus-secreting appendiceal tumours (cystadenoma and cystadenocarcinoma) may result in pseudomyxoma peritoneii
- this condition may also be secondary to mucinous tumours of the ovary or gallbladder
- in this condition there is accumulation of large amounts of mucinous material within the peritoneal cavity
- condition is progressive and often fatal due to adhesion formation and intestinal obstruction

CARCINOID TUMOUR

- this is a neuroendocrine tumour
- commonest appendiceal tumour
- carcinoids are usually located at tip of the appendix and are generally small (less than 1.5 cm)
- usually discovered incidentally on pathological examination following appendicectomy
- grossly often are yellow in colour
- microscopically there are insular and trabecular patterns of uniform tumour cells
- may infiltrate through muscle coat to the serosa but this has no effect on prognosis
- vast majority are benign
- metastatic disease may be associated with tumours greater than 2 cm in diameter and those located at the base of appendix with extension into the caecum

GOBLET CELL CARCINOID

- also called adenocarcinoid or mucus-secreting carcinoid
- tumour contains neuroendocrine cells as well as mucus-secreting cells
- more often symptomatic than ordinary appendiceal carcinoids
- may present as appendicitis or an intestinal obstruction due to tumour infiltration of terminal ileum

- microscopically there is a mixture of mucus-secreting goblet cells and neuroendocrine cells
- more aggressive behaviour than ordinary appendiceal carcinoids
- if the tumour is confined to appendix or mesoappendix the prognosis is good. However, if extension beyond the appendix occurs the prognosis is much more guarded
- metastatic spread may occur in up to 20% of patients
- secondary deposits occur in peritoneum, ovary or liver

Anal region

5

NORMAL STRUCTURE

- the anal canal is approximately 3.5 cm in length and extends from the upper to the lower border of the internal sphincter. At the lower border of the internal sphincter the squamous mucosa of the anal canal merges into the true skin of the anal margin
- the upper part of the canal is derived from endoderm and the lower part of the canal is derived from ectoderm
- in adults the junction of upper and lower canal is marked by a series of anal valves. The line of the anal valves is known as the pectinate or dentate line
- the anal mucosa is plum coloured above and pale below the dentate line. The mucosa below the dentate line is composed of squamous epithelium
- the lower border of the sphincter marks the start of the perianal skin
- the transitional zone represents the area 1 cm above the junction of endoderm and ectoderm
- microscopically the transitional zone includes squamous, transitional and glandular epithelium
- internal sphincter consists of smooth muscle
- an external sphincter is present which is composed of three parts – subcutaneous, superficial and deep. These all consist of voluntary muscle

CONGENITAL ANORECTAL ABNORMALITIES

Divided into 'low' and 'high' abnormalities:

Low abnormalities

- ectopic anus – opens into vulva, vagina or perineum
- covered anus – lateral genital folds fuse posteriorly and a bar of skin covers the opening of the anal canal
- stenotic anus
- anal membrane. The normally sited anus is closed by an extremely thin membrane

High abnormalities

- anorectal agenesis. Anus, anal canal and lower rectum are missing
- rectal atresia where bowel ends blindly above the pelvic floor
- cloacal persistence where rectum, urinary and genital tracts open into a common cloacal cavity. Occurs only in girls

HAEMORRHOIDS

- internal haemorrhoids arise in upper two-thirds of anal canal
- external haemorrhoids are covered by squamous epithelium of lower one-third of canal

Internal haemorrhoids

- usually two on right and one on left side of canal
- microscopically there are dilated venous plexuses with arterial branches of superior haemorrhoidal artery and loose submucosal and subcutaneous connective tissue
- veins are tributaries of internal haemorrhoidal plexus
- occasionally haemorrhoids are associated with pelvic venous obstruction and portal hypertension
- most important complication is bleeding which may result in anaemia
- other complications include prolapse out of anus, strangulation, thrombosis, necrosis and infection
- precipitating factors include heredity, straining at stool, constipation, low fibre diet and altered sphincter tone

External haemorrhoids

- covered with squamous epithelium (derived from ectoderm and possesses a somatic type of nerve supply) and therefore painful
- thrombosed anal haematomas are due to rupture and thrombosis of external vein

ANAL FISSURE

- ulcer in squamous epithelial lined part of anal canal, usually in the midline posteriorly
- more common in women
- overlies internal sphincter and subcutaneous part of external sphincter
- predisposing factors include loss of normal elasticity of mucosa, hard stools and previous haemorrhoidectomy
- non-specific fissure should be distinguished from other causes of ulceration including Crohn's disease, squamous carcinoma, syphilis and tuberculosis
- if there is any doubt as to the diagnosis, a biopsy should be performed

ANORECTAL ABSCESS

- usual implicated organisms are *Bacteroides fragilis*, *Escherichia coli* and *Streptococcus faecalis*
- usually no cause is apparent, but may be associated with an anal fissure or an infected perianal haematoma

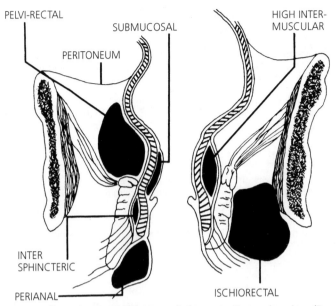

Figure 5.1 Different anatomical types of abscess in the anal region. (From Goligher 1984 with permission)

- the initial event appears to be an intersphincteric abscess arising between the internal and external sphincters. This can spread laterally to form an ischiorectal abscess. Spread downwards results in a perianal abscess
- most abscesses have an unknown aetiology, but associated conditions include diabetes, Crohn's disease, tuberculosis (TB) and AIDS

Classification of anorectal abscess

- perianal
- ischiorectal
- submucosal
- intersphincteric
- high intermuscular

ANAL FISTULA (FISTULA-IN-ANO)

- a fistula is a chronic granulating tract between two epithelial-lined surfaces
- in many cases the aetiology is unknown. Some cases may be secondary to an infected anal fistula or to infection of anal glands. Other associations include:
  - pyogenic anorectal abscess
  - foreign body

- postoperative
- Crohn's disease
- TB
- ulcerative colitis
- rectal cancer
- actinomycosis
- lymphogranuloma venereum
- during exploration and surgical treatment of anal fistulae and abscesses, it is important that tissues are sent for histological examination, in order to exclude other conditions

Classification of anal fistula

1. Intersphincteric fistula:
   - crosses internal sphincter. Does not cross external sphincter or anorectal ring. No problem with incontinence
2. Trans-sphincteric fistula:
   - passes through external sphincter and may also have high blind tract
3. Suprasphincteric fistula:
   - tract passes over top of anorectal ring and then down through levator muscle to ischiorectal fossa and then to skin
4. Extrasphincteric fistula:
   - tracks from perineal skin through ischiorectal fat and levators into rectum

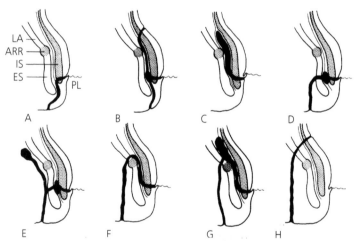

Figure 5.2   Fistula-in-ano. LA = Levator ani; ARR = anorectal ring; IS = internal sphincter; ES = external sphincter; PL = pectinate line. A = Intersphincteric; B = intersphincteric with a track passing upwards and entering the rectum; C = intersphincteric in which the track passes upwards without a perineal opening; D = trans-sphincteric; E = trans-sphincteric with a secondary track which reaches the apex of the ischiorectal fossa; F = sphincteric; G = suprasphincteric with a supralevator abscess; H = extrasphincteric

RECTAL PROLAPSE

- may be partial or complete

Partial prolapse

- only mucosa prolapses
- may occur in children due to absent sacral hollow, chronic cough, straining or diarrhoea
- in adults may be associated with haemorrhoids, a lax sphincter or cauda equina lesion
- often occurs in very elderly patients
- may be associated with solitary rectal ulcer syndrome (see Chapter 4)
- 20% develop complete rectal prolapse

Complete prolapse

- usually occurs in adults
- 85% are female
- often nulliparous
- associated with weak sphincter and incontinence
- denervation of sphincters is associated
- may be due to stretching of pudendal nerves
- complications include proctitis, ulceration, bleeding and, rarely, gangrene

DESCENDING PERINEAL SYNDROME

- descent of pelvic floor
- anterior rectal wall protrudes into bowel lumen causing rectal obstruction
- associated with lax sphincter

TUMOURS AND PREMALIGNANT CONDITIONS OF ANAL CANAL

Anal intraepithelial neoplasia (AIN)

- rare
- located in anal canal
- association with anal condylomata (viral warts) and human papilloma virus (HPV) infection
- more common in homosexual men and in women with cervical intraepithelial neoplasia (CIN)
- may coexist with Bowen's disease of the anal skin
- microscopically there is dysplasia of anal canal mucosa
- graded as mild, moderate or severe (AIN I, II, III)
- AIN III may progress to invasive carcinoma
- AIN III is more likely to be associated with HPV 16 infection than lower grades of AIN

Carcinoma of anal canal

- most arise *de novo*
- may rarely be associated with fistula or lymphogranuloma venereum
- occurs more often in women
- more common in homosexual men
- average age at presentation is 60 years
- usually presents with bleeding, pain and ulcerating mass
- most arise from transitional zone
- most are squamous carcinomas which may be either keratinising or non-keratinising
- other histological types include basaloid (cloacogenic) carcinoma and small cell undifferentiated carcinoma
- dentate line is adherent to internal sphincter and forms barrier to downward spread of tumour
- local spread of tumour is upwards into the lower third of the rectum. Therefore these often present clinically as tumours of the lower rectum
- lymph node spread is to pelvic and inguinal nodes
- prognosis depends on tumour size, differentiation, depth of tumour invasion and presence or absence of nodal metastasis

Carcinoma of anal ducts

- extremely rare
- adenocarcinoma
- may look like adenocarcinoma of rectum

Carcinoma in anorectal fistula

- patients present with anorectal fistula or recurrent anal abscess
- microscopy shows mucin-secreting adenocarcinoma

Malignant melanoma

- rare in anal canal
- arises from transitional zone
- presents as a polypoid anal mass
- melanin pigment often identified in tumour by electron microscopy or histochemical staining
- prognosis is poor
- most patients have involved lymph nodes at presentation
- blood spread is to liver and lungs
- 5-year survival less than 10%

Condylomata acuminata

- also known as viral warts
- usually sexually transmitted

- pink, red soft, multiple papillary growths
- microscopy shows acanthosis and hyperplasia of epidermis. Koilocytosis may also be seen, suggestive of viral infection
- due to human papilloma virus (HPV) infection
- may be associated with AIN or cervical intraepithelial neoplasia (CIN)

Giant condylomata acuminata (Buscke-Loewenstein tumour)

- exophytic, warty, tumour-like mass
- may be up to 10 cm in diameter
- may occur in anal canal or perianal skin
- cytologically bland, but probably represents a well differentiated verrucous carcinoma
- is locally invasive

Bowen's disease

- intraepithelial neoplasia involving perianal skin
- appears as red plaque, with scales or nodules
- microscopy reveals full thickness epithelial dysplasia
- ulceration may indicate the development of underlying invasive squamous carcinoma
- treatment is wide local excision
- may coexist with AIN or CIN
- there is frequently evidence of HPV infection

Bowenoid papulosis

- clinically similar to Bowen's disease
- younger adults
- multiple circumscribed papules
- microscopy similar to Bowen's disease, but no malignant predisposition
- due to HPV infection

Paget's disease of perianal skin (extramammary Paget's disease)

- rare
- appears as red, crusty, ulcerated patches
- microscopy shows large cells with vacuolated cytoplasm within squamous epithelium
- microscopically identical to Paget's disease of breast
- may indicate an *in-situ* carcinoma
- however, may be associated with an *in-situ* or invasive carcinoma in anal ducts
- treatment involves wide local excision

Squamous carcinoma of the anal margin

- less common than carcinoma of anal canal
- similar to other skin squamous carcinomas
- occurs usually in elderly men

- usually presents as an ulcer
- may be associated with poor personal hygiene
- microscopy reveals squamous carcinoma with epithelial nests and keratin pearls
- spread to inguinal lymph nodes
- surgery involves wide local excision
- better prognosis than carcinoma of anal canal

Basal cell carcinoma of anal margin

- rare
- presents as chronic indurated growth with central ulcer
- microscopically composed of cells with basaloid appearance
- surgery involves wide local excision

The liver

6

NORMAL STRUCTURE

- the liver develops as a diverticulum from the foregut
- the liver is connected to the vitelline veins of the yolk sac. These later form the hepatic and portal veins
- traditional right and left lobes of liver are divided by the falciform ligament
- surgical lobes are divided by a plane between the gallbladder fossa and the inferior vena cava
- the total hepatic blood flow is 1500 ml/min, 75% of which is from the portal vein
- portal vein pressure is 3–5 mmHg
- lymph forms in the space of Disse and runs with portal tracts

HISTOLOGY

- liver cells are arranged in hexagonal lobules with a central vein
- plates of liver cells are separated by hepatic sinusoids lined by endothelial and Kupffer cells which are part of the reticuloendothelial (RE) system
- portal tracts at the periphery of lobules contain branches of portal vein, hepatic artery and bile ducts

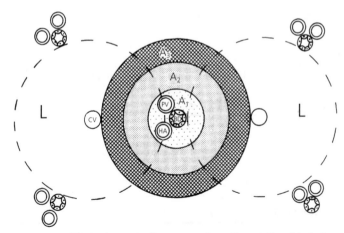

Figure 6.1 Simplified schematic diagram to show the relationship between the liver lobule (L) and the three zones of the liver acinus, A_1, A_2, A_3. CV = Central vein; PV = portal vein; BD = bile duct; HA = hepatic artery

- liver cells may be classified as centrilobular (around central veins), peripheral lobular (around portal tracts) and mid-zonal
- liver zones have also been described with the portal tracts as the centre and the centrilobular vein as the periphery:
  - zone 1 – surrounds portal tract
  - zone 3 – surrounds centrilobular vein
  - zone 2 – between zones 1 and 3
- hypoxia tends to damage zone 3 (centrilobular necrosis)
- toxins and drugs tend to damage zone 1 (peripheral lobular necrosis)
- the biliary system is composed of bile canaliculi which lie between hepatocytes
- these bile canaliculi drain to the canal of Hering, to the interlobular bile ducts, to septal ducts and hence to the right and left hepatic ducts

NORMAL FUNCTION

- formation and secretion of bile
- synthesis of albumin, globulin, clotting factors I, II, V, VII, IX, X
- synthesis of urea, glucose, cholesterol, lipoproteins
- removes toxins, ammonia, FDPs, hormones
- stores glycogen

LIVER BIOPSY

Methods

- percutaneous
  - Trucut needle
  - FNA – under ultrasound control
- open laparotomy
- laparoscopic
- transjugular
  - useful after liver transplantation
  - may be indicated if bleeding problems or ascites are present

Relative contraindications to liver biopsy

- patient uncooperative
- defective haemostasis
- hydatid disease
- severe ascites
- suspected vascular tumour

Complications (0–3%)

- bleeding
- pneumothorax
- bile leakage resulting in bile peritonitis

- perforation of gallbladder
- tumour seedling (very rare with FNA)
- septicaemia
- hepatic abscesses

Nature of biopsy

- normal – brown
- fatty change – yellow
- fragmented – cirrhosis
- jaundice – green
- haemochromatosis – dark brown
- secondary carcinoma – white
- Dubin-Johnson syndrome – black

JAUNDICE

- obvious if serum bilirubin above 35 μmol/l
- most easily seen in sclera of eyes
- bilirubin formed from haem (haemoglobin, myoglobin)
- RE system converts haem to biliverdin and then to bilirubin
- in plasma most bilirubin is bound to albumin – unconjugated bilirubin (water insoluble)
- bilirubin converted by enzyme glucuronyl transferase in hepatocytes to bilirubin mono-glucuronide and then di-glucuronide (conjugated bilirubin)
- conjugated bilirubin (water soluble) excreted into bile canaliculi
- in gut bilirubin is converted by bacteria into urobilinogen and is absorbed and re-excreted by liver (enterohepatic circulation)
- excess urobilinogen is excreted in urine

Causes of unconjugated hyperbilirubinaemia

- haemolysis. May be intravascular, e.g. haemolytic anaemia or extravascular, e.g. reabsorption of haematoma
- impaired hepatic uptake of bilirubin, e.g. in sepsis
- congenital causes
  1. Gilbert's syndrome (autosomal dominant)
     - defect in hepatic uptake of bilirubin. Patients are otherwise well. Benign condition
  2. Crigler-Najjar syndrome
     - type I (autosomal recessive). Due to absence of enzyme glucuronyl transferase. Severe jaundice and death in infancy
     - type II (autosomal dominant). Mild reduction in enzyme. Normal survival
- newborn jaundice. This is due to immature enzyme systems
- advanced liver disease. This may be due to a variety of causes

Causes of conjugated hyperbilirubinaemia

- associated with bilirubinuria, increased serum bile acids, increased serum alkaline phosphatase
- may be due to impaired secretion of bilirubin resulting in cholestasis

- Dubin-Johnson (D-J) syndrome and Rotor syndrome
- autosomal recessive conditions
- defect in excretion of bilirubin by hepatocytes
- in the Rotor syndrome the liver is normal in colour
- in D-J syndrome the liver is black in colour

Cholestasis

- may be intrahepatic or extrahepatic

INTRAHEPATIC CHOLESTASIS

- associated with hepatocellular disease, e.g. cirrhosis
- congenital atresia of bile ducts
- sex hormone administration, e.g. oral contraceptive pill
- early primary biliary cirrhosis (PBC)
- benign familial recurrent cholestasis
- recurrent jaundice of pregnancy

EXTRAHEPATIC CHOLESTASIS

- gallstones
- carcinoma of head of pancreas
- carcinoma of bile ducts
- enlarged lymph nodes at porta hepatitis
- pancreatitis
- benign bile duct stricture
- extrahepatic biliary atresia
- sclerosing cholangitis

Liver changes in jaundice

- if jaundice is due to unconjugated hyperbilirubinaemia liver appears normal
- if due to intrahepatic cholestasis microscopically there are features of underlying disease plus bile plugs within bile canalculi
- if due to extrahepatic cholestasis microscopically there are bile plugs together with oedema and inflammation within portal tract. There is also bile duct proliferation and bile infarcts may occur

Systemic effects of jaundice

- pruritus possibly due to retention of bile salts
- cardiovascular problems may occur due to bradycardia or decreased peripheral resistance
- renal complications include the hepatorenal syndrome and acute tubular necrosis
- coagulation problems occur due to lack of synthesis of clotting factors
- impaired wound healing
- sepsis may occur due to impaired RE system function

VIRAL HEPATITIS

The hepatitis viruses are hepatitis A, B, C, D, E and F. Other viruses such as cytomegalovirus (CMV) and Epstein-Barr virus (EBV) may affect the liver, but this is usually part of a systemic disease in which the liver is only one organ affected.

Hepatitis A virus (HAV)

- virus is 27 nm RNA virus
- spread by oral–faecal route
- incubation period is 15–45 days
- may be asymptomatic
- usually mild self-limiting disease
- diagnosis is by anti-HAV (IgM) in acute illness and anti-HAV (IgG) in convalescence
- no carrier state
- does not cause chronic liver disease
- rarely causes fulminant hepatitis
- no risk of malignant transformation

Hepatitis B virus (HBV)

- virus is a 42 nm DNA virus with 27 nm core
- spread by blood or blood products, mother to infant, injection or sexual transmission
- incubation period is 1–6 months
- core contains two antigens. These are known as core antigen (HBcAg) and e antigen (HBeAg)
- outer coat contains surface antigen (HBsAg). This is also known as the Australia antigen
- complete virion is called the Dane particle
- each antigen produces equivalent antibody (Figure 6.2)

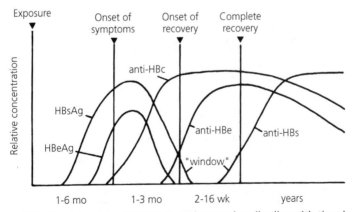

Figure 6.2 Graph to show the rises in antigen and antibodies with time in hepatitis B. (From Robbins et al. 1984, with permission)

- anti-HBs confers lifelong immunity
- persistence of HBsAg indicates risk of chronic liver disease and the development of cirrhosis
- HBeAg is associated with circulating Dane particles and indicates active infection and infectivity
- anti-HBe indicates recent disease
- healthy carriers are HBsAg positive but have no symptoms
- liver disease carriers are HBsAg positive and have chronic persistent or chronic active hepatitis
- chronic HBV infection increases risk of hepatocellular carcinoma (usually develops in cirrhotic liver)

Hepatitis C virus (HCV)

- causes 95% of post-transfusion hepatitis. Previously most of these were known as non-A non-B (NANB) hepatitis
- HCV causes 50% of sporadic cases of NANB hepatitis
- virus is a 30–60 nm diameter RNA virus
- incubation period is 14–120 days
- less infectious than HBV spread is by blood or blood products, injection, organ transplantation. Vertical spread from mother to infant has been described. Sexual transmission has been postulated
- risk groups for HCV are:
  - post-transfusion patients
  - haemodialysis patients
  - renal transplantation patients
  - thalassaemia patients
  - bone marrow or liver transplantation patients
  - health care workers
  - IV drug abusers
  - homosexuals
  - AIDs patients
- HCV usually causes a mild form of hepatitis
- can progress to chronic liver disease (50%); 20% may develop cirrhosis
- chronic HCV predisposes to hepatocellular carcinoma

Hepatitis D virus (HDV, delta agent)

- caused by 36 nm RNA virus
- infection requires coexistence of HBsAg and is either by co-infection or superinfection
- co-infection causes self-limiting disease
- superinfection causes chronic disease
- transmission is usually parenteral
- high incidence in Amazon, Middle East, Central Africa
- common in intravenous drug users
- diagnosis is by detection of hepatitis D antigen or IgM antibody

Hepatitis E virus (HEV)

- enteric (faecal–oral) transmission, usually via infected water
- 27–34 nm RNA virus

- epidemics in India, Asia, Africa
- incubation period 6 weeks
- worse in pregnant women
- self-limiting disease

Hepatitis F virus (HFV)

- not well characterised
- designation provisionally applied to 60–70 nm toga-like virus

Clinical features of viral hepatitis

- prodromal symptoms, e.g. flu-like illness, nausea, abdominal pain
- icteric phase 1–4 weeks
- usually followed by recovery

Pathology of acute hepatitis

- necrosis of hepatocytes (spotty necrosis)
- inflammation which is worse in zone 3
- enlargement of Kupffer cells
- portal inflammation
- bridging necrosis

Outcomes of viral hepatitis

- resolution
- massive necrosis
- post-necrotic scarring
- chronic persistent hepatitis
- chronic active hepatitis
- cirrhosis

TRANSMISSION OF HEPATITIS FROM PATIENT TO SURGEON

- highest risk is with hepatitis B
- protect eyes, double glove
- treat endoscopes with glutaraldehyde
- hepatitis-e-antigen-positive patient is highly infective

TRANSMISSION OF HEPATITIS FROM SURGEON TO PATIENT

- well documented
- usually only applies to hepatitis B

Current hepatitis B vaccine

- produced by recombinant techniques
- routine for health workers

Chronic hepatitis

Definition:

- chronic inflammatory liver disease which lasts for more than 6 months without improvement
- traditionally divided into chronic persistent and chronic active hepatitis. However, boundaries are not well defined

CHRONIC PERSISTENT HEPATITIS (CPH)

- abnormal liver function tests after viral infection but no progressive damage
- microscopy shows portal tracts with mild inflammatory cell infiltrate

CHRONIC ACTIVE HEPATITIS (CAH)

- this may be due to a variety of causes
- may be associated with hepatitis B, C or D
- autoimmune chronic active hepatitis. Usually female patients with positive autoantibodies
- drug induced, e.g. methyldopa
- Wilson's disease – hepatolenticular degeneration
- alcohol may cause a CAH-like picture
- in CAH get general malaise, abnormal liver function tests
- may progress to cirrhosis, usually over a long period of time
- microscopically there is piecemeal necrosis (interface hepatitis) of hepatocytes next to portal tract. May also be bridging necrosis, fibrosis and cirrhosis
- may progress to hepatocellular carcinoma

ALCOHOLIC LIVER DISEASE

- considerable individual susceptibility
- females more susceptible to effects of alcohol than males
- morphological effects of alcohol include fatty liver, alcoholic hepatitis and cirrhosis

Pathogenesis of alcohol induced liver damage

- direct cellular damage by alcohol to cytoskeleton
- increased acetaldehyde (reduced aldehyde dehydrogenase)
- damaged microfilaments and tubules in cell cytoplasm
- translation of mRNA affected
- immune damage by cytotoxins and lymphokines
- tumour necrosis factor causes fever and activates polymorphs

Clinical features

- fatty liver is usually asymptomatic
- alcoholic hepatitis presents as acute hepatitis
- in alcoholic cirrhosis get signs of chronic liver disease

Pathology

FATTY LIVER

- pale, greasy on cutting
- microscopy shows vacuolated cells containing fat

ALCOHOLIC HEPATITIS

- necrosis of hepatocytes and inflammatory cell infiltration occur
- cells contain Mallory's hyaline in a crescentic shape around cell nucleus
- get pericellular fibrosis and perivenular fibrosis around central veins

Alcoholic cirrhosis

- may get micro- or macronodular cirrhosis
- may progress to hepatocellular carcinoma

LIVER CIRRHOSIS

- there are a variety of aetiological factors in the development of hepatic cirrhosis

Alcohol

- see above

Viral hepatitis

- see above
- usually HBV or HCV

Primary biliary cirrhosis (PBC)

- usually 40–60 year age group
- usually middle-aged female (F:M=9:1)
- presents with pain, jaundice, itch, ascites, xanthelasma
- may be associated with other autoimmune diseases
- 80% progress to cirrhosis in 4 years
- median survival is 10 years
- microscopy shows lymphocytic infiltration around bile ductules in portal tracts with granulomatous reaction. Piece-meal necrosis may also be present
- serum antimitochondrial antibodies are present in most cases and are useful in diagnosis
- treated with steroids
- survival good after liver transplantation
- may progress to hepatocellular carcinoma

Secondary biliary cirrhosis

- caused by extrahepatic biliary obstruction
- damage by inflammation, ascending cholangitis
- microscopically there is pronounced bile stasis and proliferation of small ductules

Haemochromatosis (primary or secondary)

PRIMARY

- autosomal recessive condition – gene on short arm of chromosome 5 – caused by excess absorption of iron

SECONDARY

- caused by iron overload, e.g. thalassaemia

PRIMARY HAEMOCHROMATOSIS

- male:female = 10:1
- usually age 40–60 years
- clinically may present with liver disease, diabetes, skin pigmentation, heart disease and arthritis
- treatment is regular venesection
- may develop cirrhosis
- increased risk of hepatocellular carcinoma

Wilson's disease (hepatolenticular degeneration)

- autosomal recessive condition
- usually presents age 5–30 years
- gene located on chromosome 13
- excess copper in liver, basal ganglia of brain, cerebellum and eye (Kayser-Fleischer ring)
- mechanism of damage is unclear but may be due to production of free radicals
- increased risk of hepatocellular carcinoma
- may progress to cirrhosis

Alpha 1-antitrypsin deficiency

- α1-antitrypsin is a protease inhibitor
- gene is located on chromosome 14
- if deficient leads to increased α1-antitrypsin accumulation in hepatocytes
- associated with neonatal hepatitis and later cirrhosis
- may also get panlobular emphysema

Other metabolic disorders

- several other metabolic disorders which may result in cirrhosis include galactosaemia, congenital tyrosinaemia and hereditary fructose intolerance

Drugs

- drugs such as methotrexate may result in hepatic fibrosis and cirrhosis

Intestinal bypass

- may result in progressive hepatic damage and cirrhosis
- usually for morbid obesity
- may be due to chenodeoxycholate being metabolised in large bowel to lithocholate which, when absorbed, causes liver damage

Indian childhood cirrhosis

- usually Indian subcontinent, but may also be found in Caucasians
- unknown cause
- age 1–3 years
- death in 12 months

Cryptogenic

- unknown cause
- in UK this accounts for approximately 30% of cases of cirrhosis

Pathology of cirrhosis

- cirrhosis is morphologically characterised by nodules of hepatocytes surrounded by fibrous tissue septae
- may be classified into macronodular (nodules >3 mm), micronodular (nodules <3 mm) and mixed forms
- micronodular cirrhosis is typical of early alcoholic cirrhosis, Wilson's disease, haemochromatosis and primary biliary cirrhosis
- macronodular cirrhosis is typical of late alcoholic cirrhosis and hepatitis associated liver cirrhosis

Histology

- nodules of hepatocytes surrounded by fibrous tissue
- if alcohol aetiology, Mallory's hyaline may be present
- if HBV aetiology, may detect HBsAg immunohistochemically
- if PBC, there may be granulomas and paucity of bile ducts
- in secondary biliary cirrhosis, bile plugs are prominent
- special stains may show iron, copper and α1-antitrypsin in haemochromatosis, Wilson's disease and α1-antitrypsin deficiency respectively

Complications

- portal hypertension
- ascites

- liver failure
- hepatic encephalopathy
- renal complications. May be due to hepatorenal syndrome or acute tubular necrosis

PORTAL HYPERTENSION

- normal portal vein pressure is 5–7 mmHg – portal hypertension may be due to extrahepatic, intrahepatic or suprahepatic causes

Table 6.1 Causes of portal hypertension

Type of portal hypertension	Cause
Extrahepatic (prehepatic)	Portal vein thrombosis
Intrahepatic	Cirrhosis Hepatitis Congenital hepatic fibrosis Partial nodular transformation Schistosomiasis Portal tract infiltration (e.g. lymphoproliferative disease) Sarcoidosis Idiopathic portal hypertension Veno-occlusive disease
Suprahepatic	Budd–Chiari syndrome Constrictive pericarditis Right-sided heart failure
Increased hepatic blood flow	Massive splenomegaly Hepatoportal arteriovenous fistula

Extrahepatic portal hypertension

- causes include portal vein thrombosis. May be due to umbilical vein catheterisation or infection in children
- other causes include trauma, tumour, sepsis or pancreatitis
- no cause found in 50%
- liver function is good. Therefore prognosis is good

Intrahepatic portal hypertension

- most common cause is cirrhosis
- schistosomiasis may cause intrahepatic portal hypertension. This disease results in intrahepatic presinusoidal portal hypertension. Schistosome ova result in characteristic pipe-stem fibrosis
- veno-occlusive disease. This results in post-sinusoidal intrahepatic portal hypertension. Branches of small hepatic veins are obliterated. Cause is ingestion of alkaloids, e.g. in bush teas

Suprahepatic portal hypertension

- Budd-Chiari syndrome is usually due to thrombosis of main hepatic veins. Usually idiopathic
- other recognised causes of thrombosis of hepatic veins include oral contraceptive pill, tumours, hypercoagulable states

Complications of portal hypertension

- bleeding oesophageal varices (see Chapter 2)
- ascites

LIVER CYSTS

Non-parasitic

- simple – usually solitary, contain brown fluid and are lined by cuboidal epithelium
- traumatic – bile filled, solitary, no epithelial lining
- polycystic liver disease
  - associated with polycystic renal disease (90% of cases)
  - associated with spina bifida
  - many cases are asymptomatic
  - rarely rupture and haemorrhage occur
  - wall consists of loose connective tissue lined by cuboidal epithelium

Hydatid liver cysts

- due to larval or cyst stage of tapeworm *Echinococcus granulosus*
- structure of cyst (Figure 6.3)

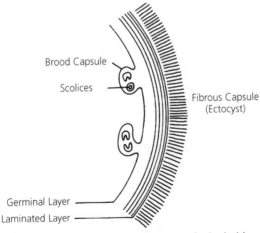

Brood Capsule

Scolices

Fibrous Capsule
(Ectocyst)

Germinal Layer

Laminated Layer

Figure 6.3 Schematic diagram of part of the wall of a hydatid cyst (see text)

- inner nucleated germinal layer
- laminated non-nucleated layer
- outside is dense host fibrous capsule
- budding of germinal layer forms brood cysts
- brood cysts contain scolices of the worm which form hydatid sand
- complications include rupture of cysts with resultant peritoneal seedlings, secondary infection, biliary obstruction and portal hypertension

LIVER ABSCESS

Pyogenic abscess

- usually occur in elderly people
- present with abdominal pain, rigors
- abscesses may be single or multiple
- in chronic abscess there is fibrous capsule with granulation tissue
- local extension to subphrenic and pleural spaces may occur
- metastatic abscesses may occur in brain or lung

CAUSES

- biliary obstruction
- portal pyaemia, e.g. appendicitis, diverticulitis
- septicaemia
- direct extension from gallbladder infection
- infection of liver cyst or tumour
- trauma
- 20% no obvious cause
- in young children may be complication of leukaemia
- causative organisms include Gram-negative bacilli, *E. coli*, *Klebsiella*, *Proteus*, staphylococcal species, streptococcal species, *Clostridium*, *Actinomyces* and *Bacteroides*; 30% have multiple organisms

Amoebic abscess

- intestinal lesion spreads to liver via portal vein
- characteristically there is anchovy sauce pus within abscesses
- diagnosis is by ultrasound-guided aspiration
- complications include pleural effusion, pneumonia, rupture into pleural space, lung, peritoneal cavity and pericardium
- open drainage rarely required
- treatment is aspiration plus metronidazole

BENIGN EPITHELIAL LIVER TUMOURS AND TUMOUR-LIKE CONDITIONS

Liver adenoma

- usually occurs in young women
- may be asymptomatic or may present with pain sometimes as an emergency due to bleeding, especially with the oral contraceptive pill (OCP)

- associated with OCP and androgenic steroids
- grossly single well circumscribed nodule
- no capsule
- microscopy shows plates of liver cells (2–3 thick). Bile ducts are absent
- may regress after stopping OCP
- major complication is bleeding with rupture
- microscopically may be difficult to distinguish from well differentiated hepatocellular carcinoma

Focal nodular hyperplasia (FNH)

- usually single nodular lesion in otherwise normal liver
- mostly asymptomatic but occasionally may get pain, rupture or bleeding
- male:female ratio = 1:2
- weak association with OCP
- grossly appears as yellow/brown mass which, on cross-section has a central stellate scar
- microscopy shows nodules of normal liver cells with central fibrous scar. Large vascular channels may be present
- stopping OCP may result in regression
- may enlarge during pregnancy

Bile duct adenoma

- rare benign lesion
- usually discovered incidentally
- microscopy shows proliferation of small bile ductules

MALIGNANT EPITHELIAL LIVER TUMOURS

Hepatocellular carcinoma (HCC)

EPIDEMIOLOGY, AETIOLOGY AND PATHOGENESIS

- rare in Western countries
- in West usually elderly patients
- male:female ratio = 9:1
- common tumour in East Asia, China, Africa
- in Eastern countries, usually younger patients with male:female ratio of 3:1
- strong association with HBV infection
- in South-East Asia 10% of population are HBsAg positive
- patients with HCC are often HBsAg positive
- in Western countries 90% arise in cirrhotic livers
- 5% of cirrhotic livers will develop HCC
- HCC is most common in post-viral cirrhosis and haemochromatosis
- mycotoxins such as *Aspergillus* may also be implicated

CLINICAL FEATURES

- usually arise in background of cirrhosis
- weight loss and abdominal pain may worsen
- serum alpha-fetoprotein (αFP) raised in 90% of HCC patients

GROSS PATHOLOGY

- massive, nodular and diffuse forms
- massive is a solitary tumour, sometimes in young non-cirrhotic patient
- nodular form occurs in cirrhotic liver
- diffuse form occurs as multiple small nodules in cirrhotic liver

HISTOLOGY

- loss of normal lobular architecture
- tumour cells often form a trabecular pattern
- solid pattern may be seen
- pseudoglandular formation may be found
- cells show pleomorphism and hyperchromasia
- giant cells and clear cells may be present
- HBsAg may be demonstrated immunohistochemically

DIAGNOSIS

- FNA under US control
- CT guided biopsy

TREATMENT

- intrahepatic chemotherapy
- surgery
- embolisation
- liver transplantation. Long-term results are poor

Fibrolamellar variant of HCC

- young patients
- no pre-existing liver disease
- well developed nodule with central scar
- histology shows trabecular pattern with massive accumulation of fibrous stroma
- better prognosis than other forms of HCC
- serum αFP usually not raised

Hepatoblastoma

- rare, occurs mainly in childhood
- age usually less than 2 years
- presents as abdominal mass and weight loss
- occasionally rupture and bleed
- serum αFP may be raised
- associated with congenital abnormalities
- grossly there is large mass with necrosis and haemorrhage
- microscopy shows epithelial and mesenchymal elements
- aggressive and spreads widely

Intrahepatic cholangiocarcinoma

- see Chapter 7

NON-EPITHELIAL TUMOURS OF LIVER

Benign

HAEMANGIOMAS

- most common benign tumour of liver
- usually asymptomatic
- usually solitary
- occasionally if large may cause symptoms

Tumours of uncertain malignant potential

INFANTILE HAEMANGIOENDOTHELIOMA

- age less than 4 years
- arteriovenous shunting may lead to cardiac failure
- may present with abdominal mass
- may rupture and bleed
- grossly usually a multinodular tumour
- microscopy shows many vascular channels
- rarely metastasises

EPITHELIOID HAEMANGIOENDOTHELIOMA

- female:male ratio = 2:1
- often multiple
- microscopically there are epithelioid cells lining vascular channels
- prognosis unpredictable

Malignant

ANGIOSARCOMA

- male:female ratio = 3:1
- associated with thorotrast injection, exposure to vinyl chloride and arsenic
- tenuous link with the OCP
- cause unknown for majority of cases
- presents with enlarged liver, ascites, pain and jaundice
- grossly often multicentric
- microscopy shows malignant endothelial cells forming vascular channels
- metastasises to lymph nodes, lungs, bones, adrenal glands
- poor prognosis

MESENCHYMAL SARCOMA

- tumour of childhood
- most patients 6–10 years
- sex incidence is equal
- usually present with abdominal mass and weight loss
- microscopy shows spindle-shaped cells
- poor prognosis

Secondary liver tumours

- reach liver by haematogenous spread
- common primary sites include pancreas, large bowel, stomach, lung and breast
- grossly well defined, multiple white nodules with central necrosis
- microscopy may or may not give clue to primary site
- recent encouraging results with resection of limited number of metastatic deposits

The biliary system

7

NORMAL STRUCTURE

- small bile ductules within the liver coalesce to form the right and left hepatic ducts
- these join to form the common hepatic duct
- the common hepatic duct joins with the cystic duct from the gallbladder to form the common bile duct (CBD)
- the lower 2 cm of the CBD is surrounded by the choledochal sphincter
- narrowest portion of CBD is at entrance to duodenum (site of stone impaction)
- gallbladder is composed of fundus, body and neck which leads to cystic duct
- gallbladder mucosa is composed of columnar epithelium with underlying connective tissue
- thick wall of muscle fibres and connective tissue
- outer serosa
- bile ducts have a cuboidal epithelial lining with underlying connective tissue

CONGENITAL ANOMALIES OF GALLBLADDER

- may be absent (agenesis)
- may be small (hypoplasia)
- duplication. May be complete (double) or partial (bi-lobed)
- may be intrahepatic
- may have long mesentery – floating gallbladder

Congenital dilatations of the bile ducts

(Figure 7.1)

TYPE 1

- dilatation of the common bile duct which may be either large sacular, small localised or diffuse fusiform

TYPE II

- diverticulum of gallbladder or common bile duct

TYPE III

- choledochocoele

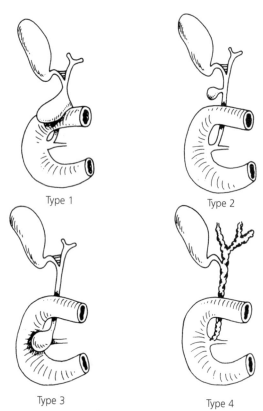

Type 1

Type 2

Type 3

Type 4

Figure 7.1   Cysts and dilatations of the bile ducts. 1 = Choledochal cyst; 2 = diverticulum of the bile duct; 3 = choledochocele; 4 = Caroli's disease. (From Olbourne 1975, with permission)

TYPE IV

- multiple intrahepatic and extrahepatic dilatation (Caroli's disease)

TYPE V

- fusiform intrahepatic and extrahepatic dilatation

Choledochal cyst

- classically presents with pain, abdominal mass and jaundice
- cause is unknown, but theories include muscle weakness and neuromuscular incoordination or reflux of pancreatic juice

- microscopically the wall of bile duct is thickened by inflammatory fibrous tissue
- treatment usually involves drainage of cyst by choledochocystojejunostomy

COMPLICATIONS

- perforation
- pancreatitis
- abscess
- cholangitis
- biliary cirrhosis
- malignant change. This is usually adenocarcinoma but occasionally squamous carcinoma

Biliary atresia

- incidence is 1/10 000 live births
- presents as neonatal jaundice
- aetiology unknown, but possibly due to viral infection *in utero*
- microscopically there is fibrous obliteration of bile ducts, cholestasis and giant cell transformation of hepatocytes
- liver biopsy may be difficult to distinguish from neonatal hepatitis
- treatment is surgical repair (Kasai operation) within 2 months of birth
- in some series long-term results are good with 85% of patients asymptomatic in 5 years

GALLSTONES

These may be cholesterol, pigment or mixed in type

Epidemiology

CHOLESTEROL OR MIXED STONES

- common
- in Europe and USA 20% of women and 8% of men have cholesterol or mixed gallstones
- in Europe and USA 80% of gallstones are mainly cholesterol
- female: male ratio is 3:1
- incidence increases with age
- obesity, oral contraceptive pill and high calorie diet predispose
- positive family history, abnormal cholesterol metabolism, total parenteral nutrition (TPN), open heart surgery, ileal resection or bypass, gastrectomy and vagotomy are associated with an increased incidence of gallstones

PIGMENT STONES

- more common in Far East
- associated with infected bile, cirrhosis and haemolytic anaemia

Pathogenesis

CHOLESTEROL AND MIXED STONES
Supersaturation of bile

- bile becomes lithogenic due to increased cholesterol concentration or reduced bile salt pool
- rate-limiting enzyme for production of cholesterol is 3-hydroxy-3-methylglutaryl coenzyme A (increased activity with age and obesity)
- bile salt pool becomes reduced with increasing age or secondary to ileal resection or disease, e.g. Crohn's disease. This is because bile salts are reabsorbed in the ileum (enterohepatic circulation)

Crystallization

- may be initiated by:
  - bacteria
  - parasites
  - epithelial cells
  - calcium crystals
  - mucin

Growth

- continues if bile remains supersaturated with cholesterol

Role of gallbladder

- stasis promotes growth, e.g. during pregnancy
- fasting reduces flow of bile
- decreased motility promotes sludge in wall

PIGMENT STONES

- supersaturation of bile with bilirubin in haemolytic anaemias

Pathology

- cholesterol stones are large, pale, smooth and often solitary
- mixed stones are multiple, faceted, laminated and variable in colour
- pigment stones are small, black and multiple; 10% of these stones are radio-opaque

Complications of gallstones

BILIARY COLIC

- due to temporary impaction of stone in cystic duct

ACUTE CHOLECYSTITIS

- obstruction of gallbladder outlet
- initial chemical inflammation due to lysolecithin being converted to cytotoxic compound

- increased luminal pressure on wall results in inflammation
- gallbladder enlarged and hyperaemic with surface fibrinous exudate
- mucosal surface is hyperaemic and ulcerated. May later proceed to gangrenous cholecystitis
- *Escherichia coli, Streptococcus faecalis, Clostridium welchii* and *Bacteroides* are commonest organisms isolated from bile

EMPHYSEMATOUS CHOLECYSTITIS

- caused by gas-forming bacteria
- associated with diabetes
- x-ray shows gas in wall of gallbladder

EMPYEMA OF GALLBLADDER

- lumen filled with pus
- patient ill with features of septicaemia

PERFORATION OF GALLBLADDER

- rare
- repeated attacks of inflammation thicken wall
- fundus has poorest blood supply and is commonest site of perforation

MUCOCOELE OF GALLBLADDER

- gallbladder mucosa secretes mucus
- if outlet is obstructed may get accumulation of mucus in lumen
- asymptomatic or may present with mass
- may perforate resulting in pseudomyxoma peritoneii

CHRONIC CHOLECYSTITIS

- chronic low grade symptoms
- gallstones nearly always present
- usually chemical inflammation
- thickening of gallbladder wall with fibrous tissue
- Rokitansky-Aschoff sinuses form due to herniation of epithelium through wall

PORCELAIN GALLBLADDER

- dystrophic calcification occurs in wall of gallbladder
- high risk of malignant change

CARCINOMA OF GALLBLADDER

- see later

OBSTRUCTIVE JAUNDICE

- may be due to formation of stones in bile duct or migration of gallbladder stones

SECONDARY BILIARY CIRRHOSIS

- see above (Chapter 7)

ASCENDING CHOLANGITIS

- classically presents with Charcot's triad of pain, temperature, jaundice
- on liver biopsy microscopy shows oedema and polymorphs in portal tracts with collection of polymorphs in ducts

LIVER ABSCESS

- (see Chapter 6)

PANCREATITIS

- (see p. 105)

GALLSTONE ILEUS

- biliary-enteric fistula between gallbladder and duodenum or colon
- most commonly causes obstruction 20 cm proximal to ileocaecal valve
- x-ray shows air in biliary tree
- usually elderly female patient

ACALCULOUS CHOLECYSTITIS

- associated with diabetes, burns, trauma, AIDS
- more common in males
- common in ICU
- causes include multiple blood transfusions, dehydration, TPN, ventilators, ischaemia
- high mortality (40%)
- perforation and gangrene common

CHOLESTEROLOSIS

- strawberry gallbladder
- mostly asymptomatic
- due to absorption of cholesterol from supersaturated bile
- grossly there are yellow flecks in mucosa
- microscopically there are lipid-filled histiocytes within mucosa of gallbladder beneath epithelium

PRIMARY SCLEROSING CHOLANGITIS (PSC)

- rare
- results in fibrous obliteration of bile ducts
- usually presents 25–45 years

- male:female ratio = 2:1
- may have immunological cause. Many cases are associated with HLA B8 or DR3 phenotypes
- over 50% have associated ulcerative colitis
- may require liver transplantation

Criteria for diagnosis

- diffuse generalised involvement of intra- and/or extra-hepatic bile ducts
- absence of previous biliary surgery
- absence of gallstones
- exclusion of cholangiocarcinoma by long-term follow up
- cholangiogram reveals beaded appearance with dilatations and strictures
- grossly ducts are thickened with narrowed lumina
- microscopy of liver biopsy shows periductal fibrosis with obliteration of small ductules which are replaced by scar tissue
- extrahepatic ducts show focal ulceration, inflammation and fibrosis

Complications

- secondary biliary cirrhosis
- oesophageal varices
- liver failure
- cholangiocarcinoma

BILE DUCT STRICTURES

There are many causes of bile duct stricture:

1. Cholangiocarcinoma – see below

2. Primary sclerosing cholangitis – see above

3. Stenosis of ampulla of Vater
   - associated with recurrent papillitis
   - cause unknown
   - microscopy shows decrease in muscle and increase in subepithelial fibrous tissue

4. Post-inflammatory stricture
   - uncommon
   - associated with gallstones, chronic pancreatitis and duodenal ulcer

5. Traumatic
   - most due to surgery (usually cholecystectomy)
   - increasing numbers in learning curve of laparoscopic cholecystectomy
   - occasionally due to penetrating injury

Presentation

- obstructive jaundice
- bile peritonitis
- biliary fistula
- cholangitis

Complications

- ascending cholangitis
- secondary biliary cirrhosis
- oesophageal varices
- liver failure

TUMOURS OF GALLBLADDER

Adenoma

- rare
- pedunculated or sessile mass with gland formation on histology
- may be divided into papillary, tubular or tubulopapillary
- may be multiple
- common with gallstones
- small risk of malignant transformation

Adenomyoma and adenomyomatosis

- an adenomyoma is a localised collection of cystic spaces in the gallbladder wall lined by glandular epithelium and surrounded by hyperplastic smooth muscle
- may be hamartomatous rather than neoplastic
- appears as nodule
- usually involves the fundus of the gallbladder
- if widespread area of gallbladder wall affected, this is termed adenomyomatosis

Carcinoma of gallbladder

- may be incidental finding at cholecystectomy
- if symptomatic usually presents late with jaundice, weight loss or abdominal mass
- 1% of gallbladder specimens contain carcinoma
- more common in females (6:1)
- usually elderly, 60–80 years
- affects whites more commonly than blacks
- gallstones are present in a high proportion of cases
- may arise in a porcelain gallbladder

PATHOLOGY

- most are infiltrating or fungating
- microscopically over 80% are adenocarcinomas
- may be papillary
- variable differentiation
- most of remainder are squamous or adenosquamous in type
- rarely oat cell or small cell undifferentiated carcinomas occur
- giant cell types may also occur

SPREAD

- direct spread to liver
- lymphatic spread to adjacent glands
- venous spread to liver

PROGNOSIS

- depends on stage
- most present at advanced stage and prognosis is poor

Miscellaneous tumours of gallbladder

- rare malignant tumours occasionally described within the gallbladder include various sarcomas, carcinosarcoma, malignant melanoma, carcinoid tumour and lymphoma

TUMOURS OF BILE DUCTS

Bile duct adenoma

- usually intrahepatic
- see p. 98

Cystadenoma

- rare
- sessile or papillary
- often intrahepatic

Biliary papillomatosis

- rare
- multiple papillomas involving intra- and extrahepatic bile ducts

Carcinoma of the bile duct (cholangiocarcinoma)

(Figure 7.2)

- May be intra- or extrahepatic in location

EPIDEMIOLOGY, AETIOLOGY AND PATHOGENESIS

- common in South-East Asia where infestation with liver flukes may be a major aetiological factor
- associated with typhoid carriers
- occurs in 4% of choledochal cysts
- occurs in 7% of cases of Caroli's disease

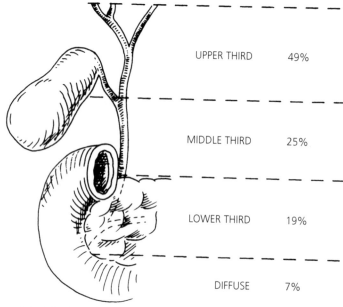

Figure 7.2 Distribution of carcinoma of the extrahepatic biliary system. (From Tompkins et al. 1981, with permission)

- more common in patients with ulcerative colitis
- may complicate primary sclerosing cholangitis (PSC)
- association with radiological contrast medium thorotrast

CLINICAL

- sex distribution equal
- usually elderly patients
- may present with mass lesion in liver
- may present with obstructive jaundice

PATHOLOGY

- intrahepatic tumour may be solitary or multiple
- firm due to extensive fibrosis
- microscopically almost all are adenocarcinomas
- characteristically get tubular structures surrounded by extensive fibrous reaction
- most are well differentiated
- may be adjacent *in situ* carcinomatous change
- papillary types are more common in distal common bile duct
- if well differentiated frozen section diagnosis is difficult

SPREAD

- direct along ducts
- lymphatic to local lymph nodes
- blood spread to liver, lungs and distant sites
- perineural infiltration is common

PROGNOSIS

- prognosis is poor
- outlook is better for extrahepatic tumours
- palliation with surgical bypass or ERCP stenting

The pancreas

8

NORMAL STRUCTURE

Embryology

- pancreas develops from ventral and dorsal outpouchings of foregut (Figure 8.1)
- ventral bud forms lower part of head and uncinate process
- dorsal bud forms body, neck, tail and upper head
- main pancreatic duct of Wirsung drains into ampulla of Vater. Accessory duct of Santorini ends separately in a minor duodenal papilla
- variations of duct anatomy are common

Arterial supply

- head of pancreas is supplied by superior and inferior pancreaticoduodenal arteries
- neck, body and tail are supplied by splenic artery

Venous drainage

- head drains via superior and inferior pancreaticoduodenal veins to portal and superior mesenteric veins
- rest of pancreas drains to splenic vein

Lymphatic drainage

- head of pancreas drains to coeliac nodes
- most of rest of pancreas drains to retroperitoneal nodes
- uncinate process drains to superior mesenteric nodes

Structure

- pancreas is composed of lobules separated by fibrous tissue septa
- lobules are composed of acini (exocrine pancreas) which consist of pyramidal cells with apices pointing towards lumen. These cells have granular cytoplasm because of numerous zymogen granules which contain pancreatic enzymes
- islets of Langerhans (endocrine pancreas) also lie within lobules
- intralobular arteries first supply islets and then exocrine acini
- acini therefore receive blood supply rich in islet hormones
- islets are distributed throughout the pancreas but are more numerous in the tail
- islets contain alpha, beta, delta and PP cells

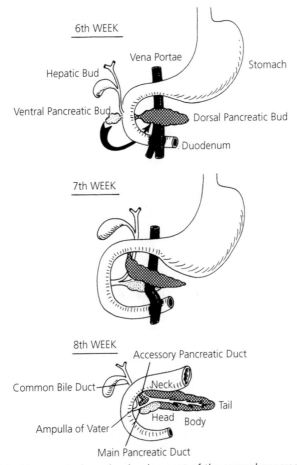

Figure 8.1 Diagram to show the development of the normal pancreas

- alpha cells produce glucagon and are mainly situated at the periphery of islets
- beta cells produce insulin and are mainly situated at the centre of islets
- delta cells produce somatostatin and are situated between alpha and beta cells
- PP cells produce pancreatic polypeptide
- in the normal adult pancreas there are no gastrin-producing cells but pancreatic endocrine neoplasms may produce gastrin (see p. 26)
- acinar cells of exocrine pancreas produce enzymes which are important in the digestive process
- these enzymes are important in:
  - protein digestion (trypsin, chymotrypsin, elastase, carboxypeptidase A, B)
  - fat digestion (lipase, phospholipase)
  - starch digestion (amylase)
  - nucleic acid degradation (ribonuclease, deoxyribonuclease)

PANCREATIC BIOPSY

Pancreatic juice cytology after secretin stimulation

- not popular

Ultrasound or CT guided FNA

- 90% accuracy in some series
- seeding of tumour cells does not occur
- complications are rare

Intraoperative biopsy

- FNA
- trucut biopsy – transduodenal
- wedge biopsy
- chronic pancreatitis may mimic malignancy and distinction on frozen section may be difficult

CONGENITAL ABNORMALITIES OF PANCREAS

Pancreas divisum

- ventral and dorsal parts of gland fail to fuse
- ducts of Santorini and Wirsung drain separate parts
- may predispose to pancreatitis

Annular pancreas

- rare
- due to failure of ventral bud to rotate properly
- get encirclement of duodenum by pancreas
- may be associated with other congenital malformations of the gastrointestinal tract
- may occur in Down's syndrome
- usually presents with vomiting in first week of life
- occasionally presents with duodenal obstruction in adult
- may predispose to pancreatitis

Ectopic pancreas

- relatively frequent congenital abnormality
- nodules in submucosa of stomach, duodenum, jejunum, ileum, Meckels' diverticulum, gallbladder and other areas
- may ulcerate or bleed
- many are asymptomatic
- microscopically there are always acinar tissue and ducts
- islets found in one-third of cases

PANCREATITIS

Marseille classification 1963

1. acute pancreatitis
2. acute relapsing pancreatitis
3. chronic pancreatitis
4. chronic relapsing pancreatitis

Cambridge classification 1984

1. acute pancreatitis
2. chronic pancreatitis

In chronic pancreatitis there are irreversible morphological changes, usually associated with loss of function.

Acute pancreatitis

This appears to be increasing in incidence, especially in males.

AETIOLOGY

Many aetiological factors have been implicated in the causation of acute pancreatitis:

- gallstones. These may be situated either in the gallbladder or in the common bile duct
- alcohol
- trauma
- post-ERCP
- pancreatic carcinoma
- pancreas divisum
- annular pancreas
- ischaemia
- hypothermia
- infection. Many organisms have been implicated including mumps, rubella, hepatitis, coxsackie virus, *Helicobacter*, TB, *Ascaris*
- drugs, e.g. diuretics, azothiaprine
- hyperlipidaemia
- hyperparathyroidism
- hereditary forms
- idiopathic. As many as 30% of cases may be idiopathic

PATHOGENESIS

- pathogenesis remains controversial
- in many cases obstruction of ampula of Vater results in bile passing from the common bile duct into the pancreatic duct. This activates trypsinogen and begins a cascade of events which include digestion of duct walls, pancreatic parenchyma and vessel walls by trypsin. Splitting of fats and formation of calcium soaps is initiated by lipase

- however, in many cases no obstructive lesion can be demonstrated
- gallstones may have migrated or biliary sludge or spasm of sphincter of Oddi may have resulted in obstruction

AUTODIGESTION

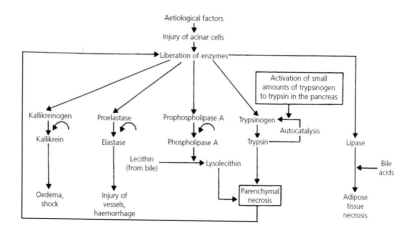

activation by trypsin

Figure 8.2 Diagram to show the pathogenesis of acute pancreatitis

- final common pathway appears to be via trypsin activation and hence cascade
- bradykinin and kallidin cause vasodilatation, increased vascular permeability and produce systemic shock
- lipase causes fat necrosis
- phospholipase A causes destruction of cell membranes

CLINICAL FEATURES

- abdominal pain, vomiting
- high serum amylase
- criteria to assess prognosis include Ranson factors, Imrie criteria, Apache scores

PATHOLOGY

- oedematous phase in which pancreas is swollen but there is no necrosis
- haemorrhagic phase. There are areas of haemorrhagic necrosis within pancreas and fat necrosis surrounding pancreas
- microscopically there is destruction of pancreatic parenchyma
- necrosis of blood vessels, thrombosis, haemorrhage
- fat necrosis, calcification
- acute inflammatory reaction

COMPLICATIONS

Pulmonary

- right to left shunting caused by microthrombi in microvasculature
- adult respiratory distress syndrome (ARDS) caused by phospholipase which damages surfactant

Shock

- hypovolaemia
- vasodilatation due to kinins
- increased vascular permeability
- myocardial depressant factor

Renal

- shock resulting in acute tubular necrosis – fibrin deposits in glomerular capillaries

Hypocalcaemia

- fall in albumin
- fat necrosis
- decreased magnesium
- shift of calcium from extra- to intracellular compartments

Hyperglycaemia

- islet cell dysfunction results in excess secretion of glucagon and decreased secretion of insulin

GI bleeding

- stress-induced erosions in stomach or duodenum
- DIC
- involvement of duodenal wall by pancreatic mass
- gastric varices due to splenic vein thrombosis
- false aneurysm of splenic artery

Skin/bone

- fat necrosis in subcutaneous tissues and in bone

Pancreatic pseudocyst

- (see p. 109)

Pancreatic abscess

- 4–25% of patients with severe acute pancreatitis
- secondary infection usually occurs in second week after acute attack
- mortality up to 30%

Pancreatic necrosis

- necrotic mass of pancreas
- diagnosed by contrast-enhanced CT scan

PROGNOSIS

- overall mortality is approximately 5%
- in very severe pancreatitis, mortality is over 15%
- may need urgent necrosectomy

Chronic pancreatitis

- this is a chronic inflammatory process of the pancreas which results in destruction of the exocrine and later the endocrine pancreas with replacement by fibrous tissue

AETIOLOGY

- alcohol – causes 75% of cases of chronic pancreatitis in Europe
- gallstones
- idiopathic
- hyperparathyroidism
- other miscellaneous causes include cystic fibrosis, hereditary types, haemochromatosis

PATHOGENESIS

Two major anatomical forms have been described:

1. Obstructive chronic pancreatitis:
   - pancreatic duct obstructed by gallstones or tumour
   - usually pancreatitis occurs distal to obstruction

2. Chronic calcifying pancreatitis:
   - microscopically there is dilatation of ducts and acini with calcified intra-luminal plugs
   - plugged ducts cause stenosis and atrophy

CLINICAL FEATURES

- abdominal pain
- diabetes
- weight loss, steatorrhoea, jaundice
- calcification may be seen on abdominal x-ray

PATHOLOGY

- initial increase in size of gland which later becomes atrophic
- loss of normal surface lobulation of pancreas
- fibrotic gland with stones in duct
- microscopy shows periductal fibrous tissue, atrophy of pancreatic parenchyma and infiltration by chronic inflammatory cells
- islets usually preserved until late
- grossly and microscopically may mimic pancreatic adenocarcinoma

COMPLICATIONS

- superimposed acute pancreatitis
- exocrine dysfunction with steatorrhoea

- endocrine dysfunction with development of diabetes
- obstructive jaundice
- splenic vein thrombosis with sectorial portal hypertension
- pseudocyst development (see below)

PANCREATIC TRANSPLANTATION

- two main indications are chronic pancreatitis and insulin-resistant diabetes
- problems include pancreatic thrombosis, recurrence of original disease and rejection

CYSTS OF PANCREAS

Epithelial cysts

CONGENITAL

- rare
- may be associated with polycystic disease of kidney and liver
- usually multiple
- histology shows thin fibrous capsule lined by smooth membrane of flattened epithelial cells
- mostly asymptomatic
- may be component of von Hippel-Lindau syndrome

LYMPHOEPITHELIAL CYSTS

- rare
- often multilocular
- squamous epithelial lining with lymphoid tissue in wall

RETENTION CYSTS

- behind obstructed duct
- duct may be obstructed by tumour or chronic pancreatitis

NEOPLASTIC CYSTS

- (see p. 110)

Non-epithelial cysts (pseudocysts)

- no epithelial lining
- associated with acute and chronic pancreatitis and trauma
- often multiple
- usually develop approximately 4 weeks after acute pancreatitis
- may spread beyond pancreas into lesser sac
- presents with pain, vomiting and possibly jaundice. May be palpable mass
- diagnosis is by ultrasound

- histology shows fibrous capsule with no epithelial lining
- complications include infection, perforation and haemorrhage. May be massive haemorrhage from splenic artery
- small pseudocysts may be treated with excision
- others treated by external or internal drainage

TUMOURS OF EXOCRINE PANCREAS

Benign tumours

SEROUS CYSTADENOMA

- also known as glycogen-rich or microcystic cystadenoma
- usually elderly patients with no sex predilection
- often found incidentally at autopsy
- cut surface shows multiple cysts
- histology shows cysts lined by cuboidal cells
- may be associated with von Hippel-Lindau disease

INTRADUCT PAPILLOMA

- rare
- occurs in pancreatic duct, usually in body or head
- may be multiple
- middle-aged patients
- intraduct mass may cause obstruction of duct
- histology shows papillary lesion lined by mucus-secreting epithelium

Tumours of uncertain malignant potential

PAPILLARY AND SOLID EPITHELIAL NEOPLASM (PSEN)

- also known as papillary cystic neoplasm
- usually young women
- present as abdominal mass
- periphery is solid, centre is cystic
- microscopy shows solid areas with pseudopapillae and cystic areas
- excellent prognosis after resection
- occasional cases have resulted in local recurrence and liver metastases

MUCINOUS CYSTIC NEOPLASM

- usually middle-aged females
- usually in tail or body of pancreas
- x-ray shows sunburst calcification
- grossly multilocular cyst containing mucoid material
- histology shows epithelial lining of mucus-secreting cells
- may get benign, borderline or malignant variants analogous to similar tumours in ovary
- pathologist must examine multiple histological sections to exclude invasive malignancy

- treatment is surgical excision
- prognosis is good
- metastases usually develop late and when present are restricted to abdominal cavity

Malignant tumours

DUCTAL ADENOCARCINOMA

Epidemiology and aetiology

- incidence in Western countries – 11 per 100 000 per year
- increasing incidence
- male:female ratio is 1.5:1
- usually elderly patients
- associated with cigarette smoking
- associated with benzidine and beta-naphthylamine exposure
- possible association with alcohol, coffee, diabetes, gallstones and chronic pancreatitis

Clinical features

- pain, weight loss, jaundice, vomiting
- unstable diabetes
- thrombophlebitis
- Courvoisier's sign

Pathology

- distribution is head (70%), body (15%), tail (10%), multifocal (5%)
- grossly hard, infiltrating, white coloured mass
- may be difficult grossly to distinguish from chronic pancreatitis
- microscopy shows adenocarcinoma of varying differentiation
- often there are extensive fibrous stroma
- rare morphological variants include mucinous adenocarcinoma, squamous carcinoma, adenosquamous carcinoma, clear cell carcinoma and giant cell carcinoma

Diagnosis

- ultrasound, CT scan
- cytology of pancreatic juice obtained during ERCP
- percutaneous FNA or trucut under ultrasound or CT guidance
- intraoperative FNA
- frozen section. May be difficult to distinguish well differentiated adenocarcinoma from chronic pancreatitis

Spread

- local spread
- perineural spaces
- lymphatics to local lymph nodes
- blood spread, especially to liver, lungs, bones, adrenals

Prognosis

- overall prognosis is extremely poor

ACINAR CELL CARCINOMA

- usually occurs in adults but occasionally children
- large soft necrotic tumour
- microscopy shows acinar and tubular structures with little fibrous stroma
- poor prognosis

PANCREATOBLASTOMA

- most common form of pancreatic malignancy in children
- also occurs in adults
- get epithelial and stromal components
- prognosis in infants is relatively favourable

ENDOCRINE TUMOURS OF PANCREAS

- these are neuroendocrine tumours which are also termed APUDomas
- may present with an abdominal mass, pain or jaundice
- often present with endocrine symptoms due to elaboration of hormones
- most commonly located in body and tail of pancreas as these have greatest concentration of islets
- depending on microscopic growth pattern may be categorised as:
  - Type A – solid or insular pattern
  - Type B – gyriform or ribboned pattern
  - Type C – glandular pattern
  - Type D – non-descript pattern
- benign and malignant tumours are difficult to distinguish histologically
- large tumours more likely to be malignant
- amyloid may be found in stroma
- some tumours produce multiple hormones

Insulinomas

- beta cell tumours
- most common neuroendocrine tumour of pancreas
- usually middle-aged patients with equal sex incidence
- presents with Whipple's triad
- usually solitary except if associated with multiple endocrine neoplasia (MEN) type 1
- usually small (1–5 cm) with a red/brown colour
- location helped by intraoperative ultrasound or arteriography
- 90% benign
- microscopically usually type A or B pattern
- treatment is surgical but may be difficult to locate tumour

Gastrinomas

- G cell tumours
- gastrin not normally produced in pancreas
- cause Zollinger-Ellison syndrome (multiple gastric, duodenal or jejunal ulcers)
- may be multiple, especially in association with MEN-1

- often malignant (60%)
- may occur outside pancreas, especially in duodenal wall or gastric antrum
- 20% associated with MEN-1
- microscopically usually type A or C pattern
- 90% are found in gastrinoma triangle which is formed from the gallbladder neck, the neck of the pancreas and the second part of the duodenum
- intraoperative ultrasound is useful in localisation
- may be tiny and difficult to locate
- good prognosis – 80% 20-year survival
- malignant tumours spread slowly to nodes and later liver
- usually middle-aged patients
- presents with resistant ulcer symptoms in atypical sites
- 30% have diarrhoea

Glucagonomas

- alpha cell tumours
- 1% of pancreatic-endocrine tumours
- may present with skin rash (necrolytic migratory erythema), diabetes, anaemia
- 60% are malignant
- usually middle-aged patients
- may be solitary or multiple
- solitary tumours more likely to be malignant

Somatostatinomas

- delta cell tumours
- very rare
- may be found in pancreas and duodenum
- rarely large and functional
- cause diabetes, hypochlorhydria, diarrhoea and steatorrhoea

PP cell tumours

- rare
- no specific syndrome
- pain, weight loss, GI bleeding
- if large, potentially malignant

Vipomas

- 5% of pancreatic endocrine tumours secrete VIP (vasoactive intestinal polypeptide)
- Verner-Morrison syndrome
- WDHA (watery diarrhoea, hypokalaemia, achlorhydria)
- large size
- 60% malignant
- usually solitary
- microscopically usually type A or B pattern

The kidney, ureter, urinary bladder and urethra

9

NORMAL STRUCTURE

Kidney

- the normal adult kidney measures approximately $12 \times 6 \times 3$ cm and weighs 120–170 g
- kidneys are situated retroperitoneally
- posteriorly related to the diaphragm, quadratus lumborum and psoas muscles and the posterior recess of the pleura
- situated anteriorly is the second part of the duodenum on the right and the tail of pancreas on the left
- hepatic and splenic flexures of the colon are also situated anteriorly
- kidneys are surrounded by perinephric fat and are situated within perinephric fascia. The fascia is attached to the hilum of the kidney and the renal vessels
- the renal arteries divide into three branches at the hilum, usually two in front and one behind the renal pelvis. The posterior branch passes to the upper pole of the kidney
- veins form venous arcades along the bases of the medullary pyramids and five main veins unite beyond the hilum to form the renal vein
- the lymphatics drain to para-aortic nodes at the level of the second lumbar vertebra
- kidney receives both sympathetic and parasympathetic nerve supply, the former having a vasomotor function
- the renal cortex extends towards the pelvis between the darker striated pyramids of the medulla. These pyramids open into the renal papilla, each of which projects into a minor calyx
- the cortex contains the glomeruli and convoluted tubules
- the medulla contains loops of Henle and collecting tubules
- nephron consists of glomerulus, proximal convoluted tubule, loop of Henle, distal convoluted tubule and collecting duct
- glomerulus is a network of capillaries invaginated into Bowman's capsule. It is supplied by an afferent and drained by an efferent arteriole
- the loop of Henle has a thick limb which descends from the cortex into the medulla and a thin ascending limb which joins the distal convoluted tubule
- distal convoluted tubule in contact with afferent arteriole forms the juxtaglomerular apparatus which secretes renin. This hormone initiates the renin-angiotensin system
- in the proximal convoluted tubule 80% of the filtrate is reabsorbed. Glucose, sodium chloride and sodium bicarbonate are actively reabsorbed, followed by passive reabsorption of water

- within the loop of Henle the high osmotic pressure allows the urine to be concentrated
- in the distal convoluted tubule water is reabsorbed due to the actions of antidiuretic hormone

Ureter

- the ureters are approximately 25 cm long in the adult
- they start medial to the tips of the transverse processes of the lumbar vertebrae, cross the bifurcation of the common iliac artery and sacroiliac joint, pass to the ischial spine and run anteromedially to base of bladder
- narrowest points are at pelviureteric junction of kidney, pelvic brim and at the bladder wall. These are the points where stones are likely to lodge
- the ureters are supplied by branches of renal, gonadal, common iliac and uterine or vesicle arteries
- veins drain to renal, gonadal and internal iliac veins
- lymphatics run with the ureters. The abdominal ureter drains to the para-aortic nodes and the pelvic ureter drains to the internal iliac nodes
- the mucus membrane of the ureter consists of loose fibrous tissue lined by transitional epithelium (the urothelium)
- the ureteric muscle lies in three layers. These are the inner and outer circular and the intermediate longitudinal layers

Bladder

- bladder is located within the pelvis, beneath the peritoneum
- develops from the urogenital sinus
- mucus membrane is lined by transitional epithelium with underlying lamina propria
- deep to this is submucosa and muscle layer
- wall contains detrusor smooth muscle which is arranged in spirals to give a trabeculated appearance
- trigone lies between internal urethral and ureteric orifices
- fundus is mobile and distensible
- ureters pierce wall of bladder obliquely and this prevents vesico-ureteric reflux
- bladder is supplied by the superior and inferior vesicle arteries
- veins drain to vesicle plexus at the bladder base and thence to internal iliac veins
- lymph drainage follows arteries to side walls of pelvis
- sympathetic nerve supply is inhibitory to the bladder wall and motor to the sphincter
- parasympathetic system is motor to the wall and inhibitory to the sphincter, thus facilitating emptying

Urethra

- in males the urethra is 15–20 cm in length and in females it is approximately 4 cm in length
- proximal urethra is lined by transitional epithelium and distal urethra by non-keratinising squamous epithelium

CONGENITAL ANOMALIES

Kidney

BILATERAL RENAL AGENESIS (POTTER'S SYNDROME)

- agenesis means absence of kidney and corresponding ureter
- rare. Most are stillborn
- associated with oligohydramnios
- results in pulmonary hypoplasia

UNILATERAL RENAL AGENESIS

- occurs in 1 in 1000 live births
- condition may be entirely asymptomatic
- more frequent in males
- affects left kidney more commonly
- in up to 70% of cases other congenital abnormalities, most often affecting the genital tract, are present
- contralateral kidney may undergo compensatory hypertrophy

RENAL HYPOPLASIA

- significant reduction of renal mass without evidence of parenchymal malformation
- may be bilateral
- cardiovascular abnormalities may be present
- affected kidney is susceptible to infection
- may get renal failure or hypertension
- in bilateral hypoplasia child may present with failure to thrive, polyuria and renal rickets

SUPERNUMERARY KIDNEY

- rare – most commonly located below one or other kidney

CONTRALATERAL FUSION

- occurs in 1 in 500 live births
- affects males more than females
- kidneys are usually joined at the lower poles to form horseshoe kidney
- horseshoe kidney is usually situated ectopically, anterior to the aorta and vena cava
- ureters may be partially obstructed
- many cases are asymptomatic but may have abdominal pain or fainting due to pressure on inferior vena cava. The kidney is more prone to trauma, infection, stone formation and hydronephrosis

IPSILATERAL FUSION

- rare
- both kidneys lie on the same side of the vertebrae and the upper pole of one is fused to lower pole of the other

RENAL ECTOPIA

- failure of kidney to reach its usual location
- usually ectopic kidney fails to ascend and remains medially in the iliac fossa or pelvis

RENAL DYSPLASIA

- kidney shows aberrant nephronic differentiation
- may be secondary to urinary tract obstruction

Ureter

DUPLICATION OF THE URETER, ECTOPIC URETER AND URETEROCOELE

- various permutations of ureteric duplication occur (Figure 9.1)

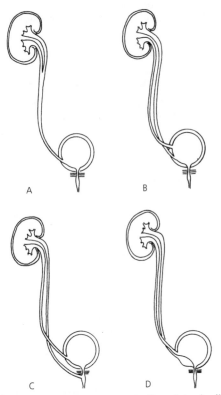

A

B

C

D

Figure 9.1   A. Partial duplication of ureter. B. Complete duplication of ureter. C. Complete duplication of ureter with ectopic ureter. D. Complete duplication of ureter with ectopic ureterocoele

SIMPLE PARTIAL DUPLICATION

- ureter can become double at any point
- usually an incidental finding and asymptomatic

SIMPLE COMPLETE DUPLICATION

- entire ureter is duplicated
- ureter draining upper pole of kidney always enters bladder below and medial to lower pole ureter
- often asymptomatic
- lower pole ureter has a direct course through bladder wall and predisposes to vesico-ureteric reflux

DUPLICATION WITH ECTOPIC URETER

- ureteric bud to upper pole of kidney may arise away from other ureteric bud
- gives rise to upper pole ureter which opens lower than the normally situated lower pole ureter. It is therefore ectopic
- common points of entry for the ectopic ureter are lower trigone and bladder neck
- in boys ectopic ureter may enter urethra
- in girls may enter the urethra distal to the sphincter and cause incontinence

DUPLICATION WITH ECTOPIC URETEROCOELE

- ureterocoele is congenital dilatation of distal ureter within the bladder
- usually associated with ectopic ureter
- ureteric opening may be narrowed causing stasis and infection or reflux
- duplication of ureter, ectopic ureters and ureterocoeles may be uni- or bilateral and can occur in any combination

CONGENITAL URETERAL VALVES

- folds of redundant mucosa
- occasionally persist and cause obstruction

Bladder

ECTOPIA VESICAE

- defect in the anterior abdominal wall and bladder wall
- symphysis pubis is frequently absent
- bladder mucosa is exposed resulting in chronic inflammation and infection
- mucosa may be replaced by granulation tissue
- adenocarcinoma may develop

PERSISTENT URACHUS

- total persistence of the urachus between the bladder and umbilicus produces a vesico-umbilical fistula
- middle segment persistence results in a urachal cyst
- persistence of the cloacal segment results in a bladder diverticulum

Urethra

CONGENITAL URETHRAL VALVES

- mucosal folds that project into the urethral lumen and cause obstruction
- more common in males

URETHRAL DIVERTICULUM

- uncommon
- mostly in women
- may be asymptomatic or may get urinary symptoms
- rarely undergo malignant change

ACUTE RENAL FAILURE

- may be due to prerenal, postrenal or renal causes
- prerenal causes include severe blood loss and hypotension
- postrenal causes include obstruction due to stones, tumours or enlarged prostate
- renal causes include glomerulonephritis, pyelonephritis, papillary necrosis, malignant hypertension, diffuse intravascular coagulation (DIC), eclampsia, arteritis, acute tubular necrosis

Acute tubular necrosis

- ischaemic tubular necrosis. Occurs after hypotension, severe trauma, surgery, bacterial infection, burns, severe vomiting and diarrhoea, myocardial infarction
- nephrotoxic acute tubular necrosis. Due to substances which are toxic to tubules including heavy metals (mercury and cis-platinum), solvents (carbon tetrachloride), drugs and poisons

CLINICAL FEATURES

- initial oliguric phase during which urine output is less than 400 ml per day. During this time the blood urea rises
- after 1–2 weeks there is a diuretic phase
- in early diuretic phase there is polyuria with loss of electrolytes, including sodium and potassium
- in late diuretic phase urinary output returns to normal and the concentrating ability of the kidneys returns

PATHOLOGY

- grossly the kidneys may be pale and swollen
- microscopically in the early stages of ischaemic acute tubular necrosis, there is patchy necrosis of the epithelial lining of proximal convoluted tubules
- rupture of basement membrane of the tubules (tubulorrhexis) occurs
- casts are seen in the distal convoluted tubules and collecting tubules
- myoglobin casts occur after crushing limb injuries
- ischaemic acute tubular necrosis may be patchy and may affect only short segments of the proximal convoluted tubules

- little change may be seen on needle biopsy
- when recovery occurs epithelial cells regenerate and mitotic figures may be seen
- in nephrotoxic acute tubular necrosis the findings are similar, although tubulorrhexis is rare and tubular damage is often more widespread

PROGNOSIS

- renal tubular epithelium has the ability to regenerate rapidly and the prognosis is good

URINARY TRACT INFECTION

- after the first year of life and up to middle age, urinary tract infections are more common in females than males
- in the neonatal period boys more commonly contract urinary tract infections than girls. This is due to the higher incidence of congenital urogenital abnormalities in boys
- sex distribution becomes even again in old age due to obstruction of bladder neck by benign nodular hyperplasia of the prostate

Aetiology and pathogenesis

- *Escherichia coli* accounts for 75% of non-hospital and up to 50% of hospital urinary tract infections
- less common pathogens are *Proteus, Staphylococcus saprophyticus, Klebsiella,* streptococci and candidal organisms
- majority of organisms infect the urinary tract by the ascending route
- organisms may also spread to the urinary tract by the haematogenous route. These include bacteria such as *Mycobacterium* and *Salmonella,* fungi such as *Histoplasma duboisii,* viruses such as cytomegalovirus and adenovirus and parasites such as *Schistosoma haematobium*
- important factors in the development of infection include the shorter urethra in females, catheterisation of the bladder, urethral strictures, prostatic hypertrophy and neurological impairment of bladder function
- vesico-ureteric reflux is a common predisposing factor in children

Clinical features

- may present as cystitis, acute pyelonephritis or chronic pyelonephritis
- symptoms include frequency of micturition, dysuria and lower abdominal pain
- pyonephrosis or perinephric abscess may occur
- chronic pyelonephritis may lead to chronic renal failure

Pathology

CYSTITIS

- the bladder mucosa initially becomes hyperaemic and friable
- microscopy shows acute and chronic inflammation, often with denudation of the urothelial lining

ACUTE PYELONEPHRITIS

- grossly kidneys are swollen and cortical abscesses may be seen on the external surface
- on sectioning, yellow abscesses containing pus are seen. These may radiate outwards from renal pelvis through the medulla to the cortex
- infection may burst through the renal capsule into the perirenal space to form a perinephric abscess

CHRONIC PYELONEPHRITIS

- grossly there is coarse corticomedullary scarring overlying distorted calyces, i.e. both the renal substance and the pelvicalyceal system are involved
- scars are irregular and if bilateral are asymmetrical
- histologically there is atrophy of tubules with thyroidisation and replacement by fibrous tissue and a chronic inflammatory cell infiltrate is present
- glomeruli tend to be resistant to damage although glomerular and periglomerular fibrosis may occur
- islands of foamy macrophages may be found, especially in cases of E. coli or Proteus infections. This is termed xanthogranulomatous pyelonephritis

RENAL PAPILLARY NECROSIS

- serious complication of pyelonephritis
- probably ischaemic basis
- tips of renal papillae become necrotic and slough off into the pelvicalyceal system
- predisposing factors include pyelonephritis, diabetes, urinary tract obstruction usually due to prostatic enlargement, sickle cell disease and analgesia abuse (especially phenacetin)
- if necrosis is widespread mortality is high

GENITO-URINARY TUBERCULOSIS

- usually blood-borne from focus in lung, pharynx, intestine or bone
- usually appears years after primary lesion in the lung
- predisposing factors include malnutrition, diabetes, measles infection and steroid administration
- most cases are due to the human variety of Mycobacterium tuberculosis
- blood-borne organisms lodge in kidneys and spread to other parts of urinary tract
- microscopy shows characteristic caseating granulomas
- tubercle bacilli may be demonstrated by Ziehl-Neelsen stain
- progression leads to destruction of renal parenchyma as granulomas become confluent
- renal involvement may be uni- or bilateral
- in late stages the kidney may be replaced by calcified fibrous tissue
- healing by fibrosis may result in stricture formation
- fibrosis at pelvi-ureteric junction causes obstruction and hydronephrosis
- bladder becomes contracted by fibrous tissue causing urinary frequency
- treatment is with antituberculous therapy

SCHISTOSOMIASIS

- the world's leading cause of haematuria
- caused by infestation with one of the species of trematode flukes
- three principal species to infest humans are *S. haematobium, S. mansoni* and *S. japonicum. S. haematobium* has a predilection for the pelvic veins and causes urinary schistosomiasis (bilharziasis). The other two species reside in portal vein tributaries and cause hepatic schistosomiasis
- patients with urinary schistosomiasis complain of general malaise, pyrexia and haematuria
- damage to bladder is caused by eggs which release soluble antigens resulting in an inflammatory reaction
- eggs become surrounded by a granulomatous reaction
- may get bladder polyps or ulcers
- commonest sites of infection are trigone and ureteral orifices
- later as fibrosis occurs bladder contracts and calcification occurs
- fibrosis causes ischaemia and chronic mucosal ulcers
- may get fibrosis of wall of ureter with obstructive uropathy, hydronephrosis and renal failure
- bladder transitional epithelium undergoes metaplasia to squamous epithelium
- malignant bladder tumours may occur
- the most frequent carcinoma to complicate schistosomiasis is squamous carcinoma
- other complications include secondary infection with stone formation

UNUSUAL INFLAMMATORY CONDITIONS OF THE BLADDER

Malakoplakia

- rare condition
- usually long history of urinary tract infections
- most common cultured organism is *E. coli* but *Proteus, Klebsiella* and streptococcal organisms may also be isolated
- yellow plaques develop in the bladder, ureter and renal pelvis
- may bleed and cause haematuria
- histologically plaques consist of sheets of large macrophages with granular cytoplasm and interspersed chronic inflammatory cells
- most specific histological feature is the presence of Michaelis-Gutmann bodies. These are small, round, laminated bodies within and between macrophages. They contain calcium and may be identified using the von Kossa stain
- in late stages may be extensive fibrosis

Hunner's ulcer (ulcerative interstitial cystitis)

- presents with frequency, dysuria and lower abdominal pain
- both men and women may be affected, but more common in women
- urine is sterile
- at cystoscopy there are ulcerated linear cracks in bladder mucosa
- histologically there is non-specific inflammaton and ulceration which extends deeply into the bladder wall
- mast cells are often present in inflammatory infiltrate

Emphysematous cystitis

- gas-filled blebs are seen on mucosa
- may be associated with diabetes
- most common infecting organism is *E. coli*

Encrusted cystitis

- mucosal lesions have a gritty appearance and may be calcified
- due to infection by urea-splitting organisms
- microscopically mucosa contains fibrin and necrotic calcified debris

PROLIFERATIVE AND METAPLASTIC LESIONS OF THE BLADDER

- von Brunn's nests. These are nodular thickenings of the bladder epithelium which result in nests of transitional epithelium within the lamina propria
- nests may develop lumina and appear as cyst-like spaces lined by transitional epithelium within the lamina propria. This is termed cystitis cystica
- metaplasia of the cyst lining to mucus-secreting columnar cells results in cystitis glandularis
- squamous metaplasia may result from long-standing inflammation and this may predispose to the development of squamous carcinoma

URINARY STONES

- annual incidence of urinary stones is 7 per 10 000 of the population
- prevalence is 3–4% of the population
- calcium and uric acid stones are commoner in males than females
- stones formed on an infective basis are more common in females than males
- cystine stones are equally distributed between the sexes
- in USA and UK 75% of stones are composed of calcium salts. This is usually a mixture of calcium oxalate and calcium phosphate. Mixed phosphate stones formed in infected urine account for approximately 15% of stones
- uric acid stones account for approximately 7% of stones
- cystine and other rarer types account for approximately 3% of stones

Aetiology

CALCIUM STONES
- usually a mixture of calcium oxalate and calcium phosphate
- patients with calcium stones may have hypercalciuria due to hypercalcaemia
- more commonly patients have idiopathic hypercalciuria
- may have hyperoxaluria
- many have no identifiable biochemical abnormality
- primary hyperparathyroidism is the most common cause of hypercalcaemia

- other causes include sarcoidosis, Paget's disease, vitamin D intoxication, Cushing's syndrome and malignant tumours
- idiopathic hypercalciuria is defined as an increased urinary calcium in the presence of normal serum calcium
- may be due to increased intestinal absorption of calcium, or to a defect in calcium reabsorption by renal tubules
- hyperoxaluria may be primary or secondary to a variety of causes such as ethylene glycol ingestion, gastrointestinal disease and pancreatobiliary disease

URIC ACID STONES

- may be a result of various causes of hyperuricosuria such as gout, high dietary protein intake, lymphoproliferative disorders and uricosuric drugs such as diuretics
- in many cases there is no increase in urinary uric acid concentration. In these patients there is an unexplained low urinary pH. At low pH uric acid becomes insoluble and stone formation may occur

INFECTIVE STONES

- composed of magnesium ammonium phosphate and calcium carbonate
- occur in urine infected by urea-splitting organisms such as *Proteus* and staphylococci
- often result in staghorn calculi

CYSTINE STONES

- occur in the autosomal recessive condition cystinosis
- characterised by a defect in transport of cystine across lysosomal membranes
- cystine accumulates in several organs, including the kidney

Gross and radiological appearance of stones

- majority of renal stones contain calcium and are radio-opaque
- pure uric acid stones are radiolucent
- stones with a high calcium oxalate content may be jagged in outline, whereas uric acid stones are smooth
- cystine stones are soft
- staghorn calculi are large and assume the shape of the renal pelvis and pelvicalyceal system

Complications of renal stones

- ureteric colic
- infection, especially if causing obstruction
- may develop acute pyelonephritis, chronic pyelonephritis, pyonephrosis and perinephric abscess
- may develop renal failure
- ureteric obstruction causes acute renal failure in patients with only one functioning kidney

Outcome

- stones less than 5 mm in diameter are likely either to pass spontaneously or to require only Dormia basket removal. Other treatment modalities available include laser, percutaneous nephrolithotomy and ultrasound stone disintegration
- recurrence of urinary stones is common

OBSTRUCTIVE UROPATHY

- obstruction may occur at the level of the prepuce (phimosis), urethra, bladder, ureters or pelvis of kidney
- ureter proximal to obstruction becomes dilated (hydroureter) as does the renal pelvis (hydronephrosis)
- stasis predisposes to infection which may result in pyonephrosis
- persistent obstruction causes atrophy of the renal parenchyma accompanied by fibrosis
- obstruction in the urethra or bladder neck causes changes within the bladder. The bladder muscle undergoes hypertrophy with resultant trabeculation. Blockage at the level of the urethra or bladder may result in bilateral hydronephrosis and hydroureter
- complete obstruction causes irreversible damage to the kidney in a few weeks. After relief of obstruction a massive diuresis may occur causing severe electrolyte disturbances
- causes of obstruction include urethral valves, stones, tumours, benign and malignant lesions of the prostate, retroperitoneal fibrosis and post-radiotherapy
- in retroperitoneal fibrosis dense fibrous tissue forms within the retroperitoneal space. This may surround the ureters and lead to obstruction. Retroperitoneal fibrosis may be associated with mediastinal fibrosis, sclerosing cholangitis, Riedel's thyroiditis and fibromatosis
- if both ureters become obstructed this leads to obstructive uropathy and finally to renal failure

BLADDER DIVERTICULA

- congenital bladder diverticulum may be secondary to obstruction of the bladder outflow during intrauterine life, e.g. due to a posterior urethral valve or to a developmental abnormality when the mesonephric ducts fuse with the cloaca
- acquired diverticula arise secondary to bladder neck obstruction. This is most commonly due to benign nodular hyperplasia of the prostate
- diverticula may obstruct ureter causing hydroureter and hydronephrosis
- urinary stasis within the diverticula results in infection and stone formation
- epithelium undergoes metaplasia from transitional to squamous
- carcinoma may develop and this is often squamous in type

BLADDER FISTULA

- vesicovaginal fistulas may be caused by a prolonged second stage of labour or may be secondary to malignancy of the bladder, especially following radiotherapy and trauma

- vesico-enteric fistulas may be caused by diverticular disease, colonic carcinoma, Crohn's disease, tuberculosis and perforating injury
- vesicocutaneous fistula may be secondary to bladder surgery

CYSTIC LESIONS OF THE KIDNEY

- renal cell carcinoma and other neoplasms such as Wilm's tumour may occasionally show extensive cystic degeneration

Cystic dysplasia

- renal dysplasia is a developmental abnormality almost invariably associated with cyst formation
- the term dysplasia in this context does not denote a premalignant condition
- may be unilateral or bilateral
- kidney may be completely or segmentally affected
- congenital abnormalities of the lower urinary tract are also present in many, e.g. posterior urethral valves, ectopic ureter and ureterocoele
- cases with total involvement of both kidneys may be stillborn or die shortly after birth
- unilateral involvement usually presents in infancy as a loin mass
- grossly kidney is enlarged, cystic and irregular
- microscopically between cysts, abnormal differentiation of the renal tissue is seen. Primitive tubules are surrounded by primitive mesenchymal tissue
- immature glomeruli and foci of immature cartilage are also characteristic microscopic findings

Polycystic disease of the kidneys

INFANTILE FORM

- inherited as autosomal recessive condition
- four types are recognised: perinatal, neonatal, infantile and juvenile
- pathogenesis not known
- many cases are associated with congenital hepatic fibrosis
- most cases result in stillbirth or early neonatal death
- in other forms patients live longer but die in childhood from renal failure or hepatic complications
- affected neonates have massively enlarged kidneys which produce palpable masses and abdominal distension
- both kidneys are affected
- the kidney has sponge-like appearance with cysts extending through cortex and medulla in a radiating pattern
- microscopically cysts are lined by cuboidal epithelial cells
- in the liver, fibrosis of the portal tracts with proliferation and focal dilatation of bile ducts occurs

ADULT FORM

- inherited as autosomal dominant condition
- most common cystic renal disease
- most cases are linked to a mutant gene on the short arm of chromosome 16

- most patients present age 30–50 years
- presents with hypertension, haematuria, urinary tract infection or progressive renal failure
- may get chronic flank pain or acute flank pain due to haemorrhage into a cyst
- may be associated with liver, pancreatic and pulmonary cysts
- associated with berry aneurysms on the circle of Willis
- death from subarachnoid haemorrhage occurs in 10%
- kidneys are greatly enlarged weighing up to 4 kg each. On cut section the kidney is seen to be a mass of cysts without apparent intervening parenchymal tissue
- microscopically the cysts either have no epithelial lining or are lined by flattened cells
- the intervening tissue is atrophic due to pressure from the cysts
- progress is variable but renal failure usually occurs

Simple cysts

- very common in elderly patients
- commonly asymptomatic
- may present as an abdominal mass or as an incidental finding during radiological investigation or laparotomy
- may be single or multiple
- usually situated in the cortex and contain clear fluid
- may get acute pain due to haemorrhage into cyst
- renal cysts may also occur in von Hippel-Lindau disease, in tuberous sclerosis and in patients on long-term renal dialysis

RENAL ARTERY STENOSIS

- cause of secondary hypertension
- kidney becomes small and atrophic. If unilateral, may get compensatory hypertrophy of contralateral kidney
- two common causes are atheroma and fibromuscular dysplasia
- atheroma is more common cause in the elderly. Atheromatous plaque is usually situated at or near the ostium of renal artery
- fibromuscular dysplasia is the more common cause of renal artery stenosis in patients under 40 years
- medial fibromuscular dysplasia is the most common type. This appears as alternating ridges of stenosis with intervening thinned areas of arterial wall which form small aneurysms
- a typical 'string of beads' appearance is seen on arteriography
- microscopically there are foci of proliferation of fibrous tissue and smooth muscle within the arterial wall

RENAL TUMOURS

Renal cell adenoma

- usually a well defined cortical nodule
- may be found as an incidental finding in up to 15% of autopsies
- may be multiple

- rarely cause symptoms
- on cut section pale, yellow and discrete
- upper size limit is controversial but some authorities suggest that a tumour up to 3 cm should be regarded as an adenoma
- microscopy usually shows papillary arrangements of tumour cells
- cells show little or no atypia
- renal cell adenoma is difficult to distinguish from well differentiated renal cell carcinoma. Lesions are usually regarded as adenomas if they are less than 3 cm in diameter but occasionally small tumours of 2-cm diameter or less may metastasise

Oncocytoma of the kidney

- male to female ratio is 3:1
- usually presents in adults
- often asymptomatic and detected as an incidental finding on radiological investigation or at autopsy
- tan in colour on cut section and often with a central scar
- radiology shows 'spoke and wheel' appearance
- microscopically tumour cells have deeply eosinophilic granular cytoplasm and do not show pleomorphism
- electron microscopy shows numerous mitochondria within cytoplasm
- usually benign behaviour with excellent prognosis
- rarely metastasise

Angiomyolipoma

- rare usually benign renal tumour
- may mimic renal cell carcinoma on gross inspection
- may be solitary or multiple and bilateral
- often asymptomatic
- may present with chronic flank pain, haematuria or a palpable intra-abdominal mass
- microscopically tumour consists of thick-walled blood vessels, fat and smooth muscle
- tissues are well differentiated
- tumour is almost always benign, although in rare cases a sarcoma has developed
- approximately half occur sporadically and half are associated with tuberous sclerosis
- in tuberous sclerosis, tumours are usually small, multiple and bilateral
- in general population tumours are often solitary and large

Renal cell carcinoma

- most common renal neoplasm
- renal cell carcinoma (clear cell carcinoma, hypernephroma) accounts for approximately 3% of all tumours in adults
- annual incidence is approximately 4 per 100 000
- peak incidence is sixth to seventh decade
- two to three times more common in men than women

- develops in two-thirds of patients with von Hippel-Lindau disease
- more common in patients with tuberous sclerosis
- slightly more common in horseshoe kidneys and polycystic kidneys than in normal kidneys
- most cases arise from cells of the proximal convoluted tubules

CLINICAL FEATURES

- haematuria, flank pain and palpable mass are commonest presenting symptoms
- presentation may be due to secondary deposits, in lung, bone, brain or other organs
- non-metastatic effects of malignancy are common. These include pyrexia, hypertension, polycythaemia (due to erythropoietin production), hypercalcaemia, hepatic dysfunction, leukaemoid reaction, ectopic hormone production and amyloidosis

GROSS PATHOLOGY

- usually relatively well circumscribed spherical mass, often situated at one pole, more commonly the upper pole
- predominantly cortical location
- on sectioning mass may appear to be encapsulated due to compression of the surrounding renal tissue
- satellite nodules may be present
- cut surface has variegated and lobulated appearance and is often yellow in colour (due to intracytoplasmic lipid). Areas of haemorrhage and necrosis and cystic degeneration often occur
- renal vein is often invaded by tumour which can extend into the inferior vena cava and rarely as far as the right atrium of the heart

HISTOLOGY

- recent morphological classification is Mainz classification (1986)
- this divides renal cell carcinomas arising from the tubules into clear cell, chromophil and chromophobe types
- clear cell is most common type. The cells contain abundant clear cytoplasm due to the presence of glycogen and lipid
- may be sarcomatoid areas in clear cell carcinoma
- chromophil renal cell carcinoma is second most common type. This is also known as papillary renal cell carcinoma
- as well as papillary areas, may also contain tubular areas
- chromophobe renal cell carcinoma recognised only recently
- typically shows prominent cytoplasmic membranes and pale flocculent cytoplasm
- on electron microscopy there are numerous cytoplasmic vesicles
- renal cell carcinomas may be graded as 1 to 4 depending on nuclear features

GENETICS OF RENAL CELL CARCINOMA

- in recent years, genetic abnormalities have been well characterised in renal cell carcinoma
- in clear cell carcinoma, loss of genetic material on the short arm of chromosome 3 is the most frequent and consistent abnormality

- in chromophil renal cell carcinoma, various abnormalities may be found. The most common is a gain of chromosomes, especially trisomy or tetrasomy of chromosomes 17 and 7
- chromophobe renal cell carcinoma is often characterised by chromosomal losses

SPREAD, STAGING AND PROGNOSIS

- staging is by the TNM or Robson method as shown in Table 9.1
- extension into perinephric fat often occurs
- renal vein is involved by tumour in 20% of cases
- blood-borne spread is to lungs, bone, liver, opposite kidney, adrenal and brain
- lymphatic spread to local lymph nodes is common
- overall 5-year survival after nephrectomy is 40%
- recurrence or metastases may develop years after removal of primary tumour
- resection of solitary metastasis may improve survival

Table 9.1 Comparison of TNM and Robson system of staging renal cell carcinoma

TNM	Extent of disease	Robson stage	Frequency at diagnosis (%)
T1	Tumour within capsule (small) (<2.5 cm)	I	33
T2	Tumour within capsule (large)		
T3	Tumour in perinephric fat	II	12
N1–N3	Tumour in regional nodes	III	24
V1	Tumour in renal vein		
V2	Tumour in vena cava		
T4	Adjacent organ invasion	IV	31
M1	Distant metastases		
N4	Tumour in juxtaregional nodes		

Adapted from Sufrin (1982).

Collecting duct carcinoma of kidney

- rare
- recently described
- arises from collecting ducts and not tubules
- grossly is situated in renal medulla
- infiltrative borders
- microscopically composed of duct-like structures and abundant fibrous stroma

Wilms' tumour (nephroblastoma)

- accounts for 80% of renal tumours in childhood
- most frequently occurs in children aged 2–4 years

- rarely seen in adults
- slight preponderance in females
- commonest presentation is with abdominal mass or pain
- may be bilateral
- may be associated with a variety of congenital abnormalities. These include urinary tract abnormalities such as ureteric duplication and horseshoe kidney
- associated with Beckwith-Wiedemann syndrome and Drash syndrome
- risk of Wilms' tumour arising in children with aniridia is 30%
- proportion of tumours are familial
- associated with a genetic abnormality on short arm of chromosome 11
- grossly tumours are large and may breach capsule of kidney with invasion of perirenal fat or adrenal
- invasion of renal vein is common
- microscopically extremely variable. Consist of immature epithelial, mesenchymal and blastemal elements
- divided into favourable and unfavourable categories depending on presence or absence of anaplasia

SPREAD AND STAGING

- staging system is shown in Table 9.2
- metastases occur to lungs, liver and brain

PROGNOSIS

- depends on tumour stage and the histological features (anaplasia)
- benefit with combined surgery, radiotherapy and chemotherapy
- presence of anaplastic elements in the tumour and involvement of lymph nodes are poor prognostic signs

Table 9.2 Staging of Wilms tumour (Medical Research Council's Working Party 1978)

Stage	Extent of disease
Stage I	Tumour confined to kidney and completely resected
Stage II	Tumour extending beyond the capsule of the kidney by local infiltration or extension along the renal vein or involvement of the para-aortic nodes but complete macroscopic removal achieved
Stage III	Tumour extending beyond the capsule of the kidney and not completely resected or the operative field contaminated with tumour spilled at operation
Stage IV	Haematogenous metastases
Stage V	Bilateral renal involvement

Nephroblastomatosis

- persistence of nodules of primitive renal blastemal tissue beyond 36 weeks' gestation
- found in 12–15% of Wilms' tumour
- if present in association with Wilms' tumour there is an increased risk of development of tumour in the contralateral kidney

Clear cell sarcoma (bone metastasising renal tumour of childhood)

- rare, highly malignant tumour of childhood
- resistant to conventional Wilms' tumour chemotherapy
- 4% of paediatric renal tumours
- more common in males than females
- most present at age 2 years or younger
- tend to metastasise early with a predeliction for bony involvement
- microscopy shows cells with clear cytoplasm
- poor prognosis but aggressive treatment with chemotherapy and radiotherapy has resulted in an improved outlook

Rhabdoid tumour of kidney

- highly malignant tumour of childhood
- differs from Wilms' tumour in that it presents at a younger age, shows marked male predominance and is not associated with aniridia or any other syndromes
- microscopically there are cells with abundant eosinophilic cytoplasm
- highly aggressive. Patients usually die within 12 months of diagnosis

Mesoblastic nephroma

- most common renal neoplasm in first 3 months of life
- uncommon after 6 months
- usually present with abdominal mass
- usually benign
- microscopy shows spindle-shaped cells
- good prognosis

TUMOURS OF THE URINARY BLADDER

Transitional cell carcinoma

- this is the commonest tumour of the bladder
- most are papillary lesions
- often multiple and may affect other parts of urinary tract
- divided into invasive and non-invasive, depending on whether there is invasion across the basement membrane into the subepithelial tissue
- diagnosis is by histological examination or by cytological examination of urine

EPIDEMIOLOGY AND AETIOLOGY

- fifth commonest malignancy in men
- 7% of all cancers in men and 2.5% of cancers in women
- male to female ratio is 3:1
- rare before the age of 50 years but shows an increasing incidence with increasing age
- accounts for 90% of epithelial tumours of urinary bladder in Western countries
- cigarette smoking is an aetiological factor in the development of bladder transitional cell carcinoma
- industrial exposure to aromatic amines is also a factor
- occupations which have a recognised risk include the manufacturing of dye stuffs, tyres and other rubber goods
- drugs such as cyclophosphamide and phenacetin have been implicated in some cases

CLINICAL FEATURES

- painless haematuria is the commonest presentation
- irritating symptoms such as frequency, urgency and dysuria may also be present

PATHOLOGY

- commonest macroscopic appearance is a papillary growth with multiple fine or coarse fronds
- microscopically there are papillary formations of transitional epithelial cells. May also show a solid growth pattern
- occasionally spindle cell and giant cell variants occur. These have a more aggressive behaviour
- transitional cell carcinomas are graded I to III depending on the degree of differentiation
- grade I tumours are rarely invasive
- grade II and III tumours are often aggressive with deep invasion of the bladder wall
- may contain squamous and glandular elements as a minor component

STAGING

- may be done clinically and histologically. Computed tomography, magnetic resonance imaging, ultrasound and bimanual palpation under anaesthesia at the time of cystoscopy help in clinical staging. TNM system of staging is given in Figure 9.2.

SPREAD AND PROGNOSIS

- transitional cell carcinomas spread directly through the bladder wall
- positive correlation between histological grade and degree of local spread
- outside bladder wall may infiltrate side walls of pelvis, prostate, uterus and vagina
- lymphatic spread is to iliac and para-aortic nodes
- blood-borne metastases occur most commonly in lungs and liver
- grade I tumours have an excellent prognosis
- high grade carcinomas are more aggressive with 10-year survival of 30%

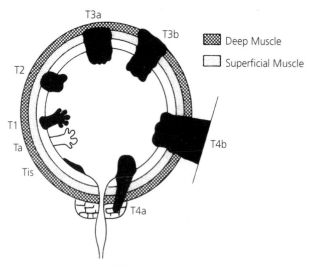

Figure 9.2 T grading of the TNM staging system for bladder tumours: Tis is flat carcinoma-*in-situ*; Ta is papillary carcinoma which has not invaded across the basement membrane into the lamina propria of the papillary cores; T1 is a carcinoma which has invaded the lamina propria

Carcinoma *in situ*

- can occur in the absence of other urothelial tumours
- more common in males
- typical symptoms are dysuria, pain, frequency and haematuria
- often associated with prior or synchronous transitional cell carcinoma
- may be multifocal and extensive throughout bladder and other parts of urinary tract
- at cystoscopy usually appears as red, velvety patch which may mimic cystitis
- microscopically there is full thickness dysplasia of surface transitional epithelium without papillary formations or invasion through basement membrane
- substantial number of patients will develop invasive cancer if untreated

Squamous carcinoma of the bladder

- 5% of epithelial bladder tumours in Western countries
- much more common in countries such as Egypt where it accounts for majority of bladder cancers. This is because schistosomiasis is endemic in these countries
- associated with conditions causing chronic inflammation and infection such as *Schistosoma haematobium* infestation, bladder calculi and long-standing in-dwelling catheters
- squamous metaplasia is risk factor in development
- prognosis is poor

Adenocarcinoma of the bladder

- rare
- may arise from urachal remnants in bladder or from areas of cystitis glandularis
- may also occur in association with ectopia vesicae and schistosomiasis (although much rarer than squamous carcinoma)
- possibility of secondary spread from an adjacent organ such as prostate or rectum must be excluded
- prognosis is poor

Inverted papilloma

- rare benign tumour
- predominantly elderly males
- mainly found around trigone
- presents with haematuria or urinary obstruction
- characteristically sessile or pedunculated with a smooth surface
- benign lesion but occasionally recurs

Nephrogenic adenoma

- rare benign lesion
- metaplastic and not a true neoplasm
- usually occurs in bladder but occasionally in the urethra and ureter
- more common in males
- often associated with cystitis, history of genitourinary operation, trauma or stones
- may be papillary, sessile or polypoid
- microscopy shows small tubules and papillae lined by cuboidal epithelium

Miscellaneous tumours of the bladder

- small cell carcinoma is a rare and highly aggressive primary bladder carcinoma
- embryonal rhabdomyosarcoma is a malignant tumour of skeletal muscle which generally occurs in infants and children. It may form a polypoid mass resembling a bunch of grapes
- phaeochromocytoma is a rare neuroendocrine tumour of the bladder wall. Histology is similar to phaeochromocytoma of adrenal medulla. The diagnosis is suggested by raised serum or urinary catecholamines or their breakdown products
- malignant melanoma can occasionally occur as a primary bladder neoplasm
- occasionally mesenchymal tumours such as haemangioma, neurofibroma, leiomyoma and various sarcomas occur in the bladder wall
- primary malignant lymphomas can occasionally arise within the bladder

Transitional cell carcinoma of the renal pelvis

- accounts for less than 10% of renal tumours
- may be associated with transitional cell carcinomas elsewhere in urinary tract
- causes obstruction and hydronephrosis

- associated with abuse of analgesic compounds containing phenacetin. Also associated with urinary stones and Balkan nephropathy
- grossly papillary lesions
- microscopically identical to transitional cell carcinoma of urinary bladder

Transitional cell carcinoma of the ureter

- commoner in distal half of ureter
- causes ureteric obstruction and hydronephrosis
- microscopically identical to those tumours arising in bladder or renal pelvis

Carcinoma of the urethra

- rare
- occurs in elderly patients
- most common in females
- may be squamous or transitional in type
- proximal tumours are usually transitional in type and distal tumours are usually squamous
- adenocarcinomas occasionally occur

The male genitalia

10

TESTIS AND EPIDIDYMIS

Normal structure

- the average size of the adult testis is $4 \times 3 \times 2.5$ cm
- the testis is covered by a dense layer of connective tissue, the tunica albuginea
- anteriorly and laterally the testis is lined by the visceral layer of the tunica vaginalis. This is continuous with the parietal layer
- fibrous septa extend from the tunica albuginea into the testis separating it into approximately 250 lobules
- each lobule consists of 1–4 convoluted seminiferous tubules
- these connect with the efferent ducts which drain into the epididymis
- seminiferous tubules have a basement membrane and contain two cell types. These are the Sertoli (supporting) cells and the spermatogenic cells
- the stroma between the seminiferous tubules contains interstitial (Leydig) cells
- the blood supply of the testis is from the spermatic arteries which arise from the aorta. A smaller supply comes from the arteries of the vas
- venous drainage is via the pampiniform plexus of the spermatic cord. The right spermatic vein enters the vena cava and the left spermatic vein drains into the left renal vein
- lymphatics from the testis drain to the para-aortic nodes
- the epididymis is attached to the dorsomedial portion of the testis and connects the efferent ductules of the testis with the vas deferens
- the upper portion of the epididymis (globus major) connects to the testis via numerous efferent ductules. The lower pole (globus minor) is continuous with the vas deferens
- the ducts of epididymis are lined by pseudostratified columnar epithelium
- lymphatic drainage is to external iliac and hypogastric nodes
- blood supply is from the internal spermatic artery and the artery of the vas

Maldescended testis

- a maldescended testis is one which has failed to reach the normal low scrotal position
- a maldescended testis may be found at some point along the line of normal descent (cryptorchidism)
- less commonly the testis may be positioned outside the normal line of descent (ectopic testis)

- incidence of testicular maldescent is 1.5% at age of 3 months
- if normal descent has not occurred by 1 year the testis is likely to remain undescended
- in the majority of cases of maldescent the testis is found in the superficial inguinal pouch or high scrotum
- in 20% of cases it is in the inguinal canal
- in 10% it is intra-abdominal (Figure 10.1)
- in maldescended testes impairment of testicular function, which may result in infertility, is common
- testicular maldescent is associated with a greater than average incidence of malignant testicular tumours
- in cases of unilateral maldescended testis both the normally and the abnormally placed testis are at increased risk of malignant transformation
- orchidopexy before the age of 6 years protects against the development of malignancy but, if this is delayed until puberty, there is no protection
- commonest malignant tumour in maldescended testis is seminoma
- small benign Sertoli cell tumours are also common
- other complications of maldescended testis include hernia formation, torsion and trauma
- current surgical management is early orchidopexy which may be performed laparoscopically
- computed tomography scanning may be helpful in localising an impalpable undescended testis
- maldescended testis may be part of a variety of syndromes, including Klinefelter's, Prader-Willi and prune belly syndrome

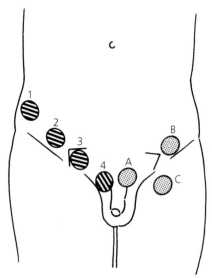

Figure 10.1 Common positions for maldescended testis: arrested descent (on the left): 1 = intra-abdominal; 2 = inguinal canal; 3 = superficial inguinal pouch; 4 = high scrotum; ectopic testis (on the right): A = penile; B = superficial inguinal; C = femoral

Inflammatory lesions of the testis and epididymis

PRIMARY EPIDIDYMITIS AND ORCHITIS (EPIDIDYMO-ORCHITIS)

- inflammation of the epididymis and/or testis which is not part of a generalised systemic infection
- commonly occurs in association with infection elsewhere in the urinary tract, e.g. cystitis, urethritis and prostatitis
- may follow trauma or instrumentation of the urinary tract
- in patients aged over 35 years *Escherichia coli* and *Pseudomonas* are the commonest organisms
- in patients aged less than 35 years, sexually transmitted organisms such as *Neisseria gonococcus* and *Chlamydia* are common
- grossly the epididymis and testis may be swollen and tense
- microscopically tubules and surrounding tissues contain polymorphs and other inflammatory cells
- if condition becomes chronic the tubules become obliterated by fibrous tissue
- fibrous obstruction of the epididymis may result in infertility
- in tuberculous epididymitis the epididymis is replaced by a caseous mass
- microscopically characteristic caseating granulomas are seen in tuberculous epididymitis
- epididymo-orchitis is a common complication of mumps infection in adults
- in mumps the testis is more often affected than the epididymis
- epididymo-orchitis may also occur in patients with brucellosis, enteric fever, infectious mononucleosis and malaria

SPERM GRANULOMA

- foreign body giant cell reaction to extravasated sperm
- occurs in the epididymis or spermatic cord
- may be asymptomatic or may present as a painful nodule
- may be single or multiple
- often follows trauma or infection
- may occur post-vasectomy
- grossly, lesion comprises a white or yellow nodule
- microscopically sperm are seen in interstitial tissues surrounded by a foreign body giant cell histiocytic reaction

VASIITIS NODOSA

- benign ductular proliferation that results in nodularity of vas deferens
- may follow vasectomy
- may coexist with sperm granuloma

GRANULOMATOUS ORCHITIS

- granulomatous inflammation of the testis
- may be due to tuberculous, fungal, or other infection
- idiopathic granulomatous orchitis is where no apparent cause is found
- usually occurs in middle-aged to elderly
- may be history of trauma or infection
- clinically presents with scrotal mass and may be confused with malignancy

- on cut section, the testis has a rubbery consistency and is pale. Areas of necrosis may be present
- microscopically the testis is diffusely involved. Tubules and/or interstitium contains numerous granulomas with giant cells

SYPHILITIC ORCHITIS

- may be congenital or acquired
- in congenital orchitis, both testes are enlarged at birth
- acquired orchitis occurs in the tertiary stage of syphilis
- presents with painless testicular enlargement
- microscopy shows interstitial inflammation and fibrosis with tubular atrophy
- gummas may form in testis. These consist of central areas of necrosis with a surrounding inflammatory infiltrate

MALAKOPLAKIA

- uncommon chronic inflammatory disease
- may also occur in bladder and other parts of genitourinary tract
- grossly testis is enlarged with brown-yellow appearance
- microscopy shows abundant macrophages containing Michaelis-Gutmann bodies

Testicular torsion

- may be intravaginal or extravaginal
- extravaginal torsion occurs in neonates and in patients with an undescended testis. The entire testis, including the tunica vaginalis, twists on the spermatic cord
- surgical fixation of the contralateral testis is advised
- intravaginal torsion which is most common usually occurs in patients between 12 and 25 years
- the underlying defect is a high insertion of the tunica vaginalis on the cord
- abnormality is often bilateral
- maldescended testes are more susceptible to torsion than descended testes
- 50% of patients with unilateral torsion are subfertile
- initially the veins are occluded causing the testis to become swollen and cyanotic
- later arterial occlusion occurs with subsequent infarction
- presentation is with sudden acute scrotal pain
- there is often a history of warning attacks of pain and swelling
- treatment is by bilateral surgical fixation as soon as possible
- torsion of the hydatid of Morgagni (appendix testis) may also occur

Hydrocoele

- collection of serous fluid between the parietal and visceral layers of the tunica vaginalis
- congenital hydrocoele occurs when a patent processus vaginalis within the spermatic cord communicates with the peritoneal cavity
- most cases of acquired hydrocoele are idiopathic but may also be associated with hernias, scrotal trauma, infection or tumours

- filariasis is a common cause of hydrocoele in tropical areas
- complications include rupture, herniation into dartos muscle, haematocoele and fibrosis with adhesion formation

Haematocoele

- accumulation of blood in the space between the visceral and parietal layers of the tunica vaginalis
- may follow trauma or tapping of a hydrocoele
- may be idiopathic
- late fibrosis and calcification may result in compression of the testis

Epididymal cyst

- common multilocular cysts, usually occurring in middle age
- contain clear fluid and are translucent

Spermatocoele

- dilatation of efferent ductule in the region of the rete testis or epididymis – fluid is white and cloudy due to the presence of spermatozoa

Varicocoele

- varicosity of the pampiniform venous plexus of the spermatic cord
- most cases are idiopathic
- mostly found in young adults
- most occur on the left side
- unilateral cases in elderly men may be due to a renal tumour which has invaded the renal vein and occluded the spermatic vein drainage
- symptom is dragging pain in the scrotum
- long-standing varicocoele may cause testicular atrophy and infertility

Testicular tumours

GERM CELL TUMOURS

- the complexity of testicular tumours has been clarified by the classification published by the British Testicular Tumour Panel (Table 10.1)
- seminomas, teratomas and yolk-sac tumours all arise from germ cells
- there is an association between germ cell tumours and maldescended testes
- usual presentation is with hard painless enlarged testis
- some present with symptoms of metastases
- alpha-fetoprotein (AFP) is a product of the yolk sac and liver in fetal life. Elevated serum levels are found in pure yolk-sac tumours of the testis and in malignant teratomas with a yolk-sac component
- beta-human chorionic gonadotrophin (HCG) is produced by the normal placenta. Elevated serum levels are found in some patients with germ cell tumours, especially malignant teratomas
- the risk of a second primary testicular neoplasm in a patient with a previous testicular tumour is 2%

Table 10.1 Classification of testicular tumours and the percentages seen in 2739 cases referred to the Testicular Tumour Panel (Pugh 1976)

	%
Seminoma	39.5
Teratoma	31.7
Combined tumour	13.5
Malignant lymphoma	6.7
Sertoli cell/mesenchyme	1.2
Interstitial (Leydig) cell	1.6
Yolk sac tumours	1.9
Metastases	0.9
Miscellaneous	0.8
Uncertain	2.2

SEMINOMA

- commonest tumour of the testis
- incidence is approximately 1.5 per 100 000 males per year
- peak age of presentation is 30–40 years
- occurs more commonly in patients with a maldecended testis
- in patients with a unilateral maldescended testis, both testes are at risk of malignant transformation
- teratomatous elements may coexist in a mixed germ cell tumour

Pathology

- testis is symmetrically enlarged
- there may be an associated hydrocoele
- on cut section the tumour is white or yellow in colour
- bands of fibrous tissue impart a lobulated appearance
- microscopy shows sheets, groups and trabeculae of tumour cells separated by fibrous bands
- cells are uniform in size and the cytoplasm is clear
- there is a stromal lymphocytic infiltrate and granulomas may also be present
- immunohistochemical staining for placental alkaline phosphatase may be useful in diagnosis

Spread

- invades and destroys the surrounding normal testis either directly or by spreading along seminiferous tubules
- distant metastatic spread occurs by lymphatics to common iliac and para-aortic nodes. Later, thoracic nodes and supraclavicular nodes are involved
- blood-borne metastases occur to lungs, liver and bone

Staging and prognosis

- clinical staging of testicular tumours used by the Royal Marsden Hospital is given in Table 10.2
- the majority of patients present with stage I or II disease
- prognosis for stage I disease is excellent and few patients die of their disease

Table 10.2 Royal Marsden staging classification of testicular tumours

Stage	Extent of disease
I	No evidence of disease outside the testis
II	Infradiaphragmatic node involvement: IIa Maximum diameter of metastases <2 cm IIb Maximum diameter of metastases 2–5 cm IIc Maximum diameter of metastases >5 cm
III	Supra- and infradiaphragmatic lymph node involvement: a, b and c as for stage II Mediastinal nodes noted M+ Neck nodes noted N+ 0 = Negative lymphogram
IV	Extension of tumour to extralymphatic sites: a, b and c as for stages II and III Lung substage: L_1 metastases <3 in number L_2 metastases >3 in number, <2 cm diameter L_3 metastases >3 in number, >2 cm diameter

Adapted from Peckham (1981).

- stages IIa and IIb also have an excellent prognosis
- patients with stage II disease require radiotherapy to the lymph nodes in the abdomen and chemotherapy is often given prior to radiotherapy
- stages III and IV require chemotherapy and radiotherapy treatment

SPERMATOCYTIC SEMINOMA

- occurs in an older age group than classical seminoma with a peak incidence of 45–50 years
- microscopically there are sheets of cells which can show marked pleomorphism and a high mitotic rate
- a lymphocytic infiltrate is absent
- prognosis after orchidectomy is excellent
- does not require radiotherapy treatment
- very rarely undergoes sarcomatous transformation

TERATOMA

- tumour containing tissue derived from more than one germ cell layer
- slightly less common than seminoma
- occurs in a younger age group with a peak incidence at 20–30 years
- occurs more commonly in patients with maldescended testes
- majority present with testicular swelling

- may also present with testicular pain due to haemorrhage or necrosis
- presentation may occasionally be with secondary deposits, usually in lung or retroperitoneum
- teratomas are divided by the British Testicular Tumour Panel into teratoma differentiated (TD), malignant teratoma intermediate (MTI), malignant teratoma undifferentiated (MTU) and malignant teratoma trophoblastic (MTT)

Gross appearance

- unlike seminoma the testis may be asymmetrically enlarged
- cut surface may be haemorrhagic with necrotic areas and cyst formation

Teratoma differentiated (teratoma mature, teratoma immature)

- most common teratoma found in children
- rare in adults
- composed of mature tissues of many types
- although no malignancy is seen, some immature tissue in the form of immature glands, stroma or neuroepithelium may be present
- in adults especially, it is essential histologically to examine the tumour extensively to look for malignant areas which would bring the tumour into the MTI category
- prognosis is good but metastases may rarely occur

Malignant teratoma intermediate (embryonal carcinoma and teratoma, teratocarcinoma)

- differentiated tissues are present together with unequivocally malignant elements
- yolk sac areas may be present and are often associated with an elevated serum alpha-fetoprotein (AFP)
- trophoblastic tissue may be found and may be associated with increased serum levels of beta human chorionic gonadotrophin (βHCG)
- prognosis gets worse with increasing amounts of malignant tissue

Malignant teratoma undifferentiated (embryonal carcinoma)

- microscopically entirely composed of malignant elements with a complete absence of differentiated tissue
- consists of masses of cells resembling a carcinoma. Cellular pleomorphism and mitoses are prominent
- may get yolk sac areas or trophoblastic areas

Malignant teratoma trophoblastic (choriocarcinoma)

- grossly extensive haemorrhage and necrosis are common
- usually found in combination with MTU
- to make diagnosis it is essential to demonstrate that syncytiotrophoblast and cytotrophoblast are both present with a papillary pattern. This finding, even if present in a small proportion of a tumour, puts the lesion into the MTT category
- elevated serum HCG levels are frequently found
- associated with very poor prognosis

Spread and staging

- local spread is directly into the testis, epididymis and cord
- metastases occur to lungs, liver, abdominal and mediastinal lymph nodes
- histologically metastatic deposits may exhibit poorer differentiation than the primary tumour
- clinical and pathological staging is the same as for seminoma

Prognosis

- embryonal carcinoma and choriocarcinoma have a worse prognosis than the other tumours
- the pathological stage of the tumour is an important prognostic factor
- prognosis has markedly improved with the introduction of *cis*-platinum and etoposide into chemotherapeutic regimens
- patients with stage I disease have an excellent prognosis with 90% being cured by radical orchidectomy alone
- patients with stage II disease are treated by surgery and chemotherapy and have a good prognosis
- serum levels of βHCG and AFP are useful in monitoring recurrence and response to therapy. Elevation of the serum levels may indicate tumour recurrence or metastases

COMBINED SEMINOMA AND TERATOMA

- 10% of testicular tumours are composed of a mixture of both seminoma and teratoma (combined germ cell tumour)
- microscopically there are areas of classical seminoma and of various types of teratomas
- behaviour and prognosis of combined germ cell tumour is variable and depends on the type of the teratomatous element

SERTOLI CELL TUMOUR (ANDROBLASTOMA)

- occurs at any age but commonest under age 40 years
- also occur in childhood and infancy
- usually presents as testicular swelling
- gynaecomastia may occur due to elaboration of hormones
- microscopically is composed of small tubular structures
- 10% of cases behave in a malignant fashion. The remainder are benign with an excellent prognosis
- microscopic examination may not be able to predict which tumours are likely to behave in a malignant fashion

INTERSTITIAL CELL TUMOUR (LEYDIG CELL TUMOUR)

- arise from the interstitial cells (Leydig cells) of the testis
- presentation is usually with a testicular mass
- microscopically is composed of sheets of cells with abundant eosinophilic cytoplasm
- may present with features due to hormone elaboration such as feminization with loss of body hair, loss of libido and gynaecomastia
- 10% of these tumours are malignant
- microscopic examination may not be able to predict which tumours behave in a malignant fashion

YOLK SAC TUMOUR (ENDODERMAL SINUS TUMOUR)

- commonest testicular tumour of childhood
- presents as a testicular mass and is often associated with raised serum AFP
- microscopy shows tubular and papillary areas
- the characteristic microscopic feature is the presence of Schiller-Duval bodies. These are composed of a central vascular structure surrounded by cuboidal cells
- immunohistochemical staining of tumour for AFP may be useful in establishing a diagnosis
- spreads locally to testis, epididymis and cord
- lymphatic metastasis is to para-aortic nodes
- haematogenous spread occurs to multiple sites, especially lung
- when the tumour is localised to the testis orchidectomy is often curative
- even when distant metastases are present, combination chemotherapy produces good results

Carcinoma-*in-situ* of the testis (intratubular germ cell neoplasia)

- may be recognised in testicular biopsies performed during investigation of infertility
- seen within testicular tubules adjacent to invasive germ cell tumours, both seminomas and teratomas
- also found in a small proportion of maldescended testes, in infertile patients and in the contralateral testis in cases of testicular germ cell tumour
- risk of development of invasive tumour is 50% within 5 years
- positive immunohistochemical staining with placental alkaline phosphatase may be useful in establishing a diagnosis

Lymphoma and leukaemia

- malignant lymphoma involving the testis may be a manifestation of disseminated disease in elderly patients
- primary lymphoma of the testis can occur and is often bilateral
- usually arise in elderly patients
- they are usually high grade B-cell non-Hodgkin's lymphomas
- the most common primary testicular neoplasm in the elderly
- the prognosis is good and they often remain confined to the testis
- testicular infiltration by leukaemic cells may occur, especially in acute lymphoblastic leukaemia in children

Paratesticular tumours and tumour-like lesions

- the adenomatoid tumour is a common benign neoplasm which can occur in the epididymis or spermatic cord
- it may invade the testis giving a false impression of malignancy
- microscopically adenomatoid tumour consists of numerous slit-like spaces lined by bland flat cells
- adenomatoid tumour is a benign neoplasm of mesothelial origin
- the commonest paratesticular sarcoma is the embryonal rhabdomyosarcoma which usually occurs in infants and children

- leiomyosarcomas, fibrosarcomas and other sarcomas occur occasionally in the paratesticular region in older patients
- fibrous pseudotumour (fibrous periorchitis) is a reactive paratesticular lesion which clinically may mimic a neoplasm
- microscopically it is composed of spindle-shaped cells with scattered inflammatory cells

THE PROSTATE

Normal structure

- the normal adult prostate weighs approximately 20 g
- the prostate is traversed by the prostatic urethra which is approximately 2.5 cm in length. Posteriorly the ejaculatory ducts enter the urethra at the verumontanum
- the median lobe of the prostate lies posteriorly between the urethra and the ejaculatory ducts
- the two lateral lobes are below and lateral to the medial lobe
- benign nodular hyperplasia develops in periurethral prostatic tissue
- the peripheral zone is the site of origin of most prostatic cancers
- microscopically the normal prostate consists of glands embedded in a fibromuscular stroma
- the glands are lined by two layers of epithelial cells and drain into the excretory ducts which enter the floor of the urethra
- the blood supply of the prostate is from the inferior vesicle, internal pudendal and middle rectal arteries
- venous drainage is to periprostatic venous plexus
- lymphatic drainage is to hypogastric, sacral, vesicle and external iliac nodes

Prostatic biopsy

- most commonly a needle biopsy is used
- perineal or transrectal approach may be used
- biopsy may be performed under radiological guidance
- complications include profuse bleeding and bacteraemic shock. Bacteraemia after transrectal biopsy occurs commonly and antibiotic cover is required

Prostatitis

ACUTE BACTERIAL PROSTATITIS

- associated with urinary tract infections
- may get systemic features of infection as well as local symptoms
- on rectal examination the prostate is swollen and tender
- the common causative organisms are those which cause urinary tract infections, i.e. *Escherichia coli*, *Proteus*, *Klebsiella*, *Enterobacteria* and *Pseudomonas*
- microscopically there is polymorph infiltration and small abscess formation
- treatment is antibiotics

CHRONIC PROSTATITIS

- may be caused by bacterial infection or may occur without infection
- referred pain in various areas (suprapubic, perineal, low back, scrotal, penile, inner thigh) is a common symptom
- on rectal examination the prostate may be tender and may be hard simulating a carcinoma

GRANULOMATOUS PROSTATITIS

- may be idiopathic or associated with other diseases
- other diseases include tuberculous and fungal infections, sarcoidosis or vasculitic processes
- may occur post-biopsy
- microscopy shows granulomatous inflammation

Benign nodular hyperplasia (BNH) of the prostate

EPIDEMIOLOGY, AETIOLOGY AND PATHOGENESIS

- most common urological disease of men
- autopsy studies show that 50% of men aged between 50 and 60 years and 80% aged over 70 years have BNH of the prostate
- less than 10% require treatment
- aetiology and pathogenesis are related to changes in androgen and oestrogen metabolism with increasing age
- testosterone is metabolised into 5-alpha-dihydrotestosterone (DHT) in peripheral tissues. The concentration of DHT in prostatic tissue of patients with BNH is increased. This may be one factor which results in BNH
- 5 alpha-reductase inhibitors inhibit the conversion of testosterone to dihydro-testosterone and result in decreased prostatic weight

CLINICAL FEATURES

- symptoms include frequency, poor stream and nocturia
- sequelae of bladder outlet obstruction include bladder distension, trabeculation, sacculation, stasis and infection with stone formation
- hydroureter, hydronephrosis and renal failure may eventually occur

PATHOLOGY

- BNH often involves the periurethral area of the prostate and results in obstructive symptoms
- on rectal examination the prostate may be enlarged or may be of normal size, depending on the area of gland affected
- on cut section the prostatectomy specimen shows many nodules of varying sizes with surrounding compressed prostatic tissue
- microscopy shows hyperplasia of the fibromuscular and glandular elements
- glands are lined by two cell layers
- areas of squamous metaplasia, infarction and chronic inflammation are common

PROGNOSIS

- treatment of BNH is usually surgical (TURP)
- recently developed treatments for BNH include self-expanding stents, local hyperthermia and dilatation of the prostatic urethra with cylindrical balloons
- treatment with 5-alpha-reductase inhibitors or anti-androgen therapy is possible

Prostatic cancer

- clinical prostatic cancer gives rise to prostatic symptoms
- occult cancer is one which presents with metastatic disease
- latent cancer is unsuspectedly found at autopsy
- incidental cancer is found during microscopic examination of prostate removed for BNH

EPIDEMIOLOGY, AETIOLOGY AND PATHOGENESIS

- the incidence of prostatic cancer has increased in the past decade, probably due to earlier detection
- primarily affects males over 50 years. At autopsy almost 70% of men over 80 years have microscopic foci of latent carcinoma
- many prostatic cancers are asymptomatic
- little is known of the aetiology of prostatic cancer
- androgens are essential for maintenance and growth of adenocarcinoma cells
- growth may be controlled by castration or oestrogen therapy
- there may be a familial association
- obesity and alcohol abuse may be risk factors
- a possible link between previous vasectomy and development of prostatic cancer has been suggested but is unproven

CLINICAL FEATURES

- most carcinomas arise in the peripheral zone of the prostate and give rise to urinary obstruction late
- invasion through rectal mucosa may cause confusion with a primary rectal carcinoma
- digital rectal examination is limited in the diagnosis of prostatic cancer
- normal, hyperplastic and malignant prostatic epithelium produces acid phosphatase
- prostatic acid phosphatase can be distinguished in the laboratory from other acid phosphatases
- prostatic acid phosphatase (PAP) and prostate-specific antigen (PSA) are useful in the detection of prostate cancer
- raised circulating levels of PSA and PAP are found in patients with adenocarcinoma
- slightly raised levels are also found in BNH, prostatitis, and following needle biopsy or transurethral resection
- very high serum levels are strongly indicative of prostatic carcinoma
- serial estimation of circulating PSA levels are useful in monitoring the response to treatment

PATHOLOGY

- may be diagnosed by transrectal needle core biopsy or FNA
- on sectioning a prostatectomy specimen, cancer may be detected as a firm gritty area
- microscopically the vast majority of prostatic cancers are adenocarcinomas and most arise from the acini of the peripheral zone
- well differentiated adenocarcinomas are difficult to distinguish from BNH
- in adenocarcinoma the normal double cell layer of glands is replaced by a single cell layer

- prominent nucleoli may be a useful microscopic feature in diagnosing prostatic adenocarcinoma
- in poorly differentiated adenocarcinomas the acini are poorly formed and sheets of tumour cells are seen
- Gleason's is the most commonly used grading system
- ductal adenocarcinoma is a variant which arises from large ducts and which commonly results in obstructive symptoms
- foci of prostatic intraepithelial neoplasia (PIN) may be found adjacent to prostatic adenocarcinoma

SPREAD

- direct spread occurs into the seminal vesicles, bladder or rectum
- lymphatic spread is to nodes along the internal and common iliac arteries and to the para-aortic nodes
- bony metastases occur in the pelvis, lumbosacral spine and long bones
- bony metastases are often osteosclerotic
- distant metastases may also occur to the liver and lungs

STAGING AND PROGNOSIS

- staging is by the TNM system which is shown in Table 10.3
- T category is assessed by clinical examination, urography, endoscopy and by manual palpation
- computed tomography (CT) scanning aids assessment of pelvic nodes. The M status is assessed by serum levels of PSA and PAP, chest x-ray and bone scan

Table 10.3 TNM classification of prostatic cancer

Stage	Extent of disease
Tis	Preinvasive carcinoma (carcinoma-*in-situ*)
T0	No tumour palpable. Incidental finding at operation or biopsy
T1	Intracapsular tumour surrounded by palpably normal gland
T2	Tumour confined to gland. Smooth nodule deforming the gland contour but lateral sulci and seminal vesicles not involved
T3	Tumour extending beyond the capsule with or without the involvement of the lateral sulci or seminal vesicles
T4	Fixed tumour or infiltration of adjacent structure
N0	No evidence of regional node involvement
N1	Single homolateral regional lymph node
N2	Contralateral or bilateral node involvement or multiple regional nodes affected
N3	Fixed regional nodes
N4	Involved juxtaregional nodes
M0	No distant metastases
M1	Distant metastases

- prognosis depends on histological grading and stage
- Gleason system of histological grading is used
- this system designates five grades ranging from small uniform glands (grade I) to infiltrating anaplastic tumours (grade V)
- tumour heterogeneity is accounted by assigning a primary pattern for the dominant grade and a secondary pattern for the non-dominant grade. The Gleason score is derived by adding the two scores
- the higher the score the worse the prognosis
- the principal factors associated with metastases are tumour volume, seminal vesicle invasion, capsular invasion and histological grade
- treatment of prostatic adenocarcinoma is controversial with four major options, i.e. radical prostatectomy, radiotherapy, androgen deprivation therapy and active surveillance (deferred treatment)

THE PENIS AND SCROTUM

Normal structure

- penis consists of two corpora cavernosa and a corpus spongiosum which contains the urethra
- corpora are capped distally by the glans penis
- each corpus is enclosed in a fascial sheath (tunica albuginea) and all are surrounded by a fascial envelope (Buck's fascia)
- the proximal ends of the corpora cavernosa are attached to the pelvic bones while the corpus spongiosum is connected to the perineal membrane through which emerges the membranous urethra
- the penis and urethra are supplied by the internal pudendal arteries
- lymphatic drainage from the skin of the penis is to the superficial inguinal nodes
- lymphatics from the glans penis drain to both inguinal and external iliac nodes
- the scrotum consists of skin, dartos muscle and several layers of fascia
- lymphatics drain to inguinal nodes

Congenital and developmental abnormalities

- congenital urethral stricture occasionally occurs in male infants
- back pressure may cause dilatation of urethra, hypertrophy of bladder muscle and hydronephrosis

POSTERIOR URETHRAL VALVES

- a pair of mucosal folds attached to the verumontanum and the anterior wall of the membranous urethra
- forms an oblique diaphragm which acts as a one-way valve
- common cause of urethral obstruction in newborn males
- treatment requires surgical resection of the valves

URETHRAL DUPLICATION

- rare condition
- may be complete or partial
- most are asymptomatic but most common complication is infection

EPISPADIAS

- congenital absence of the upper wall of the urethra
- the urethra opens onto the dorsum of the penis proximal to the glans
- frequently get urinary incontinence
- may get other congenital abnormalities such as bladder exstrophy and renal agenesis

HYPOSPADIAS

- urethra opens on the underside of the penile shaft or on the perineum
- occurs in 1 in 500 boys
- frequently associated with chordee (bowing of penis)
- due to failure of development of the distal urethra which is replaced by fibrous tissue
- often associated meatal stenosis
- high incidence of cryptorchidism and inguinal hernia

Miscellaneous conditions

PEYRONIE'S DISEASE

- usually affects middle-aged to elderly men
- firm cords, nodules or plaques of dense fibrous tissue form in the tunica albuginea
- calcification and ossification may occur in this fibrous tissue
- cause is unknown
- in some cases coexists with Dupytren's contracture or plantar fibromatosis
- may be related to coital trauma and urethral instrumentation
- patients complain of painful curvature of the penis on erection
- usually the dorsal surface of the penis is affected
- may resolve spontaneously or may require surgical treatment

PRIAPISM

- prolonged painful penile erection unrelated to sexual stimulation
- may be idiopathic or secondary
- secondary causes include genital trauma, haemostasis, neurological defects, drugs and alcohol

FOURNIER'S GANGRENE OF THE SCROTUM

- rare condition
- necrotising fasciitis of the subcutaneous tissue and muscle of the scrotum
- affects men in the fourth and fifth decades
- sudden marked oedema of the scrotum
- rapidly progresses to gangrene of the skin
- patient is systemically ill
- diabetes, local trauma, local surgical procedures, alcoholism, immunosuppression and obesity are predisposing factors
- microscopy shows polymorph infiltration with extensive vascular thrombosis and necrosis
- serious life-threatening condition which requires prompt therapy

- infective agents are usually a combination of staphylococcal and streptococcal species and anaerobic bacteria
- treatment is radical surgical debridement

Cancer of the penis

- uncommon in Western countries but more common in Uganda and Mexico
- occurs in the 40–70 year age group
- associated with poor penile hygiene and lack of circumcision
- some cases may have a viral aetiology (human papilloma virus)
- erythroplasia of Queyrat (Bowen's disease of the glans penis) may predispose to the development of penile carcinoma
- penile carcinoma presents grossly as an infiltrating, ulcerated or nodular area
- the majority of cancers arise on the glans or prepuce
- microscopically almost all are squamous carcinomas
- inguinal lymph nodes are enlarged in many cases, either due to associated infection or to metastatic carcinoma
- vascular spread is via prostatic plexus, pelvic veins and vertebral plexus
- verrucous carcinoma is an extremely well differentiated form of squamous carcinoma
- rare malignant tumours which occur on the penis include basal cell carcinoma, malignant melanoma and various sarcomas

Carcinoma of the urethra

- patients with transitional cell carcinoma of the urinary bladder have an increased incidence of carcinoma of the urethra
- this probably represents multifocal tumours arising in unstable epithelium
- distal carcinomas may be squamous in type
- tumours in the anterior urethra tend to spread via lymphatics to the inguinal nodes whereas tumours in the posterior urethra spread to iliac nodes

Carcinoma of the scrotum

- first cancer linked to occupational exposure to a carcinogen
- association with chimney sweeps noted by Percival Pott (1775). Tumour sometimes referred to as Pott's cancer
- usually affects elderly men and presents as an ulcerated nodular lesion which often becomes secondarily infected
- microscopically squamous carcinomas
- spread occurs to inguinal lymph nodes
- overall prognosis is poor
- rare malignant tumours which occur primarily on the scrotum include basal cell carcinoma, malignant melanoma and various sarcomas

The breast

11

NORMAL STRUCTURE

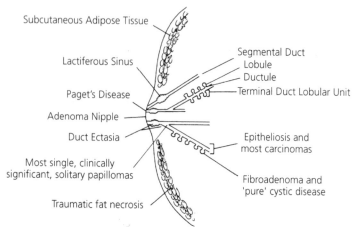

Figure 11.1 General structure of the female breast with the position of some pathological conditions

- the breast consists of 10–15 segments with each segment containing lobules, ductules, subsegmental ducts, segmental ducts, lactiferous sinuses and collecting ducts
- a lobule consists of acini surrounded by vascular connective tissue
- a lobular unit is defined as a lobule together with a central ductule
- the nipple and the first few centimetres of the collecting ducts deep to the surface are lined by keratinising stratified squamous epithelium
- the remaining ducts have two cell layers, an inner layer of cuboidal epithelial cells and an outer layer of myoepithelial cells

PREOPERATIVE BIOPSY

- preoperative biopsy to confirm malignancy means that frozen section diagnosis is now rarely, if ever, indicated
- trucut needle biopsy is used in some centres

- FNA has gained increasing popularity
- FNA is highly accurate in experienced hands
- with FNA problems may occur in the diagnosis of lobular carcinoma
- invasive malignancy cannot be distinguished from *in situ* malignancy on FNA
- stereotactic guided FNA may be used for impalpable mammographically detected lesions

CONGENITAL ABNORMALITIES OF THE BREAST

- amazia or absent breast is rare and usually affects males
- polymazia or accessory breast is common, especially in the axilla
- absent nipple may occur
- supernumerary nipples along the milk line are common

INFLAMMATORY CONDITIONS OF THE BREAST

Breast abscess

- may be associated with breast feeding
- most common organism is *Staphylococcus aureus*
- clinically the breast is swollen and tender
- subareolar abscesses may result in formation of a fistulous tract
- microscopy shows marked polymorphonuclear infiltrate
- inflammatory carcinoma may need to be excluded by FNA or rarely biopsy
- treatment is antibiotics

Tuberculosis

- rare in Western countries, but more common in Asian women
- presents with multiple, chronic abscesses
- sinuses are typical
- associated with pulmonary tuberculosis
- microscopy shows caseating granulomatous inflammation
- treatment is with antituberculous drugs

Actinomycosis

- rare
- multiple abscesses are characteristic
- sinuses are common
- penicillin is usual treatment

Mammary duct ectasia

- involves large and intermediate ducts of breast
- dilated ducts with inspissated secretions are surrounded by inflammatory cells
- aetiology is unknown but may begin with periductal inflammation

- clinical features include a yellow or green nipple discharge and palpable dilated ducts deep to the nipple
- there may be nipple inversion
- may be recurrent sinus or fistula formation

PATHOLOGY

- dilated ducts
- debris and foam cells are present in duct lumina
- periductal chronic inflammation occurs in which plasma cells are often conspicuous
- in late stages ducts become surrounded by fibrous tissue

Mondor's disease

- superficial thrombophlebitis on breast surface
- thoraco-epigastric vein is usually involved
- presents as tender cord when arm is raised
- self-limiting

TRAUMATIC LESIONS OF THE BREAST

Haematoma

- may be due to seat-belt injury
- if long-standing, fibrous scarring and calcification may ensue

Fat necrosis

- associated with trauma
- more common in obese women with large breasts
- usually presents with painless lump which may mimic carcinoma
- white chalky gross appearance
- microscopy shows fat necrosis with histiocytic and giant cell reaction
- may be diagnosed by FNA, thus avoiding unnecessary surgery

BENIGN BREAST LESIONS

ANDI

- Aberrations of Normal Development and Involution

Breast cysts

- common
- may occur at any age, although most common age 30–50 years
- often multiple and bilateral and of variable size

- often have a bluish colour when viewed prior to opening (blue-domed cyst)
- smooth wall
- contains straw-coloured or browny green fluid
- may be drained by FNA but fluid often reaccumulates
- microscopy shows flattened epithelial lining or may get apocrine cells
- if rupture occurs, inflammatory reaction and fibrosis may ensue
- often associated with other types of benign breast disease
- patients with breast cysts and a family history of cancer have a slightly increased risk of breast cancer development

Adenosis

- condition of glandular elements
- microscopy reveals increase in size and/or number of lobular acini
- presents with painless lump
- usually age 25–50 years
- pale, rubbery on gross appearance
- microcalcification may be present
- probably no risk of malignant transformation unless other changes are superimposed
- the double cell layer of epithelial and myoepithelial cells is generally preserved
- three variants occur

BLUNT DUCT ADENOSIS

- dilatation of acini
- double cell layer preserved

SCLEROSING ADENOSIS

- associated stromal fibrosis and often calcification
- double cell layer is preserved

MICROGLANDULAR ADENOSIS

- proliferation of small glands
- double cell layer may be lost
- may be mistaken histologically for tubular carcinoma

Radial scar and complex sclerosing lesion (CSL)

- often detected mammographically as a spiculated mass which may mimic carcinoma
- microscopy shows central fibrous core with enclosed tubules
- radial scar measures 9 mm or less, whereas CSL measures 10 mm or more
- microscopically may be confused with tubular carcinoma
- no predisposition to carcinoma but may mimic carcinoma on mammographic, gross and microscopic examination

Epithelial hyperplasia (epitheliosis)

- get proliferation of epithelial cells within confines of ducts or lobules
- may be difficult to distinguish microscopically from carcinoma *in situ*

CLASSIFICATION

Ductal

- without atypia
- atypical ductal hyperplasia (ADH)

Lobular

- atypical lobular hyperplasia (ALH)

DEFINITIONS

Ductal hyperplasia without atypia

- increase in number of epithelial cells within ducts or lobules
- may be divided into mild or moderate and florid

ADH

- has some but not all features of ductal carcinoma *in situ* (DCIS)
- either cytological or architectural criteria of DCIS is fulfilled but not both
- criteria of DCIS may be fulfilled but do not occupy at least two duct spaces

ALH

- identical microscopic picture to lobular carcinoma *in situ* (LCIS) but less than one half of acini in a lobule are filled, distorted and distended

RISK OF CARCINOMA

- mild ductal hyperplasia without atypia – no risk
- moderate and florid ductal hyperplasia without atypia – risk × 2
- ADH – risk × 4
- ALH – risk × 4
- ADH or ALH and positive family history – risk × 11

Fibroadenoma

- benign breast lesion with both epithelial and stromal components
- arises in lobules
- usually occurs in young women
- clinically presents as mobile breast lesion

PATHOLOGY

- grossly usually well circumscribed with a grey white cut surface
- microscopy shows glandular component with a double cell layer embedded in abundant fibrous tissue
- may be *pericanalicular* (no compression of tubules) or *intracanalicular* (tubules compressed with slit-like lumina) types
- usually diagnosed by FNA
- no subsequent risk of carcinoma
- many show spontaneous regression especially after the menopause

Phyllodes tumour

- may be benign, malignant or borderline malignant based on pathological features
- may be any site
- usually occur age 30–70 years
- usually well circumscribed
- on sectioning may contain clefts or cystic cavities
- microscopically differentiated from fibroadenoma by presence of hypercellular stroma
- signs of malignancy include pleomorphism and mitotic activity within stromal component and overgrowth of stromal component
- behaviour unpredictable but may get haematogenous metastasis

PAPILLARY LESIONS OF BREAST

Intraduct papilloma

- may occur in large subareolar ducts when they are usually solitary
- these present with bloody nipple discharge
- may be found in peripheral ducts where they are often multiple and associated with other benign breast lesions
- microscopy shows papillary fronds of connective tissue covered by a double layer of epithelial and myoepithelial cells
- solitary lesions probably have no malignant potential, whereas multiple lesions may have a small risk of subsequent malignant development

Papillary carcinoma

- may be invasive or non-invasive
- non-invasive papillary carcinoma has the structure of a papilloma, but the epithelium qualifies for the designation carcinoma *in situ*

Juvenile papillomatosis

- occurs in young women
- pathology reveals cyst formation, epitheliosis and papilloma formation
- may be an association between juvenile papillomatosis, family history of breast cancer and breast cancer risk elevation

Adenoma of nipple

- rare benign lesion
- presents as lump behind nipple
- microscopically benign with a variety of growth patterns

CARCINOMA *IN SITU* OF THE BREAST

Ductal carcinoma *in situ* (DCIS)

- occurs in breast ducts and may spread into lobules (cancerisation of lobules)
- microscopically malignant cells are seen within ducts, but there is no invasion through the basement membrane
- may present with breast lump
- may present with nipple discharge
- microcalcification is common and therefore the lesion is often found on mammography during breast cancer screening
- increasing in incidence due to being detected in screening programmes
- there are several microscopic subtypes of DCIS, the most common being comedo, cribriform, micropapillary and solid
- comedo DCIS has central areas of necrosis within ducts
- recent tendency is to grade DCIS as high or low grade, depending on nuclear features
- comedo DCIS tends to be high nuclear grade, whereas cribriform and micropapillary tend to be low grade
- DCIS (especially low grade) may be difficult to distinguish microscopically from florid epitheliosis and ADH
- DCIS is often found at the edge of invasive tumours
- DCIS is often multifocal
- less than 5% of cases have involvement of axillary lymph nodes
- comedo type DCIS has a high risk of tumour invasion and recurrence
- with complete excision, prognosis is excellent
- if not adequately excised, risk of tumour recurrence
- need to sample lesions adequately to exclude microinvasive carcinoma

Lobular carcinoma *in situ* (LCIS)

- arises in acini of lobules
- may be an incidental finding
- produces no symptoms
- difficult to detect on mammography
- on microscopic examination acini are filled and distended by a monotonous population of small regular cells
- may be associated with infiltrating lobular carcinoma
- multicentricity and bilaterality is often a feature of LCIS
- risk of subsequent development of invasive carcinoma in ipsilateral or contralateral breast

INVASIVE BREAST CANCER

- 14 000 deaths annually in England and Wales
- unusual before age 30 years
- in the UK one in 12 women develop breast cancer
- the triple approach which combines clinical, mammographic and cytological (FNA) parameters is important in the preoperative diagnosis of breast cancer

Aetiology

- aetiology is unknown but hormonal and familial factors are thought to be important. It has been proposed that prolonged or strong oestrogen stimulation results in cancer development on a genetically susceptible background

HORMONAL FACTORS

- breast cancer is associated with early menarche, late menopause, nulliparous women and first child over 35 years
- an early first pregnancy confers some protection from the development of breast cancer
- breast cancer may coexist with ovarian cancer which is also associated with the above factors
- oophorectomy before age 35 years reduces the risk of breast cancer
- exogenous oestrogens may be associated with an increased risk of breast cancer

FAMILIAL FACTORS

- 15% of patients may have a positive family history
- women who have a first degree relative with breast cancer have a risk two to three times that of the general population
- up to 10% of cancers may be hereditary. These often occur in young women and may be bilateral
- the gene responsible for the hereditary form of breast cancer has been identified on chromosome 17q and named BRCA1
- a second gene has been localised to chromosome 13q and named BRCA2
- these two genes probably account for approximately two-thirds of familial breast cancer
- patients with ataxia telangiectasia have an increased risk of breast cancer

MISCELLANEOUS FACTORS

- ionising radiation and high consumption of animal fats have been found in some studies to be associated with the development of breast cancer

Classification of breast cancer

(Tables 11.1 and 11.2)

LOBULAR CARCINOMA

- approximately 12% of invasive breast cancers in UK are lobular in type
- macroscopic appearance varies from well-defined mass to ill-defined indurated area
- no classical mammographic features and may be difficult to detect
- may be difficult to diagnose on FNA
- microscopy shows single file (Indian file) arrangement of regular cells
- tumour cells may be arranged around benign duct in a targetoid pattern
- tumour cells often contain intracytoplasmic lumina
- adjacent LCIS may be present
- tumour is often multifocal and may be bilateral
- prognosis is better than classical ductal carcinoma

Table 11.1 Clinical classification of breast cancer

Stage	Extent of disease
TNM system	
Tis	Carcinoma-*in-situ*
T0	No evidence of primary tumour
T1	<2 cm
T2	2–5 cm
T3	5 cm
T4	Extension to chest wall or skin:
	(a) chest wall
	(b) skin oedema, or infiltration, or ulceration
	(c) both chest wall and skin
N0	No nodes palpable
N1	Mobile axillary nodes
	(a) not considered involved by tumour
	(b) considered involved by tumour
N2	Fixed axillary nodes
N3	Palpable supraclavicular nodes
M0	No distant metastases
M1	Distant metastases
Manchester system	
Stage I	Tumour confined to breast. Not adherent to pectoral muscles or chest wall. If skin adherence, this must be smaller than size of tumour
Stage II	Primary tumour as in stage I, with the addition of mobile ipsilateral lymph nodes
Stage III	Skin involvement larger than tumour; tumour fixed to pectoral muscles but not to chest wall. Fixed nodes in axilla
Stage IV	Distant spread either blood- or lymph-borne. Invasion of skin wide of breast. Palpable supraclavicular nodes. Involvement of opposite breast. Bone, brain, lung, liver involvement

DUCTAL CARCINOMA

- most common type of invasive breast cancer
- usual macroscopic appearance is of scirrhous or stellate tumour
- seen as spiculated mass on mammography
- microscopy shows glandular formation in the case of well-differentiated tumours
- there may be associated DCIS
- poorer prognosis than other invasive breast carcinomas

Rarer types of invasive breast cancer

MEDULLARY CARCINOMA

- well circumscribed and soft on sectioning
- solid, syncytial growth pattern with well defined edge and a marked lymphocytic infiltrate
- no associated DCIS
- better prognosis than classical ductal carcinoma

Table 11.2   Classification of breast cancer

1. Lobular
   (a) *in-situ*
   (b) invasive
2. Ductal
   (a) *in-situ*
   (b) invasive
      (i)   not otherwise specified (the most common type)
      (ii)   medullary carcinoma with lymphoid stroma
      (iii) pure mucoid
      (iv)   tubular
      (v)   squamous
      (vi)   adenoid cystic
      (vii) apocrine
      (viii) lipid-rich
      (ix)   juvenile
      (x)   carcinomas with noteworthy clinical manifestations
             inflammatory carcinoma
             Paget's disease of nipple
3. Uncertain – either ductal or lobular
4. Mixture of ductal and lobular
5. Carcinoma arising in a pre-existing benign tumour
6. Carcinosarcoma
7. Unclassified

Adapted from Azzopardi (1979).

MUCINOUS CARCINOMA

- soft with a mucoid character on sectioning
- microscopy shows small groups of bland tumour cells with abundant extracellular mucin
- no associated DCIS
- good prognosis

TUBULAR CARCINOMA

- usually small and stellate in appearance, less than 1.5 cm diameter
- commonly asymptomatic and detected by mammography at breast screening
- difficult FNA diagnosis
- microscopically extremely well differentiated tumour with good tubule formation and abundant sclerosis
- mammographically, grossly and microscopically may be difficult to distinguish from radial scar and complex sclerosing lesion
- excellent prognosis

INVASIVE CRIBRIFORM CARCINOMA

- variant of tubular carcinoma
- microscopy shows cribriform arrangement of tumour cells
- excellent prognosis

ADENOID CYSTIC CARCINOMA

- rare in breast
- identical microscopic appearance to salivary gland counterpart
- good prognosis

SQUAMOUS CARCINOMA

- rare primary breast carcinoma
- often has cystic component
- poor prognosis

INFLAMMATORY CARCINOMA

- clinically there is oedema and redness of breast
- due to extensive lymphatic permeation by tumour
- poor prognosis

Prognostic factors in breast cancer

LYMPH NODE STATUS

- most important predictor of outcome
- prognosis depends on number and level of nodes involved
- may be micrometastases in nodes which are difficult to detect by conventional microscopy
- a score of 1–3 is given depending on the number of nodes involved
- overall 10-year survival for node negative patients is 75%, whereas for node positive patients it is 25–30%

TUMOUR SIZE

- independent correlation with prognosis
- size of tumour should be measured by pathologist
- larger tumours are more likely to have lymph node metastases
- tumours picked up as part of screening programme tend to be smaller

HISTOLOGICAL GRADE

- tumours may be graded as I, II or III depending on three factors: the degree of tubule formation within the tumour, the degree of nuclear pleomorphism and the number of mitotic figures
- each parameter gets a mark of 1, 2 or 3 depending on agreed criteria. These are added together to give a score out of 9
    - 3–5 = grade I – well differentiated
    - 6–7 = grade II – moderately differentiated
    - 8–9 = grade III – poorly differentiated
- A Nottingham prognostic index (NPI) may be calculated based on the above three parameters. This gives a guide as to the likely prognosis. NPI = 0.2 × size of tumour plus grade plus lymph node score

SPECIAL HISTOLOGICAL SUBTYPES

- Special histological subtypes of breast cancer such as tubular carcinoma, cribriform carcinoma, mucinous carcinoma, medullary carcinoma and adenoid cystic carcinoma tend to have a better prognosis than the usual type of ductal carcinoma

OTHER FACTORS

- Other factors such as vascular invasion, necrosis, stromal lymphocytic infiltration, hormone receptor status and proliferation index may be of prognostic significance

Paget's disease of nipple

- presents as nipple eczema, ulceration, discharge or bleeding
- usually unilateral
- associated with underlying infiltrating carcinoma or DCIS
- requires histological confirmation of diagnosis as eczema may result in a similar clinical picture
- microscopically epidermis is infiltrated by large cells with prominent nucleoli (Paget's cells)
- treatment is mastectomy as underlying invasive or *in situ* carcinoma is invariably present

Breast sarcomas

- rarely a variety of sarcomas may arise primarily within the breast
- these are usually large tumours with a poor prognosis
- a sarcoma may arise from stromal overgrowth in a phyllodes tumour
- mammary angiosarcoma is the most common primary breast sarcoma
- it usually occurs in young women and has an extremely poor prognosis
- microscopy shows vascular formation by pleomorphic tumour cells

Post-mastectomy angiosarcoma (lymphangiosarcoma, Stewart-Treves syndrome)

- rare complication of radical mastectomy, usually occurring more than 10 years after surgery
- occurs in areas of lymphoedema
- presents as subcutaneous haemorrhagic nodules on the arm
- very aggressive behaviour with dismal outcome
- microscopically similar to primary mammary angiosarcoma

LESIONS OF THE MALE BREAST

Gynaecomastia

- male breast enlargement
- may be unilateral or bilateral
- microscopy shows glandular elements and fibrous tissue
- most common around puberty and in old age, i.e. times of greatest physiological hormone imbalance
- exogenous hormones (oestrogens) and drugs, e.g. digoxin, cimetidine may be aetiological factors
- neoplasms such as testicular Leydig and germ cell tumours, adrenal tumours, pituitary tumours and hepatocellular carcinoma may be associated causes

- more common in Klinefelter's syndrome
- more common with hepatic and renal disease, hyperthyroidism and Cushing's syndrome

Male breast cancer

- rare, accounting for approximately 0.7% of all breast cancers
- usually occurs in elderly men
- may be associated with oestrogen therapy, Klinefelter's syndrome and a positive family history
- microscopically usually typical ductal carcinoma
- usually subareolar location
- presents as hard mass
- prognosis is poor

Heart

12

NORMAL STRUCTURE

- heart consists of two atria and two ventricles which are separated by a fibromuscular septum

Right atrium

- superior and inferior vena cavae drain into
- atrium contains an atrial appendage
- the smooth part of the atrial wall is derived from the sinus venosus
- the remaining part of the atrium is trabeculated and is derived from the primitive atrium
- the coronary sinus opens near the septal cusp of the tricuspid valve
- the interatrial septum has a depression (the fossa ovalis) with a prominent margin (limbus fossa ovalis)

Right ventricle

- separated from right atrium by atrioventricular groove containing right coronary artery
- most of the luminal surface is coarsely trabeculated (trabeculae carneae)

Tricuspid valve

- separates right and left atria
- composed of three cusps, the septal, inferior and anterior cusps
- attached by chordae tendineae to papillary muscles

Pulmonary valve

- composed of three cusps, two anterior and one posterior

Left atrium

- lies immediately anterior to lower oesophagus
- most of luminal surface is smooth
- contains an atrial appendage
- four pulmonary veins drain into left atrium

Left ventricle

- thick walled chamber
- contains two papillary muscles, the anterior and posterior, which are attached to the chordae tendineae of the mitral valve cusps

Mitral valve

- contains two cusps, a larger anterior and a smaller posterior
- usual circumference is 12 cm

Aortic valve

- usual circumference is 7.5 cm
- usually contains three cusps, one anterior and two posterior
- biscuspid aortic valves are relatively common

Wall

- the wall of the heart consists of three layers, the endocardium, the myocardium and the pericardium (epicardium)

ENDOCARDIUM

- innermost layer
- lined by a single layer of endothelial cells with subendocardial connective tissue

MYOCARDIUM

- thickest layer composed of branching network of cardiac muscle fibres with cross striations and central nuclei

PERICARDIUM

- composed of layer of flattened mesothelial cells with underlying fibrofatty connective tissue

Conducting system of heart

- the sinoatrial (SA) node, the pacemaker of the heart, lies at the junction of the superior vena cava with the right atrium
- the atrioventricular (AV) node lies just deep to the endocardium of the right atrium
- the AV bundle of His lies adjacent to the atrioventricular septum
- the bundle of His divides into left and right branches which end in Purkinje fibres

CONGENITAL HEART DISEASE

- incidence 6 per 1000 live births
- cause is unknown but in most cases is probably multifactorial with both environmental and genetic factors

Associations

- Down's syndrome is associated with AV canal defects and patent ductus arteriosus (PDA)
- Turner's syndrome is associated with coarctation of aorta, aortic stenosis and atrial septal defects (ASDs)
- Ehlers-Danlos' syndrome is associated with aortic dissection
- Marfans' syndrome is associated with aortic dissection and mitral valve prolapse
- osteogenesis imperfecta is associated with aortic incompetence
- Friedreich's ataxia and Duchenne muscular dystrophy are both associated with cardiomyopathies
- maternal alcohol abuse is associated with ventricular septal defect (VSD), ASD and PDA
- maternal ingestion of anticonvulsants may be associated with PDA, pulmonary and aortic stenosis and coarctation of the aorta
- maternal sex hormones are associated with transposition of the great arteries, Fallot's tetralogy and VSD
- maternal ingestion of thalidamide is associated with Fallot's tetralogy and septal defects
- maternal rubella infection is associated with septal defects, PDA and pulmonary artery stenosis
- maternal diabetes may be associated with VSD, coarctation of the aorta and transposition of the great arteries

Embryology

(Figure 12.1)

Acyanotic congenital heart disease with left-to-right shunt

ATRIAL SEPTAL DEFECT (ASD)

(Figure 12.2)

A) Secundum defect

- 90%
- defect at site of fossa ovale in mid portion of septum
- usually presents in adulthood with atrial fibrillation or right ventricular failure

B) Primum and endocardial cushion defects

- 5%
- failure of septum primum and atrioventricular endocardial cushions to meet - often associated with cleft mitral or tricuspid valve
- usually presents in childhood with heart failure and arrhythmias

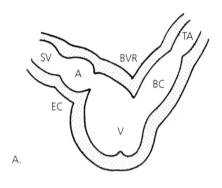

A.

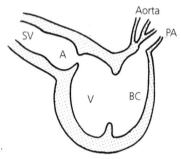

B.

Figure 12.1 Development of the heart. TA = truncus arteriosus; BC = bulbus cordis; V = ventricle; A = atrium; SV = sinus venosus; BVR = bulboventricular ridge; EC = endocardial cushions; PA = pulmonary artery

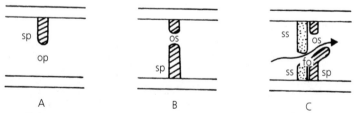

A   B   C

Figure 12.2 Development of the atrial septum. sp = Septum primum; op = ostium primum; os = ostium secundum; ss = septum secundum; fo = foramen ovale

C) Sinus venosus defect

- 5%
- high ASD near orifice of SVC

ATRIOVENTRICULAR DEFECTS

- due to maldevelopment of endocardial cushions
- usually large atrial primum defect with VSD and deformity of AV valves
- associated with Down's syndrome

VENTRICULAR SEPTAL DEFECT (VSD)

- interventricular septum has a membranous part (derived from endocardial cushions), a bulbar part and a muscular part
- 90% of VSDs involve the membranous part of the septum
- small VSD may be asymptomatic
- large VSD usually presents with left ventricular failure and repeated chest infections
- if pulmonary hypertension develops a right to left shunt forms

PERSISTENT DUCTUS ARTERIOSUS (PDA)

- ductus arteriosus in the fetus connects the left pulmonary artery to the descending thoracic aorta
- ductus usually closes after first few days of life
- a small PDA is often asymptomatic
- large PDA presents with cardiac failure
- may have characteristic machinery murmur
- later pulmonary hypertension develops and a right to left shunt may occur
- cyanosis of lower but not upper extremities (differential cyanosis)
- indomethacin therapy may result in closure
- may require surgical closure

COMPLICATIONS OF LEFT TO RIGHT SHUNTS

- cardiac failure
- infective endocarditis may occur especially with high pressure 'jet' shunts, e.g. VSD and PDA
- pulmonary hypertension may occur and pulmonary arterioles may be narrowed by intimal thickening and medial hypertrophy
- later reversal of shunt may occur, resulting in cyanosis (Eisenmenger syndrome)
- paradoxical embolism may occur into systemic circulation

Acyanotic congenital heart disease without left-to-right shunt

PULMONARY VALVE STENOSIS

- quite common
- valve cusps may be fused
- get right ventricular hypertrophy which may be asymptomatic or may present with fainting attacks

INFUNDIBULAR PULMONARY STENOSIS

- fibrous stricture forms at the entrance to the infundibulum

PULMONARY ARTERY STENOSIS

- there are several variants

EBSTEINS' ANOMALY

- abnormal tricuspid valve which results in a small right ventricle and incompetent tricuspid valve
- patients have low cardiac output and may have Wolff-Parkinson-White syndrome
- prognosis is poor

AORTIC STENOSIS

- fused valve cusps
- may be bicuspid or unicuspid valve
- infant presents with left ventricular outflow obstruction
- valve may become calcified in adults

SUPRAVALVULAR AORTIC STENOSIS

- aorta stenosed above the aortic valve
- may be associated with characteristic facies, mental retardation and hyper-calcaemia
- associated with William's syndrome (autosomal dominant)

SUBVALVULAR AORTIC STENOSIS

- uncommon
- may get membranous or muscular type

MITRAL VALVE LESIONS

- most common is congenital stenosis
- presents with heart failure

COARCTATION OF THE AORTA

- more common in males
- usually area of coarctation is distal to the origin of the left subclavian artery
- may be associated with bicuspid aortic valve, PDA, VSD
- may occasionally be associated with aneurysm of circle of Willis
- may be associated with Turner's syndrome
- may be postductal or preductal

Postductal type (adult)

- may be asymptomatic or may present with high blood pressure in the upper extremities but with weak pulses or low blood pressure in the lower extremities
- later heart failure or aortic dissection occurs

- left ventricular hypertrophy occurs
- collateral circulation develops between the precoarctation arterial branches and the postcoarctation arteries

Preductal infantile type

- associated PDA which is critical to supply blood to the aorta to sustain circulation to the lower parts of the body
- associated with ASD or VSD
- presents in early infancy with heart failure

CORONARY ARTERY ANOMALIES

- may get anomalous origin of left coronary artery from pulmonary artery. Affected patients may die as neonate from myocardial infarction
- may get coronary artery fistula or aneurysm. A fistula develops between the right coronary artery and the right ventricle or atrium. Presentation is with cardiac failure

AORTIC ARCH ABNORMALITIES

- double arch may occur where both embryological aortic arches persist. A small arch lies anteriorly to the left and a larger arch lies posteriorly to the right. This forms a ring behind the trachea and oesophagus
- an interrupted aortic arch may occur where there is discontinuity in the aortic arch

Cyanotic congenital heart disease

TETRALOGY OF FALLOT

- most common form of cyanotic congenital heart disease
- four features:
  - VSD
  - obstruction to right ventricular outflow tract due to subpulmonary stenosis
  - an aorta that overides the VSD
  - right ventricular hypertrophy
- right to left shunt occurs causing central cyanosis
- heart is often enlarged and may be 'boot-shaped'
- complications include polycythaemia, cerebral abscess and chest infection
- complete surgical repair is possible for classical tetralogy

TRANSPOSITION OF THE GREAT ARTERIES

- spiral septum of truncus arteriosus develops abnormally
- aorta arises from the right ventricle and pulmonary artery arises from the left ventricle
- condition is incompatible with neonatal life unless there is a concominant PDA, ASD or VSD
- cyanosis from birth
- more common with diabetic mothers
- emergency treatment involves creation of an ASD with balloon atrial septostomy
- later more definitive procedures such as total correction are needed
- without surgery, most infants die within the first months of life

TOTAL ANOMALOUS PULMONARY VENOUS CONNECTION

- no connection between pulmonary veins and left atrium
- pulmonary veins may drain into the right atrium, superior or inferior vena cava or other systemic veins
- survival only if ASD is present
- usually severe cyanosis from birth

PULMONARY ATRESIA

- often associated with VSD, PDA or aorto-pulmonary collaterals
- needs urgent palliative shunt, e.g. Blalock-Taussig

TRICUSPID ATRESIA

- complete occlusion of the tricuspid valve orifice with no connection between right atrium and right ventricle
- right ventricle is hypoplastic
- ASD or PDA is present which maintains circulation
- usually cyanosis from birth
- requires palliative or reparative surgery

TRUNCUS ARTERIOSUS

- failure of spiral septum between the aorta and pulmonary artery
- single great artery that receives blood from both ventricles
- usually associated VSD and other defects
- early cyanosis
- high infant mortality
- requires surgical correction at an early age

ISCHAEMIC HEART DISEASE (IHD)

- most common predisposing condition is atheroma of the proximal coronary arteries
- rarely due to atheroma of the ascending aorta which occludes the coronary ostia
- other rarer causes include vasculitis of coronary arteries
- ischaemia is worsened by hypotension, exercise, anaemia

EPIDEMIOLOGY

- approximately 30% of all male deaths and 22% of all female deaths in UK
- mortality is particularly high in Scotland and N. Ireland
- less common in non-industrialised countries
- more common with increasing age
- incidence increases in women after menopause (protective effect of sex hormones)

RISK FACTORS

- hyperlipidaemia:
  - especially familial hypercholesterolaemia
  - increased dietary cholesterol
  - increased low density lipoproteins (LDL)
  - decreased high density lipoproteins (HDL)

- hypertension
- cigarette smoking
- diabetes mellitus
- positive family history
- obesity
- reduced exercise
- stressful life style with type A personality
- diet
  - high fat and high meat diet
  - excess saturated fatty acids
- oral contraceptives

Moderate alcohol consumption may be protective

Angina pectoris

- stable or typical angina is pain relieved by rest
- Prinzmetal (variant) angina is probably associated with coronary artery spasm and comes on at rest
- unstable or cresendo angina is a pattern where pain occurs with increasing frequency, often at rest and is of long duration

Myocardial infarction (MI)

- two forms:
  - transmural which affects a localised area
  - subendocardial which affects the subendocardial region over a large area
- transmural infarction is usually a result of haemorrhage into an atheromatous plaque or thrombus formation on an ulcerated atheromatous plaque
- subendocardial infarction is usually due to a global reduction in myocardial perfusion. The subendocardial myocardial fibres have the most tenuous blood supply and are therefore most susceptible to infarction

DISTRIBUTION OF CORONARY ARTERIES

- right coronary artery supplies the posterior wall of the left ventricle, the posterior third of the interventricular septum and the adjacent part of the right ventricle
- left anterior descending coronary artery supplies the anterior wall of the left ventricle, the anterior two-thirds of the interventricular septum and the adjacent right ventricle
- left circumflex artery supplies the lateral wall of the left ventricle

MACROSCOPIC APPEARANCE OF MYOCARDIAL INFARCTION

- after 12 hours infarcted area is pale with a hyperaemic border
- at 7–10 days the infarct is yellow in colour with a dark hyperaemic rim
- later scar tissue forms and the area of infarction has a grey colour

HISTOLOGY OF MYOCARDIAL INFARCTION

- coagulation necrosis with eosinophilia of myocardial fibres at 4–12 hours
- neutrophil infiltration occurs and is most prominent at 2–3 days

- lymphocytes replace neutrophils at 7 days
- necrotic cells are replaced by connective tissue and at 4 weeks the area of infarction is replaced by hypocellular scar tissue

COMPLICATIONS OF MYOCARDIAL INFARCTION

- sudden death
- arrhythmias
- left ventricular heart failure with pulmonary oedema
- rupture of ventricular wall producing cardiac tamponade
- rupture of ventricular septum producing VSD
- rupture of papillary muscle producing acute mitral valve incompetence
- a ventricular aneurysm may form due to replacement by scar tissue. This usually involves the anterior wall of the left ventricle
- mural thrombus and embolism, especially in areas of ventricular aneurysm
- pericarditis
- deep venous thrombosis and pulmonary embolism

PROGNOSIS

- worse for left main stem coronary artery disease
- survival improved by coronary artery bypass for left main stem or triple vessel disease
- 20% of patients with myocardial infarction die in the first month
- streptokinase and aspirin reduce mortality

BYPASS GRAFTS

- may use internal mammary artery or vein grafts
- some patients are suitable for stenting

Chronic ischaemic heart disease

- insidious development of congestive heart failure due to ischaemic myocardial damage
- usually elderly
- may have history of angina and MI
- get atheroma of coronary arteries and scar tissue formation within left ventricle

RHEUMATIC FEVER AND RHEUMATIC HEART DISEASE

- rheumatic fever usually affects children and usually follows a pharyngeal infection with group A beta-haemolytic streptococci
- incidence has markedly decreased in Western countries

AETIOLOGY AND PATHOGENESIS

- antibodies to M protein of *Streptococcus* cross-react with antigens on valves and myocardium
- group A beta-haemolytic *Streptococcus* is the commonest organism
- initial attack of rheumatic fever usually occurs 1–5 weeks after streptococcal infection

CLINICAL FEATURES

- diagnosis of rheumatic fever requires evidence of a preceding group A streptococcal infection plus two major Jones' criteria or one major and two minor Jones' criteria
- major Jones' criteria are:
  - carditis
  - polyarthritis
  - Sydenham's chorea
  - erythema marginatum
  - subcutaneous nodules
- minor Jones' criteria include:
  - raised ESR
  - fever
  - arthralgia
  - a prolonged PR interval on ECG

PATHOLOGY

- chronic rheumatic heart disease is characterised by deforming fibrosing cardiac valvular disease
- produces permanent dysfunction and often cardiac failure decades after initial acute attack of rheumatic fever
- most commonly affected valves are mitral and aortic
- occasionally tricuspid valve is affected
- may cause either valvular stenosis or incompetence, but usually stenosis
- in acute attacks of rheumatic fever pancarditis with inflammation affects endocardium, myocardium and pericardium
- microscopy shows Aschoff bodies with areas of fibrinoid necrosis surrounded by inflammatory cells, including activated histiocytes called Aschoff cells
- in late stages of chronic rheumatic heart disease valves become thickened, fibrotic, calcified and vascularised
- get fusion of leaflets and chordae tendineae
- due to mitral stenosis left atrium may become dilated with mural thrombus formation
- aortic valve also commonly becomes fibrosed and calcified

INFECTIVE ENDOCARDITIS

- most commonly occurs in middle-aged or elderly patients
- most common organisms are streptococcal or staphylococcal species (especially *Streptococcus viridans* and *Staphylococcus aureus*)
- usually affects heart valves but occasionally can involve other parts of endocardium
- often affects already abnormal valve
- may be divided into acute and subacute forms
- often may complicate congenital heart disease or valvular heart disease, especially rheumatic in type
- diabetes, immunosuppression (including transplant patients and AIDS), alcohol and drug abuse are also predisposing factors
- source of organism may be from transient bacteraemia, e.g. following endoscopy, catheterisation or tooth extraction
- if known valvular abnormality, then antibiotic prophylaxis is required prior to minor procedures

- treatment is antibiotics and without treatment mortality is high
- clinical features include fever, PUO, fatigue, Osler's nodes, splinter haemorrhages, Roth's spots, rigors, cardiac murmurs and cardiac failure

PATHOLOGY

- large friable vegetations
- may involve previously abnormal valve
- microscopically vegetations consist of platelets, fibrin and polymorphs
- bacteria can be seen in cases of bacterial endocarditis
- later organisation with fibrosis occurs

COMPLICATIONS

- perforation or erosion of the underlying valve producing sudden incompetence
- may get valvular stenosis
- myocarditis or pericarditis
- dehiscence of artificial valves with paravalvular leak
- systemic emboli to brain, spleen, kidney
- vasculitis
- arthritis
- glomerulonephritis

FLOPPY MITRAL VALVE SYNDROME

- common cause of pure mitral incompetence
- microscopically there is myxomatous change of valve which prolapses into left atrium during systole
- many cases are idiopathic
- may occur in Marfan's syndrome, Ehlers-Danlos' syndrome and polycystic renal disease
- may get superimposed infective endocarditis

CALCIFIC AORTIC STENOSIS

- most frequent valvular abnormality
- usually elderly patients
- may complicate bicuspid valve
- get fibrosis and calcification

OTHER DISEASES WHICH MAY AFFECT HEART VALVES

- Marfan's syndrome (mitral incompetence)
- Ehlers-Danlos' syndrome (mitral incompetence)
- osteogenesis imperfecta (mitral incompetence)
- cystic medial necrosis (aortic incompetence)
- syphilis (aortic incompetence)

- dissecting aortic aneurysm (aortic incompetence)
- rheumatoid arthritis (aortic incompetence)
- ankylosing spondylitis (aortic incompetence)
- chest trauma
- carcinoid syndrome. In this syndrome the right side of the heart may be affected. Substances such as 5HT and bradykinin may produce a fibroblastic reaction involving the pulmonary and tricuspid valves
- systemic lupus erythematosus (SLE). May get small sterile vegetations, especially involving the mitral and tricuspid valves (Libman-Sacks endocarditis)
- non-bacterial thrombotic endocarditis (marantic endocarditis) may occur in debilitated patients

CARDIOMYOPATHY

- heart muscle disease of unknown cause

Dilated cardiomyopathy

- gradual development of cardiac failure associated with dilatation of heart
- may be genetic influence
- usually affects age 20–60 years
- develop left ventricular failure
- arrhythmias are common
- sudden death may occur
- in some cases alcohol abuse, vitamin deficiency or viral infection may be implicated
- grossly dilatation of all chambers of heart which is large and flabby
- mural thrombi are common
- microscopy shows non-specific fibrosis
- poor prognosis without cardiac transplantation

Hypertrophic obstructive cardiomyopathy (HOCM)

- most common in young males
- often familial with autosomal dominant transmission
- presents with dyspnoea, angina and sudden death
- may get atrial fibrillation with mural thrombus formation and embolism
- grossly get disproportionate thickening of the interventricular septum
- ventricular cavities are decreased in size
- microscopic changes are non-specific but get disorganisation of myocardial fibres (myofibre disarray) with bizarre nuclei

Restrictive/obliterative cardiomyopathy

- rigid left ventricular wall which fails to relax during diastole thus impeding filling
- amyloid infiltration of heart, radiation fibrosis, constrictive pericarditis, endo-myocardial fibrosis, Loeffler's endomyocarditis and endocardial fibroelastosis may produce similar disease

CARDIAC TUMOURS

- primary tumours of the heart are very rare
- most common is the myxoma
- 90% of myxomas occur in the atria, usually the left
- more common in females
- clinically may obstruct atrioventricular valves and may cause death
- PUO or weight loss may be presenting features
- may get systemic embolism
- grossly myxomas are soft gelatinous tumours
- microscopy shows stellate tumour cells in an abundant mucoid stroma
- results after surgery are excellent

PERICARDIUM

Pericarditis

- inflammation of the pericardium
- major causes are:
  1. Infectious agents
     - viruses, e.g. Coxsackie viruses. May follow respiratory tract infection. May be associated with myocarditis
     - bacteria, e.g. streptococci, staphylococci. May be a result of direct spread from empyema or pneumonia
     - tuberculosis. Microscopy shows caseous necrosis with granulomatous inflammation
     - fungi

  2. Immunologically mediated
     - rheumatic fever
     - scleroderma
     - SLE
     - postcardiotomy
     - drug induced
     - post myocardial infarction (Dressler's syndrome)

  3. Other causes
     - uraemia
     - myocardial infarction
     - trauma
     - radiation
     - neoplasia
     - post cardiac surgery
- clinically get chest pain, fever, cardiac failure
- may get characteristic pericardial friction rub
- in constrictive pericarditis the heart is encased in dense fibrocalcific tissue which limits cardiac output. May be secondary to tuberculosis infection

Pericardial tumours

- rare
- most common are metastases, especially from lung cancer
- benign lipomas rarely occur
- malignant mesotheliomas may occur
- occasionally various sarcomas occur

Blood vessels

13

NORMAL STRUCTURE

- all blood vessels consist of three layers:
  - an inner tunica intima (TI)
  - a middle tunica media (TM)
  - an outer tunica adventitia (TA)

Large elastic arteries, e.g. aorta

- TI – single layer of endothelial cells with underlying subendothelial layer consisting of collagen, elastic fibres, fibroblasts and smooth muscle cells
- TM – numerous elastic fibres together with smooth muscle cells and fibroblasts
- TA – thin connective tissue layer

Medium sized muscular arteries, e.g. coronary and renal

- TI – endothelial cells with underlying subendothelial layer consisting of elastic tissue and internal elastic lamina
- TM – many layers of smooth muscle cells, collagen and a few elastic fibres
- TA – external elastic lamina and thin layer of connective tissue

Arterioles

- TI – endothelium and internal elastic lamina
- TM – 1–5 layers of smooth muscle cells
- TA – loose connective tissue

Venules and small veins

- TI – endothelial cells
- TM – thin bundles of smooth muscle fibres
- TA – well developed loose connective tissue

Large veins, e.g. inferior and superior vena cava

- TI – endothelial cells
- TM – thin bundles of smooth muscle fibres
- TA – collagen and elastic fibres and smooth muscle cells

LOWER LIMB ISCHAEMIA

Acute

- embolism
- thrombosis
- trauma
- aortic dissection

Chronic

- causes intermittent claudication
- atheroma
- Buerger's disease (thromboangiitis obliterans)
- vasculitides
- entrapment syndromes
- Raynaud's disease and syndrome

UPPER LIMB ISCHAEMIA

Acute

- thrombosis
- embolism
- trauma
- aortic dissection

Chronic

- unusual
- atheroma of great vessels
- cervical rib
- thoracic inlet syndrome
- Buerger's disease
- vasculitides
- Raynaud's disease and syndrome

ARTERIOSCLEROSIS

- group of disorders that have in common thickening and loss of elasticity of arterial walls
- three morphological variants:
  1. atheroma or atherosclerosis
  2. Monckeberg's medial calcific sclerosis
  3. arteriolosclerosis

Atheroma

- most common cause of morbidity and mortality in Western world
- aorta, coronary and cerebral arteries are commonly affected
- myocardial infarction, cerebral infarction and aortic aneurysm are common consequences

EPIDEMIOLOGY AND RISK FACTORS

Major risk factors

- diet and hyperlipidaemia, e.g. hypercholesterolaemia
- hypertension
- cigarette smoking
- diabetes

Minor risk factors

- obesity
- physical inactivity
- male sex
- increasing age
- positive family history
- stress
- oral contraceptive
- high carbohydrate intake
- hyperuricaemia

PATHOLOGY

- atheroma is intimal lesion
- two characteristic lesions are fatty streaks and atheromatous plaque
- fatty streak is present nearly universally in children and may be a precursor of the atheromatous plaque
- fatty streaks begin as multiple yellow spots which later coalesce into streaks
- microscopy shows lipid-filled foam cells
- atheromatous plaque is white to yellow in colour and encroaches on lumen of vessel grossly (Figure 13.1)
- microscopy shows fibrous cap with underlying core containing macrophages, smooth muscle cells, lipid-laden foam cells and cholesterol clefts
- vessels characteristically involved by atheromatous plaques are abdominal aorta, around the ostia of major branches of the aorta, the coronary arteries and the cerebral arteries
- vessels of the upper extremities are usually spared

COMPLICATIONS OF ATHEROSCLEROTIC PLAQUES

- in advanced disease, atherosclerotic plaques may undergo calcification
- may get rupture or ulceration of the luminal surface which induces thrombus formation
- rupture or ulceration of the plaque may also result in the formation of cholesterol emboli

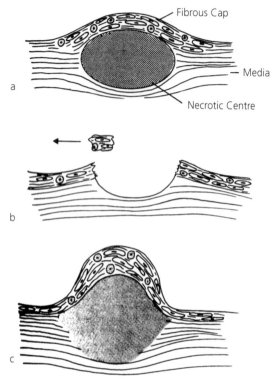

Figure 13.1 (a) Schematic diagram of a plaque of atheroma; (b) atheromatous embolus; (c) haemorrhage into an atheromatous plaque

- superimposed thrombosis may partially or completely occlude the lumen of a vessel
- haemorrhage into a plaque may occur which can encroach on the lumen
- the underlying media may undergo pressure or ischaemic atrophy causing aneurysmal dilatation

Monckeberg's medial calcific sclerosis

- characterised by calcification within media of medium-sized to small muscular arteries
- unknown aetiology
- intima and adventitia are unaffected
- no encroachment on lumen of vessels
- most commonly affected vessels are femoral, tibial, radial, ulnar arteries
- of relatively little clinical significance

Arteriolosclerosis

- hyaline arteriolosclerosis is very common in elderly patients
- more common in hypertension and diabetes
- microscopy shows pink hyaline thickening of walls of arterioles

ARTERIAL THROMBOSIS

- primary arterial thrombosis in previously normal arteries is rare

CAUSES

- direct injury
- meningococcal septicaemia
- polycythaemia
- immobility
- secondary to ulceration of atheromatous plaque
- Buerger's disease
- other arteritides

INTIMAL HYPERPLASIA

- may cause stenosis of small and medium-sized blood vessels or vascular grafts
- due to intimal smooth muscle proliferation

ARTERIAL EMBOLISM

- thrombus in blood vessel lumen may dislodge and form an embolus
- sources include a mural thrombus on the heart, an atheromatous plaque and an aortic aneurysm
- embolus may lodge in vessels of distal extremities, in cerebral circulation and at bifurcation of major arteries
- paradoxical embolus is where venous embolus passes through septal defect in the heart into arterial circulation
- rarely systemic arterial embolus may be from cardiac myxomas, infective endocarditis, prosthetic heart valves, intravenous catheters or caval filters
- other types of embolism include amniotic fluid embolism, air embolism and fat embolism

ENTRAPMENT SYNDROMES

- in popliteal artery entrapment of the medial head of the gastrocnemius muscle compresses the popliteal artery against the lateral aspect of the medial femoral condyle
- coeliac artery compression may be by the median arcuate ligament of the diaphragm

- subclavian artery compression may be due to a cervical rib compressing the artery against the scalenus anterior muscle. This may be associated with the subclavian steal syndrome

ARTERIOVENOUS FISTULAS

- abnormal communications between arteries and veins may be congenital or acquired

Congenital

- usually involve limbs and may be local or diffuse
- with local lesions get warm pulsatile mass, with surrounding varicose veins
- with diffuse lesions may be limb overgrowth
- large arteriovenous fistulas may be associated with cardiac failure

Acquired

- secondary to penetrating injuries
- secondary to infective or inflammatory necrosis of vessel wall
- spontaneous, e.g. Ehlers-Danlos' syndrome
- rupture of arterial aneurysm into adjacent vein
- iatrogenic fistulas may occur secondary to operative procedures

Arteriovenous fistulas may be of clinical significance in that they may result in high output cardiac failure or can rupture, resulting in massive haemorrhage

VASCULITIS

Temporal arteritis (giant cell arteritis)

- cause is unknown
- occurs in elderly patients
- presents with headaches and blindness
- tenderness over temporal artery
- may have polymyalgia rheumatica
- often have markedly elevated ESR
- affects arteries of medium and small size, especially cranial arteries
- genetic predisposition with increased prevalence of HLA-DR4 antigen
- requires prompt steroid treatment
- diagnosis is by clinical suspicion and temporal artery biopsy
- microscopy shows giant cell infiltration and granulomatous reaction in wall of artery

Takayasu's arteritis

- cause unknown
- affects aortic arch and origins of great vessels

- weakening of the pulses in the upper extremity (*pulseless disease*)
- usually in females, aged 15–40 years
- may present with neurological symptoms and signs with weak pulses and low blood pressure
- grossly there is thickening of aortic arch and narrowing of lumina of great vessels
- microscopy shows lymphocytic infiltration, often with giant cells
- in late stages there is extensive fibrosis of media and intima with narrowing of lumen

Buerger's disease (thromboangiitis obliterans)

- usually young males who are heavy smokers
- usually begins before age 35 years
- usually affects the legs, less commonly the arms
- thrombosing, inflammatory lesion of intermediate and small arteries and often adjacent veins and nerves
- microscopy shows polymorph infiltration with thrombus formation
- clinically there are cold and painful extremities
- ultimately may result in gangrene

Raynaud's syndrome

- paroxysmal pallor or cyanosis of digits of the hands or feet

PRIMARY RAYNAUD'S SYNDROME (RAYNAUD'S DISEASE)

- exaggerated vasoconstrictor response in normal digital arteries
- usually young, otherwise healthy women

SECONDARY RAYNAUD'S SYNDROME (RAYNAUD'S PHENOMENON)

- arterial insufficiency of the extremities secondary to other disorders
- ischaemia, ulceration and gangrene may occur
- secondary to connective tissue diseases (e.g. SLE, scleroderma), atheroma, drugs, polycythaemia, Buerger's disease
- may be first manifestation of any of these conditions

Polyarteritis nodosa (PAN)

- necrotising vasculitis, chiefly involving small and medium-sized muscular arteries
- usually disease of young adults
- main arteries affected are renal, coronary, mesenteric
- vascular thrombosis may complicate vasculitis
- microscopy shows fibrinoid necrosis with polymorph infiltration
- in late stages there is organisation with fibrosis
- clinical signs and symptoms may be varied
- untreated disease is fatal in most cases
- treatment is steroids and cyclophosphamide
- p-ANCA in serum
- may result in aneurysm formation with rupture

Wegener's granulomatosis

- necrotising granulomatous inflammation within the upper and lower respiratory tracts
- commonly there is lung involvement
- commonly there is renal involvement in form of glomerulonephritis
- peak incidence is fifth decade
- untreated 80% die within first year
- treatment is steroids or cyclophosphamide
- c-ANCA in serum

Infectious arteritis

- direct invasion by organisms
- haematogenous spread, e.g. from infective endocarditis
- vascular infection may weaken vessel wall, resulting in mycotic aneurysm

Vasculitis associated with other disorders

- may be associated with connective tissue diseases, malignancy or systemic illnesses
- diseases associated with a vasculitis include rheumatoid arthritis, SLE, Henoch-Schonlein purpura
- malignant lymphoproliferative disorders may be associated with vasculitis

ANEURYSMS

- abnormal dilatation of artery or vein
- most involve aorta or iliac arteries
- other arteries commonly involved include popliteal, femoral, subclavian, splenic, carotid, circle of Willis
- berry aneurysms are small spherical dilatations of wall of artery
- saccular aneurysms are larger spherical dilatations
- fusiform aneurysms are spindle shaped
- dissecting aneurysms (see p. 190)
- most aneurysms are secondary to atheromatous degeneration
- other types of aneurysm include syphilitic, mycotic (infective), post-stenotic and traumatic
- in a true aneurysm the wall is the vessel itself
- in a false aneurysm the wall is surrounding connective tissue

Abdominal aortic aneurysm

INCIDENCE

- 2% of population over age of 50 years
- mostly elderly males
- male:female ratio is 4:1

AETIOLOGY

- vast majority are secondary to atheroma
- autoimmune inflammatory aneurysms also occasionally occur
- may be intrinsic weakness in the wall of the aorta
- copper deficiency which decreases collagen cross-linking may be important
- genetic predisposition
- smoking
- hypertension

PATHOLOGY

- most begin a few centimetres below origin of renal arteries
- occasionally extend above renal arteries
- occasionally thoracoabdominal aneurysm occurs
- aneurysm often contains organising thrombus
- inflammatory aneurysm may be stuck to adjacent retroperitoneal structures
- microscopy shows atheroma within wall of aorta
- in inflammatory aneurysm, inflammation and fibrosis extends to the adventitia and into the surrounding tissues

COMPLICATIONS

- rupture with massive retroperitoneal haemorrhage
- thrombus formation with distal embolism
- occlusion of vessel by thrombosis. May occlude ostia of vessels
- aortocaval fistula with high output cardiac failure
- aortoenteric fistula, especially into duodenum

Thoracic aortic aneurysm

- may be dissecting aneurysm (see p. 190)
- may be secondary to atheroma
- syphilitic aneurysms are now rare but may form a large saccular or fusiform aneurysm
- syphilitic aneurysms often involve the arch of the aorta and may extend proximally to produce aortic valve incompetence
- microscopically in syphilitic aneurysms there is obliterative endarteritis of vasa vasorum and a chronic inflammatory cell infiltrate in which plasma cells predominate

Popliteal artery aneurysm

- usually secondary to atheroma
- often bilateral
- there may be an associated aortic aneurysm
- presents with a pulsatile mass or distal ischaemia

Femoral artery aneurysm

- true aneurysms are secondary to atheroma and are often associated with an aneurysm elsewhere
- false aneurysms are due to trauma or to disruption of a synthetic graft

Subclavian artery aneurysm

- may be associated with cervical rib
- presents with a mass, pain or effects of embolism
- aneurysm may occur distal to obstruction by cervical rib, i.e post-stenotic dilatation

Splenic artery aneurysm

- occurs at splenic hilum
- may be due to congenital defect in the wall
- occasionally due to atheroma
- occurs more often in females
- may rupture during pregnancy
- a false aneurysm may occur secondary to pancreatitis

Mycotic aneurysm

- secondary to septic embolus which lodges in a peripheral artery
- microscopy shows acute inflammation in the wall of the artery
- acute inflammatory process results in weakening of the wall and formation of a mycotic aneurysm
- tend to occur at bifurcation of vessels
- may rupture when quite small
- often multiple
- arteries involved include aorta, coronary, splenic, mesenteric and cerebral arteries
- origin of embolus may be from vegetation in heart in infective endocarditis

Dissecting aneurysm

- blood dissects along wall of aorta within separation in the media
- male:female ratio is 3:1
- usually begins with an intimal tear, often in the ascending aorta. This allows blood to enter the media and track within

AETIOLOGY

- related to underlying degeneration of elements of the media
- may be due to Erdheim's cystic medial necrosis where fragmentation of elastic tissue within media of aorta occurs
- associated with Marfan's syndrome
- hypertension, pregnancy, trauma and bicuspid aortic valve are also associated with aortic dissection
- dissection may also be secondary to atheroma

PATHOLOGY

- separation of tunica media by blood
- 70% of intimal tears occur in ascending aorta

- most of remainder of intimal tears occur in the descending thoracic aorta
- may get re-entry tear
- microscopy shows splitting of media with fragmentation of elastic fibres and the presence of cystic spaces

CLASSIFICATION

- 3 De Bakey types (Figure 13.2)

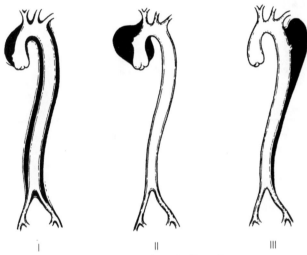

I	II	III

Figure 13.2   De Bakey classification of aortic dissecting aneurysm

COMPLICATIONS

- rupture causing haemopericardium (cardiac tamponade)
- rupture may also occur into the mediastinum, the pleural cavities or the retroperitoneum
- dissection along branches of aorta may cause ischaemia of organs
- aortic valve incompetence may result if dissection extends proximally to the root of the aorta

VEINS

Primary varicose veins

- no obvious cause
- female:male ratio is 3:1
- increases with age
- occur commonly in population
- more common in obese patients
- may have positive family history

Venous return of lower limbs depends on several factors:

- muscular pump
- competence of venous valves
- negative intrathoracic pressure
- capillary blood pressure

Primary varicose veins may be due to an intrinsic defect in the wall of the vein, causing the valves to become incompetent

COMPLICATIONS

- bleeding
- phlebitis
- dermatitis
- skin pigmentation
- chronic venous insufficiency with swelling of ankles
- ulceration

Secondary varicose veins

- secondary varicose veins are secondary to another cause and are associated with:
  - deep venous thrombosis
  - tumour in pelvis
  - pregnancy
  - tricuspid incompetence
  - constrictive pericarditis
  - congenital arteriovenous fistula
  - congenital absence of valves

Deep venous thrombosis (DVT)

- thrombosis is more common in veins than in arteries
- most common in deep veins of legs and pelvis
- increases in incidence with age
- more common in females
- not easy to detect clinically

PATHOGENESIS OF DVT

Virchow's triad is important in the pathogenesis of DVT as in the pathogenesis of thrombus formation in any vessel. The triad consists of:

1. changes in the vessel wall
2. changes in blood flow
3. changes in constituents of blood and coagulability

CONDITIONS PREDISPOSING TO DVT

- varicose veins
- recent myocardial infarction
- malignancy, especially pancreatic and lung cancer
- trauma to pelvis and legs
- postoperative period, especially following orthopaedic and major abdominal surgery

- pregnancy and post-partum
- cigarette smoking
- oral contraceptive pill
- immobility
- paraplegia
- obesity
- heart failure
- Gram-negative sepsis
- inflammatory bowel disease
- nephrotic syndrome
- polycythaemia
- Behcet's syndrome

PATHOLOGY

- platelet thrombi occur with minor endothelial injury
- fibrin deposition occurs and trapped red and white blood cells form between platelet lamellae
- thrombus occludes the vein
- thrombus propagates
- thrombus may embolise

COMPLICATIONS OF DVT

- pulmonary embolism. This is most serious complication
- post-phlebitic syndrome consisting of subcutaneous fibrosis, eczema and ulcer formation. Squamous carcinoma may rarely develop in the ulcer (Marjolin's ulcer)

Venous ulcers

- situated above medial malleolus
- due to chronic venous hypertension
- there is surrounding varicose eczema

Superficial thrombophlebitis

CAUSES

- varicose veins
- intravenous cannulae
- injection sclerotherapy
- underlying malignancy, especially pancreatic cancer

LYMPH VESSELS

Primary lymphoedema

- idiopathic (Milroy's disease)
- autosomal dominant inheritance

- if begins before age 35 years (lymphoedema congenita praecox)
- if begins after age 35 years (lymphoedema congenita tarda)

Secondary lymphoedema

- acquired obstruction due to:
  - filariasis
  - surgery, e.g. radical gland dissection
  - trauma
  - malignancy
  - radiotherapy
  - burns
  - tuberculosis
  - fungal infection
  - lymphogranuloma venereum

COMPLICATIONS

- infection
- angiosarcoma may develop many years later

Lungs, pleura and mediastinum

14

LUGS

Normal structure

- lungs develop *in utero* from primitive foregut
- left lung has an upper and lower lobe
- right lung has an upper, middle and lower lobe
- lobes are separated by interlobar fissures
- each lobe contains many bronchopulmonary segments supplied by segmental arteries and bronchi
- bronchi are lined by pseudostratified columnar ciliated (respiratory) epithelium
- lungs are enclosed within visceral pleura
- normal combined weight of lungs is 850 g in males and 750 g in females

Microstructure of lung

- acinus is the functional unit of the lung and is the part of the lung supplied by a terminal bronchiole
- each acinus contains approximately 2000 alveoli

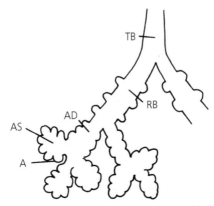

Figure 14.1 Schematic diagram of the microstructure of the lung.
TB = Terminal bronchiole; RB = respiratory bronchiole; AD = alveolar duct;
AS = alveolar sac; A = alveolus

- alveoli are lined by two types of epithelial cells, type I and II pneumocytes
- type I pneumocytes are flattened cells with long cytoplasmic processes. They facilitate rapid gas exchange
- type II pneumocytes are cuboidal cells with microvilli. They produce surfactant
- type I cells cannot proliferate after insult but type II can
- type II cells can differentiate into type I cells
- blood supply of lungs is from pulmonary arteries which accompany the bronchi
- bronchial arteries also contribute to blood supply

Bronchial and pulmonary biopsy techniques

- percutaneous fine needle biopsy may be useful for diagnosis of peripheral lung lesions. Pneumothoraces are relatively common following this procedure
- bronchoscopic biopsy is useful for central lung tumours and sarcoidosis
- bronchial brushings may be performed at bronchoscopy
- bronchial washings may be useful for diagnosis of tumours, sarcoid and AIDS infections
- pleural biopsy may be used to diagnose mesothelioma
- mediastinoscopy to biopsy paratracheal nodes
- open biopsy

Congenital and developmental abnormalities

AGENESIS

- absence of one lung

HYPOPLASIA

- often associated with other congenital abnormalities, e.g. they may be compressed by abdominal viscera if a congenital diaphragmatic hernia is present

BRONCHOGENIC CYSTS

- variant of foregut cyst
- have respiratory epithelial lining and contain cartilage within the wall
- often asymptomatic masses on chest x-ray, usually in mediastinum
- lumen filled with mucoid material
- complications include pressure symptoms on bronchus and other organs, bleeding, infection and rarely neoplastic transformation

PULMONARY CYSTS

- cyst embedded within lung parenchyma
- connects with airways
- no cartilage in walls
- complications include pressure symptoms, bleeding, infection and pneumothorax

SEQUESTRATION

- portion of lung without appropriate bronchial and vascular connections
- blood supply is from anomalous systemic arteries
- may be associated with other congenital abnormalities, especially diaphragmatic defects
- two forms of sequestration are recognised, extralobar and intralobar:
  - extralobar sequestration lies outside lung and has its own visceral pleura
  - intralobar sequestration lies within lung parenchyma

CONGENITAL ADENOMATOID MALFORMATION

- usually presents with respiratory distress shortly after birth
- in older children may present with recurrent respiratory infection
- cystic mass replaces part of lung and may be seen on chest x-ray
- surrounding lung is compressed
- microscopy shows mass of cysts lined by columnar cells
- may be associated with other congenital abnormalities

Congenital vascular anomalies

- aplasia of pulmonary artery results in the lung receiving only systemic blood, either from anomalous arteries or from collaterals from the bronchial arteries
- stenosis of pulmonary arteries or branches may be associated with cardiac abnormalities
- pulmonary arteriovenous fistula results in a shunt between pulmonary artery and vein. This is associated with polycythaemia, finger clubbing and cyanosis
- anomalous pulmonary veins result in the blood from the lungs returning to the right side of the heart rather than to the left atrium. The anomalous veins often join the inferior vena cava below the diaphragm

Pulmonary infections

BACTERIAL PNEUMONIA

Bronchopneumonia

- most common infecting organisms are staphylococcal species, streptococcal species, *Pneumococcus*, coliforms and *Haemophilus influenzae*
- often occurs postoperatively, in the elderly, in cardiac failure and in debilitated patients
- grossly there is patchy consolidation of the lungs
- microscopy shows inflammation with polymorph infiltration centred on bronchioles and adjacent alveoli

Lobar pneumonia

- grossly whole lobe is consolidated
- often young patients who present acutely with systemic symptoms and respiratory symptoms
- organisms include *Pneumococcus, Klebsiella, Legionella, Pneumophila* (Legionnaire's disease). *Pneumococcus* is most common species
- classically four phases are described:
  1. congestion. This stage usually lasts less than 24 hours. Get vascular engorgement and intra-alveolar oedema

2. red hepatization. Consistency of affected lobe resembles that of liver. Microscopically alveoli are full of neutrophils and fibrin. Get marked vascular congestion
3. grey hepatization. Grossly lungs are solid and pale. Microscopy shows diminution of congestion and accumulation of large numbers of neutrophils
4. resolution. Lung returns to normality
- complications of lobar pneumonia include:
  1. dissemination of organisms throughout lungs and to other organs
  2. septicaemia resulting in infective endocarditis, brain abscess or meningitis
  3. empyema formation
  4. suppurative pericarditis
  5. lung abscess
  6. intra-alveolar fibrosis (carnification)
  7. bronchiectasis

ATYPICAL PNEUMONIA

Causes

- *Mycoplasma pneumoniae*
- influenza virus
- respiratory syncytical virus
- Coxsackie and Echo virus
- *Pneumocystis carinii* (especially common in AIDS, see Chapter 22)

Pathology

- atypical and viral pneumonias are often characterised by inflammation within alveolar walls with lymphocytic infiltration

PULMONARY TUBERCULOSIS (TB)

- causative organisms are mycobacteria
- main two species to infect man are *Mycobacterium tuberculosis,* which is spread by inhaled droplets, and *Mycobacterium bovis,* which is spread by ingestion of infected milk. These correspond to the human and bovine tubercle bacilli respectively
- in addition atypical mycobacteria including *Mycobacterium kansasii* and *Mycobacterium avium intracellulare* may also infect humans, especially children and immunosuppressed
- organisms are strict aerobes

Incidence

- now increasing in USA (effect of AIDS and immunosuppression)
- in major American cities many patients with tuberculosis are HIV positive and many patients with AIDS have pulmonary tuberculosis
- tuberculosis is still very common in many underdeveloped countries
- in developed countries, apart from immunosuppressed subjects, tuberculosis is largely a disease of the elderly

Pathology

- tubercle bacilli are inhaled into the lung to form a non-specific inflammatory response
- organisms are phagocytosed by macrophages

- hypersensitivity reaction occurs leading to granuloma formation
- microscopy shows central caseous necrosis with surrounding histiocytic reaction. Langhan's giant cells are seen
- hypersensitivity reaction is cell mediated via T lymphocytes which liberate cytokines which are chemotactic to macrophages
- macrophages aggregate and when activated destroy bacilli
- later there is caseous destruction

Primary tuberculosis

- may be asymptomatic and evidence for this may only be found on subsequent chest x-ray
- no previous exposure and therefore no immunity
- initially a subpleural Ghon focus develops which may be present in any lobe
- microscopy shows area of consolidation with caseous centre and surrounding granulomatous reaction, including Langhan's giant cells
- hilar lymph node may also be involved in primary infection
- Ghon (primary) complex is the primary Ghon focus with involved regional lymph node
- primary tuberculosis heals by fibrosis and calcification
- occasionally there is progressive pulmonary tuberculosis with blood spread causing miliary tuberculosis

Secondary (post-primary) tuberculosis

- can arise either from reinfection or by reactivation of latent organisms
- early lesions are almost invariably found at the apex of one or other lung
- initially consolidation and later fibrosis and calcification with scar formation
- granulomas may coalesce to form caseous cavity
- super-infection with species such as *Aspergillus* may occur
- obstructed bronchus may result in bronchiectasis
- may spread throughout both lungs, causing tuberculous pneumonia
- blood spread may result in miliary tuberculosis
- swallowing of infected sputum may result in infection of alimentary tract

FUNGAL INFECTIONS

Fungal infections of the lung are associated with:

- immunosuppression
- diabetes
- malnourishment
- steroids and other immunosuppressive drugs
- AIDS
- tuberculosis
- malignant disease
- bronchiectasis
- chronic obstructive airways disease

Candidiasis

- due to infection with *Candida albicans*
- often found normally in sputum but generally represents saprophytic growth
- may cause bronchopneumonia or miliary candidiasis
- may involve lung in cases of chronic bronchitis, bronchiectasis, bronchial carcinoma or immunosuppression

Aspergillosis

- *Aspergillus fumigatus* is most common cause of human disease
- other species which may be responsible for disease in man include *Aspergillus flavus* and *Aspergillus niger*
- *Aspergillus* species may cause an asthmatic-like condition (allergic aspergillosis)
- invasive aspergillosis with pneumonia may also occur
- bronchocentric granulomatosis may also occur
- an aspergilloma may occur when *Aspergillus* species colonise a pre-existing cavity, such as a tuberculous or tumour cavity
- microscopy shows *Aspergillus* hyphae which branch dichotomously. These may be highlighted by PAS or silver stains

Cryptococcosis

- caused by yeast-like fungus, *Cryptococcus neoformans*
- fungus occurs as a saprophyte in soil
- with pulmonary involvement may be pneumonic process or may be cavity formation
- microscopically spheroid ovoid organisms with a mucoid capsule

Histoplasmosis

- two species are pathogenic in man, *Histoplasma capsulatum* and *Histoplasma duboisii*
- endemic in many parts of North America
- macroscopically may resemble tuberculosis

LUNG ABSCESS

- organisms responsible include *Pneumococcus*, staphylococcal species and *Klebsiella*
- predisposing conditions include:
  - bronchial occlusion with tumour or foreign body
  - pulmonary infarction
  - septic emboli (drug addicts)
  - pulmonary haematoma
  - bronchiectasis
  - septicaemia from primary infection elsewhere
  - immunosuppression, e.g. AIDS
- aspiration of infected oropharyngeal secretions may result in aspiration pneumonia and subsequent abscess formation
- aspiration pneumonia is most common in the right lower lobe
- bacteria responsible for aspiration pneumonia are usually mixed anaerobes

Pathology

- fibrous tissue wall with compressed adjacent lung
- microscopy shows neutrophilic infiltration
- abscess may rupture into bronchus or into pleural cavity, resulting in an empyema
- metastatic spread may occur, resulting in a brain abscess

BRONCHIECTASIS

- irreversible dilatation of bronchi
- clinically there is chronic cough productive of large amounts of mucopurulent sputum

- may also have fever and haemoptysis
- *Haemophilus influenzae* is most common bacteria to be isolated from sputum

Causes

- infections, e.g. measles, adenovirus, pertussis
- obstruction of bronchus, e.g. by tumour or foreign body
- impaired defence, e.g. cystic fibrosis, Kartagener's syndrome, ciliary dyskinesia
- autoimmunity, e.g. ulcerative colitis
- allergy, e.g. aspergillosis
- congenital, e.g. Mounier-Kuhn's syndrome

Kartagener's syndrome

- autosomal recessive syndrome
- characterised by bronchiectasis, sinusitis, situs inversus
- due to defect in ciliary motility

Cystic fibrosis

- autosomal recessive condition
- genetic defect on long arm of chromosome 7
- prenatal testing is possible
- production of hyperviscous mucus which results in infection and bronchiectasis
- also affects intestine and pancreas

Post-infective bronchiectasis

- bronchiectasis was formerly a common sequel to respiratory infections in early childhood
- most common causative organisms are measles, adenovirus and pertussis

Post-obstruction bronchiectasis

- proximal obstruction may be caused by tumours, foreign body, mucus plugs or enlarged lymph nodes

Pathology

- bronchiectasis may be described as cylindrical, saccular or follicular
- in cylindrical bronchiectasis the dilated airways maintain a uniform diameter until they reach the pleura
- in saccular bronchiectasis, the dilated airways have one or more localised dilatations
- if lymphoid follicles are prominent histologically, the term follicular bronchiectasis is used
- dilated airways are filled with a purulent exudate
- mucosal surface is congested
- bronchial walls are often thickened by fibrosis, oedema and inflammatory infiltrate

Complications

- lung abscess formation
- empyema
- cor pulmonale
- colonisation by fungi, e.g. *Aspergillus* species

- metastatic abscess formation, especially in brain
- amyloidosis

Chronic bronchitis and emphysema

- chronic bronchitis is hypersecretory in nature, whereas emphysema is a purely destructive process
- the two diseases often coexist
- most common aetiological factor is cigarette smoking

CHRONIC BRONCHITIS

- persistent excess in bronchial secretions on most days for at least 3 months in the year, over at least 2 years
- conditions such as tuberculosis and bronchiectasis must be excluded
- most common in middle-aged to elderly males
- sputum is usually white but becomes yellow-green with superimposed infection
- most important pathogenic bacteria are *Haemophilus influenzae* and *Streptococcus pneumoniae*
- may develop cor pulmonale or bronchopneumonia

Pathology

- bronchi are filled with mucus and/or pus
- mucosa is congested
- microscopy shows hypertrophy of mucus glands in wall of bronchi
- with superimposed infection, there are neutrophils within lumen of bronchi

EMPHYSEMA

- abnormal permanent increase in size of air spaces distal to terminal bronchioles with destruction of air space walls and without obvious fibrosis
- protease–antiprotease theory is thought to be important in pathogenesis of emphysema
- three patterns of emphysema may be distinguished:

  1. Centriacinar
     - chiefly affects upper lobes
     - acini around respiratory bronchioles affected
     - may get bullae formation
     - related to cigarette smoking

  2. Panacinar
     - whole of acinus affected
     - affects all lobes of lung or is worse in lower lobes
     - may be associated with centriacinar emphysema
     - associated with α1-antitrypsin deficiency, an autosomal recessive condition

  3. Paraseptal
     - peripheral part of acinus adjacent to septa or pleura affected
     - may occur alone or in association with other forms of emphysema
     - due to forces pulling on the septa
     - large bullae may form

Senile emphysema

- not true emphysema because no destruction of alveolar walls
- occurs in elderly
- decrease in alveolar surface area is normal ageing phenomenon

Compensatory emphysema

- not true emphysema since distension occurs without destruction
- occurs when part of lung is removed or collapses

Interstitial (surgical) emphysema

- in this condition, air is present in tissues that are normally airless
- air is present in interstitium of lungs
- may be due to artificial ventilation
- other causative factors are blast injuries and fractured limbs
- air in interstitium of lung may track to pleura, to hila of lungs, to mediastinum and to neck

Bullous disease of lungs

- a bulla is an emphysematous space over 1 cm in diameter
- may be inherited
- may be due to localised emphysema
- grossly an air-filled sac is present in the subpleural region, usually in the apex of a lung

Pulmonary embolism and infarction

- usually elderly patients
- majority arise in deep veins of legs and pelvis and subsequently embolise to lungs
- occasionally embolus arises from right atrium or tricuspid valve in endocarditis
- as well as blood clot, tumours, amniotic fluid, fat and air may embolise
- massive embolus which lodges in pulmonary trunk or main pulmonary artery is usually immediately fatal
- smaller emboli which lodge peripherally may result in pulmonary infarction
- multiple microemboli may result in pulmonary hypertension

CLASSIFICATION

Acute massive pulmonary embolism

- when an embolus lodges in the pulmonary trunk or main pulmonary artery marked haemodynamic changes occur with sudden right-sided heart failure

Acute minor pulmonary embolism

- pulmonary infarction is relatively rare due to dual blood supply of lungs
- infarction usually occurs only if there is pre-existing lung or cardiac disease
- infarcts are seen as wedge-shaped shadows on chest x-ray
- grossly an infarct is haemorrhagic and wedge-shaped with the base of the infarct on the pleura. An occluded pulmonary artery may be seen at the apex

- microscopically the alveoli are filled with blood
- infarcts heal by fibrous scarring

Chronic pulmonary embolism

- recurrent multiple small emboli
- causes pulmonary hypertension

Prognosis

- prognosis depends on size of embolus and presence or absence of coexistent respiratory or cardiac disease
- death may occur with large embolus
- pulmonary infarction may occur
- in most cases resolution of the embolus occurs by both fragmentation and fibrinolysis
- chronic pulmonary hypertension may occur with multiple small emboli

Wegener's granulomatosis

- aetiology is unknown
- more common in males
- organs involved include nose, paranasal sinuses, lungs and kidneys

CLINICAL FEATURES

- may present with systemic illness with fever, malaise, weight loss
- may present with nasal obstruction, pain and epistaxis
- if lung disease present, may get cough, haemoptysis and chest pain
- may get rapidly progressive glomerulonephritis

PATHOLOGY

- nasal biopsy may be diagnostic
- microscopy shows foci of necrosis with vasculitis and granuloma formation
- in lungs upper lobes are most often affected
- usually multiple nodular necrotic masses
- microscopic appearance is of necrotising granulomatous vasculitis

DIAGNOSIS

- autoantibodies against neutrophil cytoplasmic antigen (cANCA)

Adult respiratory distress syndrome (ARDS)

Life-threatening respiratory distress that occurs suddenly following a variety of unrelated pulmonary insults

SYNONYMS

- diffuse alveolar change
- shock lung
- traumatic wet lung

- blast lung
- pump lung
- stiff lung syndrome
- acute lung injury

PREDISPOSING FACTORS

- trauma, severe burns
- haemorrhagic shock
- septic shock
- mechanical ventilation with high oxygen concentrations
- radiation
- paraquat poisoning
- pulmonary infections
- drug toxicity
- aspiration
- near drowning
- air, fat or amniotic fluid embolism
- DIC
- acute pancreatitis

PATHOGENESIS

(Figure 14.2)

- mechanism is poorly understood
- clinical and pathological end result of acute alveolar injury caused by a variety of insults
- final common pathway is diffuse damage to the alveolar capillary walls
- also damage to alveolar epithelial cells (pneumocytes)
- increased capillary permeability
- interstitial and intra-alveolar oedema ensues

DIFFUSE ALVEOLAR DAMAGE

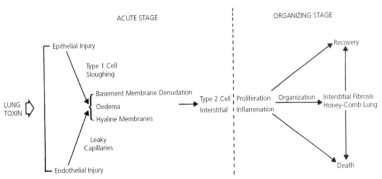

Figure 14.2 Pathogenesis of diffuse alveolar damage. (From Katzenstein and Askin 1982, with permission)

- fibrin exudation occurs
- hyaline membrane formation occurs when fibrin combines with debris from necrotic type I pneumocytes
- later interstitial fibrosis occurs
- the capillary membrane permeability defect is believed to be produced by interaction of inflammatory cells and mediators, including leucocytes, cytokines, oxygen radicals, complement and arachidonate metabolites
- type I pneumocytes are destroyed and contribute to formation of hyaline membranes
- type II pneumocytes are damaged, resulting in loss of surfactant which leads to pulmonary collapse
- in the repair stage type II pneumocytes proliferate. There is invasion by fibroblasts and subsequent fibrosis

PATHOLOGY

- in the acute stage the lungs are solid, congested and oedematous
- microscopy shows interstitial and intra-alveolar oedema
- fibrin deposition occurs in vessels and alveoli
- hyaline membranes form and line alveolar spaces
- after several days type II pneumocytes regenerate forming cuboidal cells which project into the alveolar lumen
- after a few weeks interstitial fibrosis develops
- there is often a superimposed bronchopneumonia

PROGNOSIS

(Figure 14.3)

- mortality is over 50%
- abnormal pulmonary function in survivors is common

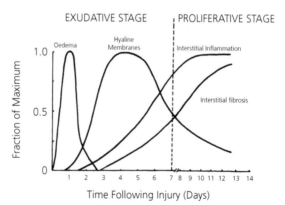

Figure 14.3 Sequence of events in 'shock lung'. From Katzenstein and Askin 1982, with permission

Pulmonary hamartomas

- may actually represent a benign neoplasm
- most common in adults, rare in children
- usually peripheral lung mass which is incidentally discovered on chest x-ray (coin lesion)

PATHOLOGY

- usually well circumscribed
- microscopy shows lobules of cartilage with fat or fibrous tissue
- at periphery slits lined by respiratory epithelium may be entrapped
- no malignant potential

Benign lung tumours

SQUAMOUS CELL PAPILLOMA

- usually middle-aged or elderly men
- often cigarette smokers
- arise in larger bronchi
- grossly warty growths
- microscopy shows connective tissue core with papillary squamous epithelial surface
- may become dysplastic and malignant

JUVENILE PAPILLOMATOSIS

- usually children aged less than 10 years
- multiple benign squamous papillomas involving respiratory epithelium, usually in larynx, trachea and large bronchi
- human papilloma virus (HPV) types 6 and 11 may be aetiological factor
- clinically may get hoarseness, stridor and airways obstruction
- malignant change, especially following radiotherapy treatment, rarely supervenes

OTHER BENIGN PULMONARY TUMOURS

- all are rare
- neurofibromas, schwannomas, lipomas and leiomyomas have occasionally been described

Malignant lung tumours

- commonest cause of death from malignant disease in males
- second most common cause of death, after breast cancer, from malignant disease in females
- peak age 65–75 years
- more common in males
- increasing in females

AETIOLOGY

Smoking

- linear relationship between number of cigarettes smoked and mortality
- passive smoking increases risk
- at least 80% of lung cancers occur in smokers
- several carcinogens in smoke are implicated, e.g. nitrosamines, polycyclic hydrocarbons
- carcinogens may inactivate p53 oncogene

Air pollution

- incidence of lung cancer is higher in urban areas

Asbestos exposure

- increased incidence of lung cancer with asbestos exposure
- there may be a long latent period between exposure and the development of lung cancer

Scarring

- occasionally lung cancers may arise within areas of scarring (scar cancers)

Industrial hazards

- contact with chromium, arsenic, nickle, beryllium
- radiation exposure

PATHOGENESIS

- chronic irritation by cigarette smoke causes squamous metaplasia
- squamous metaplasia may undergo dysplastic transformation
- squamous metaplasia and dysplasia are often found adjacent to invasive squamous carcinoma

CLINICAL FEATURES

Lung tumours may present with symptoms due to:

Local effects of tumour

- cough, haemopytsis, chest pain, dyspnoea, SVC obstruction
- pleural effusion
- Horner's syndrome
- Pancoast's syndrome
- dysphagia or hoarseness due to pressure on oesophagus or recurrent laryngeal nerve

Metastatic disease

- bone, e.g. pathological fractures or back pain
- brain, e.g. stroke, confusion, epilepsy
- liver, e.g. jaundice

Non-metastatic effects (para-neoplastic effects)

- endocrine symptoms due to elaboration of ADH, ACTH or PTH
- finger clubbing
- myaesthenia gravis-like syndrome
- peripheral neuropathy

General debility of malignant disease

- fever, weight loss, anorexia, anaemia

DIAGNOSIS

- sputum cytology
- bronchoscopy with biopsy
- bronchial brushings and washings
- percutaneous CT guided fine needle aspiration (FNA)

MORPHOLOGY

(Table 14.1)

- appear to arise from single stem cells

Table 14.1 Malignant tumours of the lung (based on World Health Organization classification (1981)

Squamous cell carcinoma
Small cell carcinoma
Oat cell
Intermediate cell type
Combined oat cell carcinoma
Adenocarcinoma
Acinar
Papillary
Bronchiolo-alveolar
Solid with mucus formation
Large cell carcinoma
Undifferentiated
Giant cell
Clear cell
Adenosquamous
Carcinoid
Bronchial gland carcinomas
Adenoid cystic
Mucoepidermoid
Other

SQUAMOUS CARCINOMA

- most common malignant neoplasm of lung
- strong association with cigarette smoking
- vast majority arise in large or medium-sized bronchi
- fungating mass in bronchial lumen on bronchoscopy
- grossly usually large hilar mass, often with hilar lymph node involvement
- distal changes include bronchopneumonia, lung abscess and bronchiectasis
- microscopically typical squamous cell carcinoma with intercellular bridges and keratin production

SMALL CELL CARCINOMA

- second most common type of lung cancer
- highly malignant
- typical oat cell carcinoma and intermediate cell carcinoma are included in this category
- associated with smoking and usually centrally located
- tumour has usually metastasised at time of presentation and is usually unresectable
- may get paraneoplastic effects due to hormone elaboration
- patients usually die with widely disseminated disease in 1–2 years
- microscopy shows darkly staining, round to ovoid cells with little cytoplasm arranged in sheets, ribbons or trabeculae
- in intermediate cell carcinoma, the cells are larger with more cytoplasm
- small cell carcinoma may be combined with other cell types such as squamous carcinoma
- may get widespread metastatic disease in absence of detectable primary tumour

ADENOCARCINOMA

- 10% of lung cancers but appears to be increasing in incidence
- relatively more common in females and in non-smokers
- usually arises in peripheral part of lung
- microscopy shows glandular formation
- WHO recognises four subtypes of adenocarcinoma: acinar (tubular), papillary, bronchioloalveolar (see below) and solid with mucus production
- however, interobserver variation is poor using this classification and it is of limited value
- adenocarcinoma may occur in areas of scarring (scar cancer)
- need to differentiate from secondary adenocarcinoma in lung from unknown primary site

BRONCHIOLO-ALVEOLAR CARCINOMA

- variant of lung adenocarcinoma
- may arise from type II pneumocytes, Clara cells or mucus-secreting cells
- grossly multiple nodules often seen
- may be bilateral
- tumour cells grow along alveolar septae, imparting a bronchiolo-alveolar pattern
- bronchial origin not usually identified
- other adenocarcinomas, including metastases, may have a focal bronchiolo-alveolar growth pattern and the characteristic growth pattern should be seen throughout the neoplasm

LARGE CELL CARCINOMA

- non-small cell carcinoma which shows no obvious attempt at squamoid or glandular differentiation
- microscopy shows sheets of large pleomorphic cells
- electron microscopy may show evidence of glandular or squamoid differentiation
- variants include giant cell and clear cell carcinoma

ADENOSQUAMOUS CARCINOMA

- tumours in which both squamous and glandular differentiation can be seen microscopically
- often peripheral tumours

SPREAD OF LUNG CANCER

Direct spread

- through lung parenchyma
- via lung lymphatics producing lymphangitis carcinomatosis
- to mediastinal structures producing SVC obstruction, dysphagia or recurrent laryngeal nerve palsy
- invasion of brachial plexus results in Pancoast's syndrome
- involvement of sympathetic nervous system may result in Horner's syndrome

Lymphatic spread

- to hilar, mediastinal or cervical lymph nodes

Blood spread

- common sites of blood-borne spread are liver, adrenal glands, bone, brain and contralateral lung

STAGING OF LUNG CANCER

(Table 14.2)

Table 14.2 Summary of TNM classification of lung cancer (T = tumour)

Classification	Extent of disease
Tis	Preinvasive (carcinoma-*in-situ*)
T0	No evidence of primary T
T1	T <3 cm in greatest dimension, surrounded by lung or visceral pleura. No evidence of invasion proximal to lobar bronchus on bronchoscopy
T2	T >3 cm, or any size of T invading visceral pleura, or any size of T associated with obstructive pneumonitis extending to the hilar region. At bronchoscopy, proximal extent must be 2 cm distal to carina
T3	T any size with direct extension to adjacent structures, e.g. chest wall, diaphragm, mediastinal contents, or T at bronchoscopy <2 cm from carina, or any T associated with obstructive pneumonitis of entire lung or pleural effusion
Tx	Not assessable
N0	No regional nodes
N1	Peribronchial and/or ipsilateral hilar nodes involved
N2	Mediastinal nodes involved
Nx	Not assessed
M0	No distant metastases
M1	Evidence of distant metastases
Mx	Not assessed

PROGNOSIS

- prognosis depends on stage of tumour
- prognosis is worse with small cell carcinoma

Rare lung tumours

CARCINOSARCOMA

- microscopically contains both carcinomatous and sarcomatous elements
- most commonly occurs in elderly men
- associated with cigarette smoking
- often present as fungating polypoid bronchial mass
- poor prognosis

PULMONARY BLASTOMA

- occur at any age with a mean age of approximately 40 years
- more common in males
- may occur in children
- usually peripheral location
- microscopy shows tubules or acini in primitive mesenchymal stroma
- prognosis is unpredictable

EPITHELIOID HAEMANGIOENDOTHELIOMA

- formerly known as intravascular bronchioloalveolar tumour (IVBAT)
- may occur in young adults
- commoner in women
- typically there are multiple small nodules in both lungs
- derived from endothelial cells
- microscopy shows epithelioid tumour cells with intracytoplasmic lumina

CARCINOID TUMOURS

- arise from pulmonary neuroendocrine cells (Kulchitsky cells)
- there is no association with smoking
- mean age is approximately 55 years, significantly lower than that of carcinoma of the lung
- most occur in large bronchus
- mucosa is usually not ulcerated
- occasionally arise peripherally
- may present with metastatic deposits or with the carcinoid syndrome

Pathology

- grossly often have a yellow colour
- microscopy shows uniform cells arranged in nests, ribbons and trabeculae
- stain positively with neuroendocrine markers
- electron microscopy shows neurosecretory granules within cytoplasm
- atypical carcinoids have atypical features with a high mitotic rate and areas of necrosis

Prognosis

- all are potentially malignant
- atypical carcinoids are much more likely to metastasise

BRONCHIAL GLAND TUMOURS

- tumours similar to those arising within salivary glands occasionally occur within lung
- adenoid cystic carcinoma, mucoepidermoid carcinoma, pleomorphic adenoma and acinic cell carcinomas may occur

PRIMARY MALIGNANT LYMPHOMA

- rare
- most are lymphomas of mucosa associated lymphoid tissue (MALTomas)
- tend to remain localised to lung
- must exclude spread from lymphomas elsewhere

MISCELLANEOUS

- rare malignant tumours which occur primarily within the lung and include malignant melanoma and various sarcomas

PLEURA AND PLEURAL CAVITY

Normal structure

- the lungs are surrounded by a thin visceral pleura which is continuous with the parietal pleura at the hilum
- two layers of pleura are in close contact and are only separated by a small amount of fluid
- both layers of pleura are composed of fibroelastic connective tissue covered by a single layer of mesothelial cells

Pneumothorax

- a pneumothorax is air within the pleural space
- air may enter the pleural space either through the chest wall or from the lung
- tension pneumothorax may occur if air can enter pleural space but not escape
- if repeated pneumothoraces, pleurodesis may be necessary

CAUSES

- due to rupture of subpleural bulla. This may occur in otherwise healthy young individuals and especially involves the apices of the lungs. Tends to involve thin males
- associated with asthma, emphysema
- artificial ventilation
- congenital pulmonary cysts
- trauma, e.g. due to fractured rib or clavicle. If blood vessels are damaged, may result in haemopneumothorax
- cystic fibrosis
- tuberculosis
- artificial pneumothorax was previously induced in treatment of chronic tuberculosis

Empyema

- accumulation of pus within pleural space
- now rare with widespread use of antibiotics
- sequel to lung infections, e.g. abscess, bronchiectasis, tuberculosis
- may be secondary to penetrating wounds
- may be associated with haemothorax
- may occur post-thoracotomy
- oesophageal rupture may result in empyema
- spread of subphrenic abscess
- rarely secondary to osteomyelitis of ribs
- more common in diabetics, alcoholics or immunosuppressed
- usually a mixture of bacteria is responsible

CLINICALLY

- rigors, weight loss and pleural effusions occur

PATHOLOGY

- pus within pleural cavity
- later fibrin deposition and organisation into fibrous tissue

COMPLICATIONS

- metastatic brain abscess
- amyloidosis
- pleural fibrosis with fibrous obliteration of pleural cavity

Chylothorax

- collection of lymphatic fluid in pleural cavity (fluid appears milky)
- due to obstruction or rupture of the thoracic duct
- rupture of thoracic duct may be due to surgical or other trauma
- obstruction of duct may be due to malignancy, infective disorders or surgery

Pleural plaques

- associated with asbestos exposure
- generally multifocal and bilateral
- usually affect the parietal pleura, particularly over the diaphragm
- microscopically composed of hyaline avascular connective tissue

Solitary fibrous tumour of pleura

- previously known as benign mesothelioma
- unrelated to asbestos exposure
- usually arise from visceral pleura
- usually are well circumscribed lesions attached to the lung by a pedicle

- may reach a large size
- microscopically composed of spindle-shaped cells
- most are benign, although occasionally exhibit malignant behaviour (10%)
- positive immunohistochemical staining for CD34 is a useful diagnostic feature

Malignant mesothelioma

- malignant tumour of mesothelial cells
- most common in pleura, although may also arise in peritoneum, pericardium or paratesticular region
- more common in men

CAUSE

- 80% associated with asbestos exposure. There may be a long latent period of 20–40 years
- amphibole asbestos fibres are most carcinogenic
- 20% have no history of exposure to asbestos

CLINICAL

- pleural mesothelioma may be asymptomatic until tumour is advanced
- presents with dyspnoea and chest pain
- often have pleural effusion which may be blood stained
- peritoneal mesothelioma presents with abdominal pain, ascites and intestinal obstruction

PATHOLOGY

- grossly the lung is encased by yellow white tumour which obliterates the pleural space and invades the interlobar fissures. There is collapse of the underlying lung. The gross appearance is characteristic
- microscopic picture is variable
- microscopy shows epithelial type, sarcomatous type, mixed epithelial and sarcomatous type and undifferentiated

DIAGNOSIS

- diagnosis is usually by pleural biopsy or by cytological examination of effusion fluid
- difficult in small biopsies
- differential diagnosis includes secondary adenocarcinoma and reactive mesothelial hyperplasia
- immunohistochemistry and electron microscopy may be of value

STAGING

(Table 14.3)

- median survival is less than 1 year
- lymphatic spread may occur to hilar lymph nodes
- blood-borne spread is rare until tumour is advanced

Table 14.3 Staging of pleural malignant mesothelioma

Stage	Extent of disease
Stage I	Tumour confined to ipsilateral pleura and lung
Stage II	Tumour involving chest wall, mediastinum, pericardium or contralateral pleura
Stage III	Tumour involving both thorax and abdomen or lymph nodes outside the chest
Stage IV	Distant blood-borne metastases

Mediastinal masses

(Table 14.4)

MEDIASTINUM

Developmental abnormalities

THYROID MASSES

- retrosternal extension of cervical thyroid
- true mediastinal thyroid

PLEURO-PERICARDIAL CYSTS

- usually asymptomatic
- usually situated in cardiophrenic angle
- unilocular containing clear fluid
- microscopy shows lining of mesothelial cells

BRONCHOGENIC CYSTS

ENTEROGENOUS CYSTS

Table 14.4 Location of mediastinal masses

Superior	Anterior	Middle	Posterior
Thyroid masses	Thymic lesions	Lymph node enlargement	Neural tumours
Lymph node enlargement	Lymphoma	Bronchogenic cysts	Thoracic meningocoele
Oesophageal tumours	Germ cell tumours	Enterogenic cysts	Oesophageal tumours
Aortic aneurysms	Pleuropericardial cysts		Aortic aneurysms
Parathyroid lesions	Paraganglioma		Paraganglioma
	Lymph node enlargement		

Lymph node enlargement

- there are many causes of mediastinal lymph node enlargement, including inflammatory conditions, infective conditions, sarcoidosis, malignant lymphoma and metastatic tumours
- lymphomas commonly found within the mediastinum include nodular sclerosing Hodgkin's disease and primary mediastinal sclerosing large B-cell lymphoma
- lymphoblastic lymphomas may present with a mediastinal mass, especially in children

Thymus

(See Chapter 15)

Germ cell tumours

- most common in males
- usually teratoma or seminoma
- usually situated in anterior mediastinum
- often asymptomatic and discovered on chest x-ray
- may present with superior vena caval obstruction
- microscopically similar to corresponding testicular tumours
- must exclude metastatic spread from occult primary testicular tumour
- malignant tumours spread to regional lymph nodes, lungs and pericardium
- seminoma is highly radiosensitive

Neural tumours

- symptoms include those secondary to pressure effects on thoracic structures
- usually situated in posterior mediastinum
- most are benign but may be malignant
- tumours found include neurilemmoma (schwannoma), neurofibroma, neurofibrosarcoma, ganglioneuroma, ganglioneuroblastoma and neuroblastoma
- most arise from thoracic sympathetic chain

Mediastinitis

- acute mediastinitis may be a result of perforation of the oesophagus. This may be secondary to tumour, trauma or chest surgery
- chronic mediastinitis may be secondary to infections, such as tuberculous and fungal infections

Idiopathic mediastinal fibrosis

- diffuse replacement of mediastinal connective tissue by dense, white collagenous, fibrous tissue
- cause is unknown but may have autoimmune aetiology

- associated conditions include retroperitoneal fibrosis, Riedel's thyroiditis and sclerosing cholangitis
- drugs, e.g. methylsergide may be causative
- symptoms may be due to compression of SVC, respiratory tract or great vessels
- steroids may be helpful
- some require surgery

The lymphoreticular system, including spleen and thymus

15

LYMPH NODES

Normal structure

- lymph node is surrounded by a thin fibrous capsule
- afferent lymphatics penetrate the capsule at various points and efferent lymphatics leave at the hilum
- lymph node contains an outer cortex and an inner medulla
- the medulla contains many interconnecting sinuses
- normal lymph node consists of lymphoid follicles, containing germinal centres, arranged around the periphery of the node
- these lymphoid follicles are composed of B-lymphoid cells (centrocytes and centroblasts)
- the interfollicular areas and the medulla are largely composed of T-lymphoid cells
- other cells found in lymph nodes include macrophages, plasma cells, dendritic reticulum cells and interdigitating reticulum cells

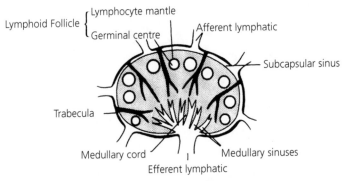

Figure 15.1 Schematic drawing of lymph node

Reactive lymphadenopathy

- many diseases may produce reactive changes in nearby lymph nodes
- many of these result in non-specific features
- reactive follicular hyperplasia involves B-cell areas of lymph node with enlarged lymphoid follicles with prominent germinal centres
- may be due to a variety of causes
- with viral infections, tend to get stimulation of T-cell areas with parafollicular hyperplasia
- this is best seen in glandular fever due to Epstein-Barr virus infection where marked parafollicular hyperplasia may simulate malignant lymphoma

Granulomatous lymphadenopathy

- granulomas within nodes may be found in a variety of diseases
- in tuberculosis there are caseating granulomas with Langhan's type giant cells. Tubercle bacilli may be demonstrated by Ziehl-Nielson staining
- sarcoidosis (well circumscribed, non-necrotising granulomas)
- Crohn's disease
- nodes draining malignant tumours
- Hodgkin's disease
- cat-scratch disease
- lymphogranuloma venereum
- *Yersinia* infections
- toxoplasmosis
- syphilis
- foreign body reaction

Hodgkin's disease

- bimodal age distribution with a peak incidence in adolescence and early adult life and a second peak after the age of 50 years
- Hodgkin's disease is more common in males, except for the nodular sclerosing subtype which is more common in females
- Reed-Sternberg cells and variants are neoplastic component but the exact lineage of these is still not proven

AETIOLOGY

- aetiology is unknown but an infective cause is suspected
- Epstein-Barr virus (EBV) has been found in the serum and also in the neoplastic cells (Reed-Sternberg cells) in Hodgkin's disease
- there is some evidence of disease clustering which would support an infective cause but data are conflicting

CLINICAL PRESENTATION

- enlarged lymph nodes, most commonly in neck or axilla
- may have constitutional B symptoms including fever, weight loss and night sweats
- often get contiguous spread between adjacent lymph node groups

PATHOLOGY

- neoplastic cells (Reed-Sternberg cells and variants) stain with antibodies against CD15 and CD30 antigens

SUBTYPES

Four subtypes of Hodgkin's disease are recognised:

1. Lymphocyte predominant
   - node contains abundant lymphocytes in nodular or diffuse pattern
   - classical Reed-Sternberg cells and variants are infrequent
   - nodular variant is now thought to represent a B-cell lymphoma

2. Mixed cellularity
   - classical Reed-Sternberg cells and variants are easily identified
   - there is a mixed infiltrate of reactive cells, including lymphocytes, eosinophils, plasma cells and histiocytes
   - second commonest subtype of Hodgkin's disease

3. Nodular sclerosing
   - most commonly affects mediastinal nodes
   - usually young females
   - microscopy shows thick fibrous capsule and nodular appearance due to fibrous bands separating the node into compartments
   - lacunar cells are often seen
   - two subtypes
   - type I. This is composed mainly of reactive cells with few neoplastic cells. This subtype has a better prognosis
   - type II. This has a lymphocyte depleted pattern with many neoplastic cells and has a worse prognosis

4. Lymphocytic-depleted
   - often elderly patients
   - contains many neoplastic Reed-Sternberg cells with few reactive cells

STAGING

(Table 15.1)

Table 15.1   Stages of Hodgkin's and non-Hodgkin's lymphomas (Ann Arbor classification)

Stage	Extent of disease
I	Involvement of a single lymph node region or involvement of a single extralymphatic organ or site
II	Involvement of two or more lymph node regions on the same side of the diaphragm alone, or with involvement of limited contiguous extralymphatic organ or tissue
III	Involvement of lymph node regions on both sides of the diaphragm which may include the spleen and/or limited contiguous extralymphatic organ or site
IV	Multiple or disseminated foci or involvement of one or more extralymphatic organs or tissues, with or without lymphatic involvement A Asymptomatic B Symptomatic

PROGNOSIS

- stage is most important
- lymphocyte predominant and nodular sclerosing type I have a better prognosis than other subtypes
- lymphocyte-depleted subtype has worse prognosis
- good prognostic factors include young age (less than 40 years) and absence of B symptoms

Non-Hodgkin's lymphoma

- occurs at any age but most common in adults
- may be nodal or extranodal
- recently all lymphomas (nodal, extranodal and Hodgkin's disease) have been combined in Revised European American lymphoma (REAL) classification (1994)
- other classifications in use include updated Kiel classification and working formulation
- spread is unpredictable and unlike Hodgkin's disease is not contiguous
- diagnosis is by immunohistochemical staining with monoclonal antibodies against B-cell or T-cell antigens or by molecular techniques to demonstrate rearrangement of immunoglobulin chain genes (B-cell lymphomas) or T-cell receptor genes (T-cell lymphomas)

AETIOLOGY

Unknown but higher incidence in:

- immunosuppressed, including transplant patients and often associated with EBV infection
- autoimmune diseases
- primary immunodeficiency syndromes
- AIDS
- some non-Hodgkin's lymphomas have characteristic chromosomal translocations, e.g. Burkitt's lymphoma (t 8/14), anaplastic large cell lymphoma (t 2/5), follicle centre cell lymphomas (t 14/18), mantle cell lymphoma (t 11/14)

CLINICAL

- usually present with painless lymphadenopathy
- may get B symptoms

B-CELL LYMPHOMAS

- most non-Hodgkin's lymphomas are of B-cell lineage
- stain positively with antibodies against B-cell antigens, e.g. CD20
- there are many subtypes but the most common are:

Small lymphocytic lymphoma

- usually elderly patients
- cells are small lymphocytes and similar to those in chronic lymphocytic leukaemia (CLL)
- often splenic, bone marrow and liver involvement
- usually relatively indolent with no treatment required
- patients usually die from unrelated causes

Follicle centre cell lymphoma

- common type of B-cell lymphoma
- usually middle-aged to elderly patients
- derived from follicle centre cells, i.e. centrocytes and centroblasts
- follicular or diffuse growth pattern
- bone marrow and spleen often involved
- progressive disease with poor long-term survival

Diffuse large B-cell lymphoma

- occurs at any age but more common in middle aged and elderly
- microscopically composed of large blasts
- may be seen in AIDS patients
- aggressive behaviour

Burkitt's lymphoma

- there are two types:
  - endemic in parts of Africa
  - sporadic in Western countries
- associated with EBV infection
- often get characteristic chromosomal translocation (t 8/14)
- often get extranodal involvement, e.g. jaws, ovaries, abdomen
- similar tumours may occur in AIDS
- aggressive behaviour but may respond to chemotherapy

T-CELL LYMPHOMAS

- much less common than B-cell lymphomas
- stain positively with antibodies against T-cell antigens, e.g. CD3
- often involve skin, e.g. mycosis fungoides and Sezary syndrome
- generally worse prognosis than B-cell lymphomas
- more common in parts of Asia

TRUE HISTIOCYTIC LYMPHOMAS

- tumours of monocytic/macrophage system
- extremely rare and many reported cases probably represent examples of T-cell lymphoma

Miscellaneous causes of lymphadenopathy

HISTIOCYTOSIS X (LANGERHAN'S CELL HISTIOCYTOSIS)

- neoplastic cell is Langerhan's cell
- electron microscopy may be useful in diagnosis by demonstration of typical Birbeck granules in Langerhan's cells
- three disease patterns:
  1. Letterer-Siwe disease
     - affects infants with widespread generalised disease
     - often get skin, lymph node, liver, spleen, bone marrow involvement
     - poor prognosis

2. Eosinophilic granuloma
   - affects bones and often presents with pathological fractures
   - microscopy shows admixture of Langerhan's cells and eosinophils
   - good prognosis
3. Hand-Schuller-Christian disease
   - less widespread that Letterer-Siwe disease
   - more indolent

Angioimmunoblastic lymphadenopathy

- nodes are infiltrated with immunoblasts
- often get systemic symptoms such as skin rash and fever
- may develop into T-cell lymphoma

CASTLEMAN'S DISEASE

- often get mediastinal involvement
- microscopy shows concentric rings of lymphocytes around blood vessels
- may be multifocal
- may get systemic symptoms

DERMATOPATHIC LYMPHADENOPATHY

- lymph node enlargement associated with chronic skin disorders
- microscopy shows parafollicular expansion due to infiltration by interdigitating reticulum cells

SILICONE LYMPHADENOPATHY

- enlargement of lymph nodes usually in axilla after silicone breast implants

DRUG-INDUCED LYMPHADENOPATHY

- phenytoin is most commonly implicated drug

AUTOIMMUNE LYMPHADENOPATHY

- benign lymph node enlargement may be found in rheumatoid arthritis and systemic lupus erythematosus
- there is also an increased incidence of malignant lymphoma in these conditions

SPLEEN

Normal structure

- spleen is surrounded by fibrous capsule from which trabeculae extend into the substance
- can get one or more accessory spleens or splenunculi
- spleen consists of white pulp and red pulp
- white pulp is composed of follicles consisting of B-lymphoid cells and adjacent T cells which are arranged around a central arteriole (periarteriolar lymphoid sheaths)
- red pulp consists of sinusoids and cords containing macrophages, red blood cells and plasma cells

Splenomegaly

- there are many causes (Table 15.2)
- may be associated with hypersplenism which results in destruction of red blood cells, white blood cells and platelets

Table 15.2 Some causes of splenomegaly

Infections	*Portal Hypertension*
Infectious mononucleosis	Liver cirrhosis
Infective endocarditis	Portal vein thrombosis
Typhoid	Right heart failure
Brucellosis	
Tuberculosis	*Storage diseases*
Malaria	Gaucher's disease
Toxoplasmosis	Niemann-Pick disease
Kala-azar	Mucopolysaccharidoses
Schistosomiasis	
	Miscellaneous
Haematological	Felty's syndrome
Hodgkin's lymphoma	Connective tissue disorders
Non-Hodgkin's lymphoma	Cysts
Leukaemia	Primary tumours
Multiple myeloma	Secondary tumours
Myelofibrosis	
Polycythaemia rubra vera	
Haemolytic anaemias	
Thrombocytopenic purpura	

Congenital anomalies

- congenital absence or agenesis of the spleen is rare and is associated with major visceral and cardiac abnormalities, including transposition
- hereditary splenic hypoplasia is rare and predisposes to infection
- lobulation of the spleen is associated with cardiovascular abnormalities
- splenunculi (accessory spleens) occur in approximately 10% of the population
- splenic gonadal fusion may occur

Effects of splenectomy

- presence of Howell-Jolly bodies (fragments of DNA within red blood cells)
- increased percentage of target cells
- increased percentage of siderocytes containing granules of free iron
- increased numbers of red blood cells containing Heinz bodies
- increased numbers of white blood cells (all types)
- initial 24-hour decrease in platelets, then marked thrombocytosis (maximum at 2 weeks)
- increased platelet adhesiveness with risk of spontaneous thrombosis
- immune defects which are more severe in young patients

- decreased phagocytic activity
- loss of mechanical filtration
- decreased opsonin
- decreased IgM
- decreased properdin titres
- impaired antibody production
- changes in T-helper cells
- B-cell dysfunction
- low IgM which persists for years
- defective complement activity
- compensatory hypertrophy of splenunculi
- prone to overwhelming postsplenectomy infection (OPSI)

OPSI (OVERWHELMING POSTSPLENECTOMY INFECTION)

- especially common in children
- overall risk is approximately 5%
- low risk after splenectomy due to trauma but much higher risk following splenectomy for haemolytic diseases such as hereditary spherocytosis and idiopathic thrombocytopenic purpura (ITP)
- mortality is high with a rapid clinical course
- DIC is frequent
- prevention with pneumococcal vaccine and lifelong prophylactic penicillin
- organisms involved include *Pneumococcus, Meningococcus, Escherichia coli* and staphylococcal species

Miscellaneous conditions of the spleen

SPLENIC ATROPHY

- normal ageing phenomenon
- associated with coeliac disease and with sickle cell anaemia (due to multiple splenic infarcts)

SPLENOSIS

- multiple foci of splenic tissue throughout abdominal and pelvic peritoneum and even in pleural cavity
- usually secondary to splenic rupture

AMYLOIDOSIS

- spleen may be affected in both primary and secondary amyloidosis, but more commonly in secondary form
- may result in 'Sago spleen' or 'lardaceous spleen'

SPLENIC INFARCTION

Causes

- embolism secondary to cardiac disease
- thrombosis of splenic artery due to atheroma, polyarteritis or sickle cell anaemia
- thrombosis of splenic vein
- common in cases of massive splenomegaly, regardless of cause

GRANULOMATOUS INFLAMMATION

- may be infective, e.g. tuberculosis
- sarcoidosis is probably most common cause in Western countries
- may occur in Hodgkin's disease

TORSION

- rare
- precipitated by developmental abnormality with folds of peritoneum entering into splenic substance

PELIOSIS

- grossly there are widespread blood-filled cystic spaces
- often associated with peliosis hepatitis
- may result in splenic rupture
- may occur in wasting diseases such as tuberculosis and disseminated malignancy

SPLENIC RUPTURE

- mostly due to trauma, either blunt abdominal trauma or surgical trauma
- usually get immediate massive haemoperitoneum, necessitating emergency splenectomy
- may get delayed rupture
- causes of spontaneous splenic rupture include infectious mononucleosis, malaria, typhoid fever, bacterial endocarditis, peliosis, malignant lymphomas and leukaemias

PERISPLENITIS

- associated with any splenic pathology which involves the capsular surface
- fibrinous exudate on the serosal surface
- later fibrous adhesions with diaphragm and adjacent organs occur

SPLENIC ABSCESS

- rare
- may be secondary to trauma
- may be due to septic emboli, especially from endocarditis
- may be due to infected haematoma
- more common in immunosuppressed patients, including AIDS patients
- may rupture resulting in subdiaphragmatic abscess, peritonitis or empyema

SPLENIC CYSTS

Pseudocysts (false or secondary cysts)

- these have no true epithelial lining
- wall is composed of dense fibrous, often calcified tissue
- cyst contains blood and necrotic debris
- rupture may result in haemoperitoneum
- usually solitary and asymptomatic
- most are probably due to previous trauma
- infection and degeneration of area of infarction are other possible causes

True cysts

- parasitic
  - most common is hydatid cyst
  - risk of rupture with haemoperitoneum and dissemination of disease
  - diagnosis usually made by ultrasound
  - treatment is careful splenectomy which is curative
- congenital cysts
  - rare
  - wall of cyst is lined by flattened, cuboidal mesothelial cells
  - may be caused by peritoneal infolding during development
  - may be multiple
- epidermoid cysts
  - rare
  - mainly seen in children or young adults
  - usually solitary, but occasionally multiple
  - uncertain origin
  - may be due to squamous metaplasia of simple cyst
  - may be due to embryonic inclusion of epithelial cells from adjacent structures
  - usually contain straw coloured fluid
  - cyst wall is fibrous tissue with stratified squamous epithelial lining
  - occasionally cause pressure symptoms or may rupture
- dermoid cysts
  - very rare
  - wall consists of keratinising squamous epithelium with skin appendage structures
  - variant of benign teratoma

Splenic tumours

BENIGN SPLENIC TUMOURS

Haemangioma

- most common primary tumour of the spleen
- often incidental finding at surgery or on imaging procedures
- occasionally large and cause pressure symptoms
- rarely may be multiple
- may be associated with haemangiomas elsewhere
- complications include thrombosis, rupture with haemorrhage, infarction, anaemia, thrombocytopenia and consumption coagulopathy
- microscopy shows blood-filled spaces lined by endothelial cells

Lymphangioma

- rare
- usually children
- usually located in subcapsular region of spleen
- cystic nodules containing yellow fluid
- may be associated with lymphangiomas elsewhere

Hamartoma

- not true neoplasm
- uncommon

- usually composed of red pulp elements with no white pulp
- usually incidental finding
- may be associated with thrombocytopenia and other signs of hypersplenism

Lipoma

- rarely occurs as a primary intrasplenic lesion

MALIGNANT SPLENIC TUMOURS

Malignant lymphoma

- lymphoma is most common malignant tumour within the spleen but is usually part of disseminated disease
- relatively rare for lymphoma to involve spleen alone
- grossly may get diffuse or nodular growth pattern
- spleen is commonly involved in low grade B-cell non-Hodgkin's lymphomas
- may also be involved in Hodgkin's disease
- lymphomas which show preferential involvement of the spleen include splenic marginal zone lymphoma and hairy cell leukaemia
- spleen may also be involved in leukaemias

Angiosarcoma

- rare
- most common primary malignant non-lymphoid tumour
- arises from endothelial cells
- often huge spleen with focal or diffuse involvement with haemorrhagic nodules
- microscopy shows vascular spaces lined by pleomorphic endothelial cells
- may get spontaneous rupture resulting in haemoperitoneum
- may get thrombocytopenia and consumption coagulopathy
- rapid clinical course with poor prognosis

Metastatic splenic tumours

- rare, although may be found at autopsy in 10% of patients with widespread metastatic disease
- primary sites include lung, breast and ovary. Malignant melanoma may also spread to spleen
- direct invasion may occur, e.g. from stomach

THYMUS

Normal structure

- arises from endoderm of third branchial pouch during sixth week of gestation
- migrates downwards into anterior mediastinum in front of great vessels
- composed of two lobes with a lobular configuration
- surrounded by a fibrous capsule
- greatest weight in proportion to body weight is at birth and greatest absolute weight is at puberty
- with increasing age there is loss of thymic parenchyma and replacement by fat

- microscopy shows lobulated appearance
  - outer dark cortex contains many lymphocytes
  - inner pale medulla contains Hassall's corpuscles which are the epithelial component of the thymus
  - in later life, thymus is predominantly composed of fat
- thymus produces T lymphocytes which are involved in cell-mediated immunity

Thymic aplasia – hypoplasia

- failure and/or arrest in development of thymus
- associated with rare immunodeficiency syndromes such as DiGeorge's syndrome, ataxia-telangiectasia and severe combined immunodeficiency
- main differential is acute thymic involution secondary to stress

Myaesthenia gravis

- thymus shows follicular hyperplasia in approximately 65% of cases
- 10% of patients have a thymoma
- thymoma may be diagnosed during investigation of myaesthenia gravis
- myaesthenia gravis is caused by reduction of acetylcholine receptors at neuromuscular junctions
- autoimmune disease
- after thymectomy many patients with myaesthenia gravis improve, especially if there is a thymoma

Ectopic thymus

- may present as mass in neck or on pleura of lung
- may be unilateral or bilateral

Ectopic tissues

- ectopic parathyroid gland may be found in a normally located thymus

Thymic tumours

THYMOMAS

- usually occur in anterior mediastinum, although occasionally occur within the posterior mediastinum, the thyroid gland or the lung
- tumours of epithelial component of thymus
- usually accompanied by many reactive T lymphocytes
- old classification was into epithelial, lymphocytic or mixed thymomas depending on relative proportions of epithelial and lymphoid components
- another classification divides these into benign thymomas, malignant thymomas and thymic carcinomas
- benign thymomas are cytologically bland and do not invade adjacent structures
- if invasion of local structures is present the term malignant thymoma is used
- if cytologically malignant the term *thymic carcinoma* is used

- recent Muller-Hermelick classification divides these tumours into medullary thymoma, cortical thymoma, predominantly cortical thymoma, mixed thymoma and well differentiated thymic carcinoma
- usually present as a mediastinal mass with pressure symptoms in middle-aged patients
- may be an incidental finding on chest x-ray
- may be found during investigation of myaesthenia gravis

Pathology

- grossly often have cystic or lobulated appearance
- microscopy shows epithelial cells and lymphoid cells in varying proportions
- many are encapsulated
- may be cystic degeneration of epithelial component
- poor prognostic features include large size of tumour, invasion of adjacent structures, the presence of epithelial atypia and the presence of metastases
- rare histological variants of thymic carcinoma include squamous carcinoma, sarcomatoid carcinoma, small cell carcinoma and anaplastic carcinoma

MISCELLANEOUS RARE TUMOURS OF THYMUS

- carcinoid tumours. These may occasionally occur as part of MEN syndromes
- thymolipoma is composed of a mixture of thymic tissue and adipose tissue
- germ cell tumours may occur in the mediastinum, within the thymus (see Chapter 14)
- malignant lymphomas may involve the thymus
- secondary deposits may occur within the thymus, especially from a lung primary

Thymic cysts

- developmental unilocular thymic cysts may originate from remnants of the third branchial pouch
- multilocular thymic cysts are acquired and are accompanied by inflammation and fibrosis. These are usually a result of acquired cystic dilatation of Hassall's corpuscles
- thymic tumours such as germ cell tumours, Hodgkin's disease and thymoma may result in multilocular thymic cysts
- other cystic lesions in the thymus include lymphangiomas and cystic degeneration of thymomas

The endocrine system   **16**

Normal structure

- thyroid gland consists of two lateral lobes united by the isthmus
- isthmus usually covers the second, third and fourth tracheal rings
- normal adult thyroid weighs 20–25 g
- pyramidal lobe is often present and extends upward from the isthmus to the hyoid bone
- accessory thyroid tissue may be found in vicinity of thyroid
- thyroid is surrounded by thin fibrous capsule
- blood supply to thyroid gland is from paired superior thyroid arteries (from external carotid) and inferior thyroid arteries (from thyrocervical trunk)
- blood drains via a venous plexus in the fibrous capsule into the internal jugular and brachiocephalic veins
- lymphatic drainage is to deep cervical nodes and also to pretracheal and retrosternal nodes
- microscopy shows follicles containing colloid, separated by vascular connective tissue
- follicles are lined by single layer of cuboidal to columnar epithelial cells
- parafollicular cells (C cells) lie between follicles. These are neuroendocrine cells and produce calcitonin which is important in the regulation of calcium metabolism

Biopsy

FNA

- useful in patients with solitary thyroid nodule
- useful to diagnose papillary carcinoma, multinodular goitre, medullary carcinoma, Hashimoto's thyroiditis, lymphoma and anaplastic carcinoma
- useful to diagnose follicular neoplasm but cannot distinguish between follicular adenoma and follicular carcinoma which requires the demonstration of capsular and/or vascular invasion
- complications of thyroid FNA are rare
- occasionally extensive haemorrhage and necrosis of thyroid neoplasm may occur following FNA
- rarely there is compression of trachea due to haemorrhage

TRUCUT

- not much used
- higher complication rate than FNA, e.g. haematoma

Causes of solitary thyroid nodule

- cysts
- tumours
- dominant nodule in a multinodular goitre
- occasional Hashimoto's disease

Causes of diffuse thyroid swelling

- Graves' disease
- multinodular goitre
- Hashimoto's disease
- occasionally tumours

Developmental abnormalities of thyroid

(Figure 16.1)

THYROGLOSSAL DUCT CYSTS AND SINUSES
- remnants of thyroglossal duct may persist anywhere along course of original duct, from foramen caecum of tongue to level of thyroid gland
- most commonly there is a midline cyst
- usually in childhood, but occasionally in adults
- usual site is anterior neck below level of hyoid bone
- cysts or ducts are lined by respiratory or squamous epithelium
- thyroid tissue may be identified in this cyst or sinus tract
- malignancy is a rare complication, and is most commonly papillary carcinoma

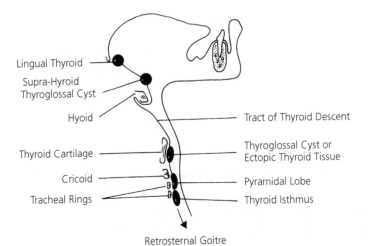

Lingual Thyroid

Supra-Hyroid Thyroglossal Cyst

Hyoid

Thyroid Cartilage

Cricoid

Tracheal Rings

Tract of Thyroid Descent

Thyroglossal Cyst or Ectopic Thyroid Tissue

Pyramidal Lobe

Thyroid Isthmus

Retrosternal Goitre

Figure 16.1 Schematic diagram to show the descent of the thyroid and the abnormalities which are found at different levels

ABSENCE HYPOPLASIA

- rare
- associated with hypothyroidism

DYSHORMONOGENETIC GOITRE

- goitre caused by enzyme defects in hormone synthesis
- usually inherited as autosomal recessive condition
- usually presents in childhood with hypothyroidism
- may be large goitre
- may be associated with congenital nerve deafness (Pendred's syndrome)
- microscopy shows intense hyperplasia with very cellular nodules. May be mistaken for malignancy

LATERAL ABERRANT THYROID

- presence of thyroid tissue lateral to jugular veins
- usually thyroid tissue is within lymph nodes
- these are usually metastases from an occult papillary thyroid carcinoma
- total thyroidectomy with careful sectioning may be required to demonstrate the primary neoplasm

LINGUAL THYROID

- relatively common
- characterised by thyroid tissue at base of tongue
- may have no thyroid at normal site and removal of the ectopic thyroid will render the patient athyroid
- rarely malignancy, especially papillary carcinoma develops

Infective thyroiditis

- rare
- bacterial thyroiditis may be seen in children, in elderly or in immuno-suppressed
- most common bacteria are staphylococci, streptococci, pneumococci and *Escherichia coli*
- thyroid involvement is usually a result of haematogenous spread
- microscopy shows neutrophil infiltration with abscess formation
- fungal and viral thyroiditis may occur in immunosuppressed
- tuberculosis may rarely affect the thyroid gland
- microscopy in tuberculosis shows caseating granulomatous inflammation

Subacute thyroiditis (de Quervain's thyroiditis)

- also known as granulomatous thyroiditis
- unknown aetiology, but many cases probably caused by virus
- systemic illness with fever, sore throat and tender thyromegaly
- may have transient thyrotoxicosis
- often get elevated ESR
- usually spontaneous recovery within weeks to months
- in late stages may get hypothyroidism

- microscopy initially shows infiltration of follicles by neutrophils and lymphocytes
- later macrophages and giant cells appear and granulomas form
- get fibrosis and follicular degeneration in late stages

Hashimoto's disease

- common cause of hypothyroidism in middle-aged females
- usually get diffuse goitre with or without nodularity
- autoimmune disease with antibodies to thyroid microsomal antigens, thyroglobulin, and TSH receptors

PATHOLOGY

- diffuse enlarged gland, sometimes with focal nodularity
- cut surface is lobulated or nodular with pale tan or grey-white colour
- microscopy shows infiltration by lymphocytes and plasma cells
- lymphoid follicles with germinal centres often occur
- thyroid follicular epithelial cells show Hurthle cell change with abundant eosinophilic cytoplasm
- in late stages there is destruction of follicles with marked fibrosis
- increased incidence of non-Hodgkin's B-cell lymphoma
- controversial whether there is an increased incidence of papillary thyroid carcinoma

Riedel's thyroiditis

- more common in females
- thyroid is replaced by fibrous tissue which extends outside the thyroid capsule to involve adjacent structures
- presents with hard mass in neck
- may be associated with dysphagia, dyspnoea or stridor
- clinically often mimics malignancy
- aetiology is unkown
- occasionally associated with mediastinal or retroperitoneal fibrosis, orbital sclerosis and sclerosing cholangitis
- may be a type of connective tissue disorder
- grossly thyroid is replaced by firm white, grey tissue which infiltrates surrounding structures
- microscopy shows fibrous tissue often with inflammatory component

Palpation thyroiditis

- result of repeated and over zealous thyroid palpation
- microscopy shows disruption of follicles with inflammatory reaction

Multinodular goitre

- also known as non-toxic goitre, simple goitre and colloid goitre
- benign non-inflammatory, non-neoplastic enlargement of thyroid gland
- may be endemic or may occur sporadically in non-endemic areas

AETIOLOGY AND PATHOGENESIS

Endemic goitre

- deficiency of iodine
- occurs in parts of world where water and soil have a low iodine content
- inborn errors of hormone synthesis and intake of natural goitrogens may also play a role
- diffuse enlargement of thyroid gland occurs at puberty representing early, compensatory stage of hyperplasia
- later get development of nodularity
- most patients are euthyroid at first due to compensatory hyperplasia but later may become hypothyroid

Sporadic goitre

- unknown cause
- occurs in non-endemic areas
- possible relative deficiency of enzymes involved in thyroid hormone synthesis
- female predominance
- almost always euthyroid
- may get dominant nodule, presenting as a solitary nodule

PATHOLOGY

- in early stages the gland is diffusely and smoothly enlarged
- later get a multinodular appearance
- haemorrhage and degeneration occurs with fibrous scarring and calcification
- may be one dominant nodule
- microscopy initially shows active hyperplastic follicles with tall epithelium and little colloid
- later involution occurs with enlarged follicles lined by flat epithelium and distended with colloid
- may be areas of haemorrhage, fibrosis and calcification

COMPLICATIONS OF MULTINODULAR GOITRE

Onset of thyrotoxicosis

- rare
- may occur after many years when one or more nodules become autonomous. This is known as toxic nodular goitre or Plummer's disease
- usually middle-aged to elderly females

Pressure symptoms

- stridor, dysphagia or dyspnoea may occur due to large size of goitre
- pressure symptoms may be secondary to haemorrhage into the gland

Malignant change

- conflicting opinions about risk of malignancy in multinodular goitre
- may be small risk of carcinoma, especially papillary carcinoma

Graves' disease

FEATURES

- diffuse thyroid enlargement
- hyperthyroidism
- eye signs (exophthalmos)
- less common features include pretibial myxoedema and thyroid acropachy
- usually females in third to fifth decades

AETIOLOGY AND PATHOGENESIS

- autoimmune disease
- association with HLA DR3
- thyroid autoantibodies
- thyroid stimulating antibodies act on TSH receptors on follicular epithelial cells. These mimic TSH action and result in hyperthyroidism
- Graves' disease and Hashimoto's disease are both autoimmune diseases and may coexist
- ophthalmopathy in Graves' disease may be due to specific immunoglobulins binding with eye muscle antigens

PATHOLOGY

- usually diffuse symmetrical enlargement of thyroid
- occasionally asymmetric with one or more nodules
- usually reddish or tan coloured
- microscopy shows small hyperplastic follicles lined by high columnar epithelium with decreased amounts of colloid
- may get small papillary projections
- may get aggregates of lymphoid cells

Neoplasms of thyroid

ADENOMAS

(Table 16.1)

- benign neoplasms
- more common in females
- usually present with solitary thyroid nodule
- almost always euthyroid although occasionally there is toxic adenoma producing hyperthyroidism

Follicular adenoma

- encapsulated
- composed of follicles of variable size. May get microfollicular or macrofollicular pattern
- surrounded by compressed 'normal' follicles
- haemorrhage and cystic change may occur
- subtypes include embryonal, fetal and solid adenomas, depending on the growth pattern. These subtypes have no clinical significance
- may get Hurthle cell change with abundant eosinophilic cytoplasm

Table 16.1 Classification of thyroid tumours

Epithelial		Non-epithelial
Benign	*Malignant*	Lymphomas
Follicular adenoma	Papillary carcinoma	Sarcomas
Atypical adenoma	Follicular carcinoma	
	Invasive	
	Encapsulated angioinvasive	
	Anaplastic carcinoma	
	Spindle cell	
	Giant cell	
	Mixed	
	Medullary carcinoma	
	Squamous carcinoma	
	Metastatic	

- must examine multiple histological sections to exclude capsular or vascular invasion
- if capsular or vascular invasion occurs then classified as minimally invasive follicular carcinoma

Papillary adenoma

- term now not used
- all considered to represent well differentiated papillary carcinoma

Atypical adenoma

- term not much used
- follicular adenomas with increased cellularity and cellular atypia
- benign behaviour
- criteria for demonstrating malignancy is same as for more usual follicular adenomas, i.e. capsular or vascular invasion

Hyalinising trabecular adenoma

- trabecular growth pattern in hyalinised stroma
- usually benign but may mimic papillary or medullary carcinoma
- occasionally malignant variants recently described

Thyroid cancer

PAPILLARY CARCINOMA

- commonest malignancy of thyroid gland
- tumour of thyroid follicular epithelial cells
- occurs in any age group with a female preponderance
- previous irradiation to the head and neck may predispose
- may be increased risk in Hashimoto's thyroiditis
- occasionally familial
- usually presents as a painless nodule in thyroid, sometimes with enlarged lymph nodes in the neck

Pathology

- often ill-defined, infiltrative tumours with hard consistency
- may be multifocal
- may be very small lesion and appear as a fibrous scar
- gritty on cutting
- cystic change may occur
- adjacent lymph nodes often involved
- microscopy shows papillary formations with fibrovascular cores
- may get solid or trabecular areas
- tumour cell nuclei are large with the chromatin around the periphery of the nucleus (orphan Annie nucleus)
- other nuclear features include crowding, overlapping and grooving
- psammoma bodies (laminated calcific spherules) often occur
- tumour may be multifocal
- often get marked stromal fibrosis
- may get cystic degeneration
- may see lymphatic permeation

VARIANTS OF PAPILLARY CARCINOMA

Occult papillary carcinoma

- less than 1 cm in size
- associated with marked sclerosis
- excellent prognosis, although occasionally get lymphatic invasion
- often discovered incidentally after thyroidectomy for unrelated disease
- may find in thyroidectomy specimen following metastatic papillary carcinoma in cervical node

Follicular variant

- follicular growth pattern but same nuclear characteristics as usual type

Diffuse sclerosing variant

- usually children and young adults
- aggressive behaviour
- extensive stromal fibrosis
- diffuse involvement of thyroid gland often with extensive lymphovascular permeation

Spread of papillary carcinoma

- usually via lymphatics to cervical nodes
- distant haematogenous metastases are rare and usually occur late in disease

Prognosis

- excellent prognosis
- prognosis worse over 40 years of age
- some studies suggest that males have a worse prognosis
- small tumours have a better prognosis
- extrathyroid extension worsens the prognosis
- distant metastases worsen prognosis whereas lymph node metastases have no effect on prognosis
- aneuploid tumours on flow cytometry may have a worse prognosis

FOLLICULAR CARCINOMA

- second commonest thyroid malignancy
- tumour of thyroid follicular epithelial cells
- peak incidence is 35–45 years
- more common in females
- may get minimally invasive and widely invasive forms

Pathology

- usually solitary
- minimally invasive tumours are well circumscribed and encapsulated
- widely invasive tumours are poorly encapsulated and may invade into surrounding tissues
- microscopy shows thyroid follicles of varying size
- cell nuclei are small and uniform without the features of papillary carcinoma
- may be focally or predominantly composed of Hurthle cells
- in follicular carcinoma get invasion of blood vessels and/or capsule
- minimally invasive follicular carcinoma cannot be distinguished from follicular adenoma on FNA

Spread

- metastases are usually blood-borne to lungs, skeleton, brain
- occasionally there is lymphatic spread to lymph nodes
- minimally invasive tumours have 10-year survival of 70–95%
- widely invasive variant has 10-year survival of 30–45%

ANAPLASTIC (UNDIFFERENTIATED) CARCINOMA

- usually elderly patients
- more common in females
- most aggressive thyroid carcinoma
- usually presents as rapidly growing hard mass in region of thyroid
- FNA is useful in diagnosis
- commonly local disease is so advanced that surgery is impossible and treatment is restricted to radiotherapy and chemotherapy

Pathology

- hard, infiltrative, necrotic tumour with areas of haemorrhage
- microscopy shows masses of spindle-shaped cells, giant cells or squamoid cells
- get frequent mitoses and marked nuclear pleomorphism
- may be difficult to distinguish from high grade lymphoma
- immunohistochemistry is useful in separation from lymphoma
- may get areas of typical papillary or follicular carcinoma suggesting that tumour has evolved from a well differentiated thyroid carcinoma

Spread

- clinical course is rapid and nodal and distant metastases are often present at presentation

Prognosis

- most present at advanced stage with involvement of adjacent neck structures
- mortality is almost 100% with a mean survival of less than 1 year

POORLY DIFFERENTIATED THYROID CARCINOMA

- clinically and morphologically intermediate between well differentiated thyroid carcinomas (papillary and follicular) and anaplastic carcinoma
- also known as insular carcinoma
- aggressive behaviour with development of metastases
- microscopy shows solid growth pattern with central necrosis

MEDULLARY CARCINOMA

- third commonest primary thyroid cancer
- tumour of parafollicular C cells
- often secrete calcitonin resulting in elevated serum calcitonin levels
- may be sporadic (80%) or familial (20%)
- familial tumours present at an earlier age than sporadic tumours and are often small and multiple
- familial tumours may be part of MEN-2 syndrome which consists of medullary carcinoma, parathyroid hyperplasia and phaeochromocytoma of the adrenal gland
- MEN-2B syndrome includes mucosal neuromas and Marfanoid habitus
- medullary carcinomas in these cases may be accompanied by and preceded by C-cell hyperplasia. This may occur at a very young age
- sporadic medullary carcinoma usually presents in middle-aged to elderly patients and is slightly more common in females
- FNA may be useful in diagnosis

Presentation

- painless mass in thyroid
- pressure symptoms
- screening MEN families
- diarrhoea
- elevated serum calcitonin
- may secrete other peptides, e.g. VIP, ACTH and prostaglandins

Pathology

- usually unencapsulated
- familial tumours are detected at an early age and may be extremely small
- familial tumours may be bilateral
- microscopy shows solid sheets of polygonal cells, often with a trabecular arrangement
- characteristically amyloid within stroma
- occasionally get spindle cell pattern
- Congo Red stain for amyloid is often positive
- immunohistochemically tumour cells are positive for CEA, calcitonin and chromogranin

Spread

- behaviour is unpredictable
- spread via lymphatics to neck nodes and via blood to lungs, bone and liver
- 5-year survival approximately 65% overall
- familial medullary carcinomas associated with MEN syndromes usually have a better prognosis as they are generally detected at an earlier stage

MALIGNANT LYMPHOMA

- must exclude metastatic spread before diagnosing primary thyroid lymphoma
- usually middle-aged to elderly females
- may occur in pre-existing Hashimoto's disease
- may present as rapidly enlarging thyroid mass and clinical differential diagnosis is anaplastic carcinoma
- most are non-Hodgkin's B-cell lymphoma
- may represent lymphomas of mucosa associated lymphoid tissue (MALTomas)
- may be high or low grade but usually confined to thyroid gland
- good prognosis
- FNA may be useful in diagnosis

MISCELLANEOUS THYROID TUMOURS

- teratomas, paragangliomas, various sarcomas and thymomas may rarely arise within the thyroid gland
- metastases may involve the thyroid gland, especially in disseminated carcinomatosis

PARATHYROID GLANDS

Normal structure

- yellow, brown in colour
- each gland usually weighs approximately 50 mg
- usually four in number, arranged in two pairs
- quite commonly there are supernumerary glands
- upper pair of glands are normally located at the middle third of the posterolateral border of the thyroid
- lower pair of glands are normally located near the lower thyroid poles, in close proximity to the inferior thyroid artery
- inferior glands arise from third pharyngeal pouch (which also forms the thymus)
- superior glands arise from fourth pharyngeal pouch
- lower glands may migrate with thymus into upper mediastinum
- parathyroid glands synthesise and secrete parathyroid hormone (PTH) which is important in calcium metabolism

HISTOLOGY

- glands are surrounded by thin fibrous capsule
- epithelial component comprises two cell types, the chief cells and the oxyphil cells
- also get stromal fat between epithelial cells
- chief cells contain pale cytoplasm and oxyphil cells contain eosinophilic cytoplasm

Primary hyperparathyroidism

- most common cause of hypercalcaemia
- usually sporadic but occasionally familial
- renal stones

- bone disease (osteitis fibrosa cystica)
- peptic ulcer disease
- pancreatitis
- psychiatric disorders and muscle weakness
- most common cause of primary hyperparathyroidism is single adenoma followed by hyperplasia involving all four glands. Rarely caused by double adenoma or parathyroid carcinoma
- part of MEN syndromes (types I and II)

BIOCHEMISTRY

- raised serum calcium and PTH
- decreased serum phosphate

Parathyroid adenoma

- most common cause of primary hyperparathyroidism
- more frequently involves lower pair of parathyroids
- may occur in ectopic parathyroids
- aetiology unknown (rarely associated with previous irradiation)
- more common in women
- very occasionally more than one gland is involved

PATHOLOGY

- may range in size from 60 mg to 300 g (commonly 200–1000 mg)
- usually soft and pliable
- tan to orange in colour
- surrounded by a thin fibrous capsule
- well circumscribed
- cells arranged in varying patterns, including solid, trabecular, alveolar and follicular
- may be composed of chief cells, oxyphil cells or transitional cells
- often get mixture of cell types
- less stromal fat compared to normal parathyroid tissue
- rim of compressed uninvolved parathyroid tissue may be present around periphery of adenoma
- may get variation of nuclear size with nuclear pleomorphism but does not indicate malignancy
- may get cystic degeneration
- massive necrosis may result in hypercalcaemic crisis

Parathyroid hyperplasia

- second commonest cause of primary hyperparathyroidism
- all four glands enlarged
- may be part of MEN syndrome
- may get chief cell hyperplasia or less commonly clear cell hyperplasia

PATHOLOGY

- all four glands enlarged but may be asymmetrical enlargement
- ectopic glands also become enlarged

- yellow, tan colour
- microscopically may affect glands focally
- usually composed of sheets of chief cells
- decreased stromal fat cells
- may get water clear cell hyperplasia (cells with abundant clear cytoplasm)
- may get cystic degeneration

Parathyroid carcinoma

- rare
- sex ratio is equal
- causes very high serum calcium
- often palpable mass in neck
- only rarely non-functional

PATHOLOGY

- firm, infiltrating mass
- usually thick fibrous capsule and thick trabeculae of fibrous tissue
- most are composed of chief cells
- may see capsular, vascular and neural invasion
- usually progresses slowly
- spread to lymph nodes, bone and lung

Prognosis

- poor
- death often caused by uncontrollable hypercalcaemia
- redevelopment of hypercalcaemia may be first sign of tumour recurrence or metastasis

Multiple endocrine neoplasia (MEN) syndromes

MEN-1 (WERMER'S SYNDROME)

- autosomal dominant inheritance
- associated with pituitary and pancreatic islet cell adenomas
- usually parathyroid hyperplasia but occasionally adenomas
- MEN-1 gene has been localised to chromosome 11

MEN-2

- autosomal dominant inheritance
- MEN-2 gene has been localised to chromosome 10

MEN-2A (SIPPLE'S SYNDROME)

- medullary thyroid carcinoma, phaeochromocytoma, parathyroid hyperplasia

MEN-2B (GORLIN'S SYNDROME)

- usually do not get parathyroid disease. Marfanoid habitas, mucosal neuromas and intestinal ganglioneuromatosis

Secondary hyperparathyroidism

- result of prolonged lowering of serum calcium level
- causes include malabsorption, vitamin D deficiency and chronic renal failure
- microscopically similar to chief cell hyperplasia

Tertiary hyperparathyroidism

- cases of secondary hyperparathyroidism who later develop hypercalcaemia
- autonomous parathyroid hyperfunction
- most commonly seen after successful renal transplantation
- microscopy shows diffuse hyperplasia

Hypoparathyroidism

- causes hypocalcaemia
- tetany and carpopedal spasm
- changes in basal ganglia of brain, in teeth and in nails
- usually occurs after thyroid or parathyroid surgery

Parathyroid cysts

- rare
- may develop on basis of cystic degeneration in hyperplastic or adenomatous gland
- associated with hyperparathyroidism or may be non-functional
- usually located in region of lower pair of parathyroids
- may also be found in upper neck or mediastinum, within thymus
- cyst wall is lined by a single layer of chief cells
- FNA yields clear fluid in which PTH can be demonstrated

ADRENAL GLANDS

Normal structure

- normally measure 5 cm in maximum diameter
- approximately 5 g in weight
- yellow in colour
- right adrenal is pyramidal shaped
- left adrenal is crescentic shaped
- each adrenal is supplied by three arteries (from the aorta, phrenic and renal arteries)
- each adrenal is drained by one vein: the right side drains into the inferior vena cava and the left side into the renal vein

HISTOLOGY
- composed of outer cortex and inner medulla

Cortex

- outer zona glomerulosa (ZG)
- middle zona fasciculata (ZF)
- inner zona reticularis (ZR)
- ZG – synthesis of mineralocorticoid aldosterone
- ZF and ZR – synthesis of cortisol and sex hormones

Medulla

- ectodermal origin – from the neural crest
- part of sympathetic nervous system
- composed of neuroendocrine cells which synthesise and secrete adrenaline and noradrenaline

Adrenal incidentalomas

- small adrenal lesion identified during routine radiological CT scan
- 1% of patients have 'incidentaloma'
- most are benign non-functioning cortical adenomas
- small benign incidental adrenal adenomas are often identified at post-mortem

Adrenal cortex

- primary lesions of adrenal cortex may be non-functional or may produce excess cortisol (Cushing's syndrome), aldosterone (hyperaldosteronism) or androgens and oestrogens
- primary lesions of the adrenal cortex include hyperplasia, adenoma and carcinoma

CUSHING'S SYNDROME

Clinical features

- truncal obesity
- muscle weakness
- osteoporosis
- electrolyte imbalance
- hypertension
- diabetes

Causes

- Cushing's disease is due to excess production of ACTH by the pituitary. This is usually due to a pituitary adenoma which is often very small (microadenoma)
- adrenal adenoma
- adrenal carcinoma
- ectopic ACTH production, e.g. oat cell carcinoma of lung, pancreatic tumour
- drugs, e.g. steroids or ACTH

Adrenal gland in Cushing's disease

- both adrenals are increased in size, weighing up to 12 g each
- grossly diffuse or nodular hyperplasia

- microscopy shows thickening of cortex in diffuse or nodular pattern with sheets of cells of ZR or ZF pattern
- a similar picture is seen in Cushing's syndrome due to ectopic ACTH production
- usual treatment is trans-sphenoidal pituitary surgery
- bilateral adrenalectomy may be followed by Nelson's syndrome (skin pigmentation with enlarging pituitary tumour)

Adrenal adenomas associated with Cushing's syndrome

- usually weigh less than 50 g, although occasionally heavier
- usually 2–4 cm in size
- yellow/brown in colour
- occasionally areas of haemorrhage
- adjacent cortex is atrophied
- contralateral adrenal is atrophied
- microscopy shows cells with pale staining cytoplasm in clusters and columns
- rarely may get black adenomas with black cut surface. This is due to accumulation of lipofuscin within cell cytoplasm

ADRENAL CARCINOMA

- rare
- usually larger than adenomas
- may present with abdominal mass
- most are non-functioning but may be associated with Cushing's syndrome
- grossly usually bulky bosselated tumours with a yellow, brown cut surface
- haemorrhage and necrosis are common
- most weigh over 100 g
- microscopy shows sheets of cells with invasion of adjacent structures and of blood vessels
- marked nuclear pleomorphism frequent
- often high mitotic rate
- others may be better differentiated and may be difficult to distinguish from adenomas
- flow cytometry to demonstrate DNA aneuploidy may be useful to distinguish carcinoma from adenoma
- tumour spread is usually via blood to lungs and liver

HYPERALDOSTERONISM

Primary

- Conn's syndrome (due to excess production of aldosterone by adrenal lesion and associated with low plasma renin)

Secondary

- excess production of renin and angiotensin II (renal artery stenosis, liver cirrhosis, heart failure, nephrotic syndrome) results in increased production of aldosterone

Conn's syndrome

- rare cause of secondary hypertension
- usually age 30–40 years

Causes

- adrenal adenoma is most common cause
- other causes include adrenocortical hyperplasia and adrenal carcinoma

ADRENAL HYPERPLASIA

- adrenal glands are increased in weight
- cause is unknown
- microscopy shows hyperplasia of ZG cells

ADRENAL ADENOMA

- often small with most being less than 2–3 cm
- may be difficult to detect
- yellow in colour
- microscopy shows clusters of clear or compact cells

ADRENAL CARCINOMA

- very rare cause of Conn's syndrome
- often yellow cut surface with areas of haemorrhage or necrosis
- microscopically similar to adrenal carcinomas described in association with Cushing's syndrome

EXCESS PRODUCTION OF SEX STEROID HORMONES

Causes

- congenital due to enzyme defect
- adrenal adenoma
- adrenal carcinoma

Congenital adrenal hyperplasia

- equal frequency in males and females
- autosomal recessive condition
- deficiency of enzyme 21-hydroxylase which results in decreased cortisol
- there is an increase in intermediate products which usually result in virilisation
- grossly adrenal glands are enlarged
- microscopy shows accumulation of cells with clear cytoplasm

Adrenal adenoma

- more often causes virilisation
- occasionally causes feminisation
- variable size but commonly large
- histological appearance similar to other adrenal adenomas

Adrenal carcinoma

- rare cause of virilisation or feminisation
- microscopically similar to other adrenal cortical carcinomas

HYPOFUNCTION OF ADRENAL CORTEX

Acute hypofunction

- adrenal haemorrhage (neonate)
- meningococcal septicaemia may result in bleeding into adrenals (Waterhouse-Friderichsen syndrome)
- anticoagulant therapy may result in bleeding into adrenals
- postpartum bleeding
- chest, abdominal trauma
- renal surgery

Chronic hypofunction (Addison's disease)

- idiopathic
- autoimmune. In this type of adrenal insufficiency lymphocytic infiltration of adrenal cortex and circulating adrenal antibodies occur
- widespread fungal infection, e.g. in association with AIDS
- tuberculosis
- metastastic tumour, most commonly from breast or lung
- sarcoidosis
- amyloid
- chronic adrenal cortical insufficiency may also be secondary to diseases of the hypothalamic pituitary axis, e.g. tumour, irradiation, infarction

Adrenal medulla

ADRENAL MEDULLARY HYPERPLASIA

- associated with MEN syndrome
- precursor of phaeochromocytoma
- medullary hyperplasia may be associated with phaeochromocytoma
- usually bilateral
- difficult to diagnose histologically and may need morphometric measurements

TUMOURS OF ADRENAL MEDULLA

Phaeochromocytoma

- rare cause of secondary hypertension
- occurs sporadically or in familial form which may be associated with MEN-2 syndrome
- most common in fourth and fifth decades, although familial cases occur at a younger age
- familial tumours may be bilateral
- also associated with neurofibromatosis and von Hippel-Lindau syndrome
- secrete catecholamines noradrenaline and adrenaline
- similar tumours may occur in an extra-adrenal location and are termed paragangliomas
- 10% of patients have bilateral tumours
- 10% of patients have extra-adrenal tumours

Pathology
- most range in size from 2 to 10 cm and most weigh 50–100 g
- usually grey in colour often with haemorrhagic areas
- turn dark brown in dichromate solution

- cystic degeneration
- microscopy shows clusters of tumour cells with granular cytoplasm separated by vascular stroma
- immunochemically there is positive staining for neuroendocrine markers
- cellular pleomorphism and vascular invasion can occur in benign lesions
- no reliable criteria of malignancy except presence of metastases
- on electron microscopy there are adrenaline and noradrenaline granules

Prognosis
- most adrenal lesions are benign
- incidence of malignancy is approximately 5%
- extra-adrenal paragangliomas are more likely to be malignant
- only reliable criterion of malignancy is metastasis
- most frequent sites of metastases are liver, lymph nodes, lungs and bone

Neuroblastomas

- 80% occur under age 5 years
- no sex difference
- often present with abdominal mass
- may also occur in extra-adrenal sites, especially along the sympathetic chain
- secrete catecholamines and breakdown products (VMA) may be found in urine
- one of 'small blue cell' tumours of childhood (also includes lymphoma, rhabdomyosarcoma, Ewing's sarcoma)
- some cases are familial
- originates from sympathetic nervous system

Pathology
- usually soft lobular tumours with areas of haemorrhage and necrosis
- microscopically composed of small round cells with hyperchromatic nuclei and little cytoplasm
- get fibrovascular stroma or may get neurofibrillary material in this stroma
- may be sheeted appearance or may have rosette formation
- marked rosette formation may imply a better prognosis
- positive immunohistochemical staining for neuron-specific enolase (NSE)
- electron microscopy shows dense-core neuroendocrine granules
- tumour spread to liver, lymph nodes, lung and bone

Prognosis
- recent improvement in prognosis with combination treatment
- good prognostic features include young age (<1 year), tumour in neck or thorax, early stage and certain histological features
- amplification of N-myc oncogene associated with advanced stage tumours and more aggressive behaviour
- occasionally spontaneous regression occurs

Ganglioneuroblastoma

- rare
- may arise in adrenal medulla or extra-adrenal sites
- usually older age group than neuroblastoma
- better prognosis than neuroblastoma
- secretes catecholamines and VMA may be found in urine
- microscopy shows mature ganglion cells with areas of typical neuroblastoma
- composite or diffuse type

Ganglioneuroma

- may arise at any age
- only rarely found in adrenal gland
- more commonly found in posterior mediastinum or retroperitoneum
- benign
- more common in females
- firm white, grey capsulated mass
- microscopy shows ganglion cells and Schwann cells
- immunohistochemically get positive staining for S-100 protein

MYELOLIPOMA OF THE ADRENAL

- rare
- non-functioning
- occasionally occurs outside adrenal
- benign
- occasionally bilateral and multifocal
- usually asymptomatic
- microscopy shows mixture of adipose tissue and bone marrow elements

ADRENAL METASTATIC DISEASE

- adrenals are common site of metastatic tumour
- found commonly at post-mortem but rarely detected ante-mortem
- lung and breast are most common primary sites
- bilateral involvement may result in adrenal cortical insufficiency (Addison's disease)

MISCELLANEOUS TUMOURS OF ADRENAL

- rare primary tumours described in the adrenal include malignant lymphoma, haemangioma, leiomyoma, schwannoma, angiosarcoma and leiomyosarcoma

The skin

17

NORMAL STRUCTURE

Epidermis

- ectodermal origin
- barrier to mechanical damage and invasion by microorganisms
- histologically composed of keratinising stratified squamous epithelium
- basal cell layer lies on basement membrane and gives rise to cells of upper layers
- epithelium contains occasional melanocytes and Langerhan's cells
- surface is covered by acellular keratin
- rete pegs project downward into dermis

Dermis

- lies beneath epidermis
- composed of connective tissues with collagen and elastic fibres
- composed of papillary dermis (between rete pegs of epidermis) and reticular dermis (deep to papillary dermis)
- contains skin appendage structures
- these include eccrine and apocrine sweat glands and sebaceous glands
- also includes hair follicles

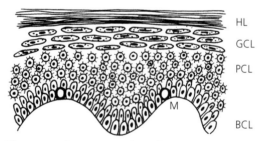

Figure 17.1 Diagrammatic representation of normal epidermis. HL = Horny layer; GCL = granular cell layer; PCL = prickle cell layer; BCL = basal cell layer; M = melanocyte

SKIN INFECTIONS

Bacterial

IMPETIGO

- usually in children
- caused by streptococci or staphylococci
- vesicles and bullae
- microscopy shows collections of neutrophils within intraepidermal vesicles

FOLLICULITIS

- caused by staphylococcal infection of hair follicles
- carbuncle occurs when several adjacent hair follicles involved

SCALDED SKIN SYNDROME

- occurs in children
- staphylococcal infection
- microscopy shows collections of neutrophils within epidermis

ERYSIPELAS

- acute cellulitis of skin caused by group A streptococci

Viral

VERRUCA VULGARIS

- common wart
- probably due to infection by human papilloma virus (HPV) types 1,2,4,26,29
- occurs on hands and face
- elevated wart-like lesion
- microscopy shows hyperplasia and hyperkeratosis of epithelium
- large vacuolated epithelial cells indicative of viral infection
- may see viral inclusion bodies

VERRUCA PLANA

- slightly elevated or flat, smooth papules
- face and hands are most commonly affected
- may be caused by HPV infection
- microscopy shows hyperplasia and hyperkeratosis of epidermis

HERPES SIMPLEX

- type I causes orofacial disease
- type II causes genital warts
- in type I primary infection occurs in childhood
- type II is usually sexually transmitted
- recurrent infections of type I manifest as cold sores

CONDYLOMATA ACUMINATA

- genital warts
- sexually transmitted
- exophytic lesions
- usually multiple
- occur in perineum, vulva, cervix, penis
- caused by HPV (most commonly types 6 + 11)
- microscopy shows hyperplasia of epidermis
- superficial vacuolated cells known as koilocytes are present

GIANT CONDYLOMATA OF BUSCHKE AND LOEWENSTEIN

- large genital warts
- viral origin (usually HPV type 6)
- may become malignant and transform into squamous carcinoma
- usually occur on penis and vulva

MOLLUSCUM CONTAGIOSUM

- caused by pox virus
- may be multiple
- most common in children
- grossly appearance is of dome-shaped pink papule with central punctum
- microscopy shows thickened epidermis
- squamous cells contain eosinophilic viral inclusion bodies (molluscum bodies)
- disappear spontaneously in a few months
- common in AIDS patients where may get hundreds of lesions

SKIN CYSTS

Epidermal cyst

- occur most commonly on face, scalp, neck and trunk
- most occur spontaneously, although occasionally arise on basis of trauma
- in Gardner's syndrome, may get multiple cysts
- grossly there is thin walled cyst containing cheesy material
- microscopically wall is composed of true epidermis
- cyst contains laminated keratin
- development of squamous carcinoma is a rare event

Pilar cysts (trichilemmal cysts)

- occur on scalp
- usually spontaneous but may be autosomal dominant pattern of inheritance
- may be multiple
- microscopically lined by squamous epithelium similar to that lining hair follicle

Dermoid cysts

- occur most commonly in head and neck region
- due to sequestration of epidermis into dermis around lines of embryological closure
- microscopically similar to epidermal cysts but contains skin appendage structures in the wall

Pilonidal sinus

- occurs in intergluteal fold
- most commonly occurs in young males
- presents with pain and discharge
- lined by squamous epithelium on surface and granulation tissue more deeply
- foreign body reaction to hair shaft material
- superimposed infection and abscess may occur

Ganglion

- subcutaneous cystic swelling
- occurs in close vicinity of joint or tendon sheath
- may be uniloculated or multiloculated
- occurs most commonly in region of wrist and foot
- microscopy shows fibrous wall with no epithelial lining

BENIGN TUMOURS OF THE EPIDERMIS

Skin tag (fibroepithelial polyp)

- common
- pedunculated lesion occurring most commonly on neck, axilla and trunk
- microscopy shows fibrovascular core with squamous epithelial lining

Basal cell papilloma (seborrhoeic keratosis)

- common benign tumour
- may be multiple
- most commonly on trunk, face and extremities
- usually middle-aged and elderly
- raised pigmented lesions which appear 'stuck on' to skin
- microscopy shows hyperkeratosis, acanthosis and papillomatosis with proliferation of basal cells
- keratin horn cysts
- very rarely, if multiple, may indicate internal malignancy

Keratoacanthoma

- may be solitary or multiple
- can be confused with squamous cell carcinoma clinically and microscopically

- usually rapid growth with spontaneous involution
- site of predilection is sun-exposed areas
- more common in females
- increased incidence in immunosuppressed patients
- may also occur in Muir-Torre syndrome (sebaceous neoplasms, keratoacanthomas, visceral malignancy)
- may be viral aetiology
- gross appearance is of dome-shaped nodule with central keratin-filled crater
- microscopy shows keratin-filled invagination
- lesion is symmetrical
- invagination of surface squamous epithelium pushes into dermis
- microscopically extremely difficult to distinguish from early invasive, well differentiated squamous carcinoma

PREMALIGNANT LESIONS OF EPIDERMIS

Solar keratosis (actinic/senile keratosis)

- caused by sun exposure
- usually multiple lesions in sun-exposed areas
- grossly scaly, erythematous lesions
- may transform into squamous carcinoma
- squamous carcinomas which arise in solar keratosis have good prognosis and do not metastasise
- microscopy shows hyperkeratosis
- squamous epithelium is atrophic with dysplasia of the basal cell layers
- solar (actinic) damage is present in the dermis

Bowen's disease

- *in situ* (intraepidermal) squamous cell carcinoma
- usually solitary
- may occur on sun-exposed or unexposed skin
- may occur secondary to ingestion of arsenic
- lesions of penis are referred to as erythroplasia of Queyrat
- grossly red, scaly raised plaque
- microscopy shows full thickness dysplasia of squamous epithelial cells
- over 20 years infiltrating squamous carcinoma develops in approximately 5% of patients
- histologically must examine multiple levels to exclude invasive malignancy

MALIGNANT TUMOURS OF THE EPIDERMIS

Squamous cell carcinoma (epidermoid carcinoma)

- usually middle-aged to elderly patients
- younger in countries such as Australia
- incidence is increasing

- occurs *de novo* or may be secondary to actinic keratosis, Bowen's disease, radiation injury, scars, chronic ulceration or sinus formation, chemical contact, e.g. organic hydrocarbons, ingestion of arsenic, immunosuppression (immuno-suppressed patients, e.g. renal transplant patients have increased incidence of squamous carcinoma)
- xeroderma pigmentosa is an autosomal recessive condition characterised by a markedly increased risk of cutaneous squamous cell carcinoma. There is increased susceptibility to sunlight and an impaired ability to repair DNA damage by UV light
- squamous carcinoma is most common on exposed parts of skin, e.g. face, but can occur anywhere
- clinically usually presents as an ulcerated lesion which fails to heal and which may bleed
- regional lymph nodes may be enlarged
- microscopy shows dysplasia of squamous epithelium with tongues of squamous cells breaching basement membrane and invading the dermis
- tumour cells produce keratin (keratin pearls) if well differentiated
- spindle cell carcinoma is a poorly differentiated variant
- a pseudoglandular pattern may occur where acantholysis of tumour cells occurs. This variant may be mistaken for adenocarcinoma
- verrucous carcinoma is a slow growing variant which has a fungating growth pattern. This variant rarely metastasises

SPREAD

- TNM system (Table 17.1)
- squamous carcinomas arising in chronic ulcers, burns and radiated areas are more likely to metastasise
- tumours arising in sun-damaged skin have a low propensity to metastasise
- tumours on pinna, lip, vulva and penis are more aggressive

Table 17.1 TNM staging system for squamous carcinoma of the skin

Stage	Extent of disease
Tis	Preinvasive carcinoma (carcinoma-*in-situ*)
T0	No evidence of primary tumour
T1	Tumour 2 cm or less in its largest dimension, strictly superficial or exophytic
T2	Tumour more than 2 cm but not more than 5 cm in its largest dimension or with minimal infiltration of the dermis, irrespective of size
T3	Tumour more than 5 cm in its largest dimension or with deep infiltration of the dermis, irrespective of size
T4	Tumour with extension to other structures such as cartilage, muscle or bone
N0	No evidence of regional lymph node involvement
N1	Evidence of involvement of movable ipsilateral regional lymph nodes
N2	Evidence of involvement of movable contralateral or bilateral regional lymph nodes
N3	Evidence of involvement of fixed regional lymph nodes
M0	No evidence of distant metastases
M1	Evidence of distant metastases

Basal cell carcinoma

- commonest malignant skin tumour
- usually occur in adults, although occasionally in children
- most common on face
- may be multiple lesions
- exposure to sunlight predisposes
- xeroderma pigmentosa predisposes
- arsenic ingestion may predispose, although squamous carcinomas more common
- radiation may predispose
- rarely basal cell naevus syndrome and Bazex syndrome may predispose
- cell of origin is basal cell of epidermis
- grossly often raised waxy nodule with tiny vessels on surface
- umbilication of surface
- ulcer with rolled pearly edges (rodent ulcer)
- occasionally pigmented or cystic lesions
- microscopy shows islands of ovoid basaloid cells with dark nuclei and little cytoplasm
- typically palisading around edge of tumour cell islands
- stroma is fibrous
- cystic degeneration
- pigmentation
- tumours may be multifocal
- can get sclerosing (morphoeic) type with dense fibrous stroma
- occasionally basosquamous carcinomas (areas of typical basal cell and squamous cell carcinoma)

SPREAD

- locally invasive
- metastases are very rare but are more common in basosquamous carcinoma
- local recurrence is common in multifocal and sclerosing types
- recurrence rate high unless clear resection margins

MELANOCYTIC LESIONS

- cutaneous melanocytes arise in the neural crest and migrate to the basal cell layer of the epidermis
- melanocytes produce melanin pigment

Benign melanocytic lesions

(Figure 17.2)

JUNCTIONAL NAEVUS

- usually appear in adolescence and early adulthood
- flat lesions which may or may not be pigmented
- microscopy shows collections of melanocytes at dermal epidermal junction
- evolve into compound and dermal naevi
- rarely become malignant

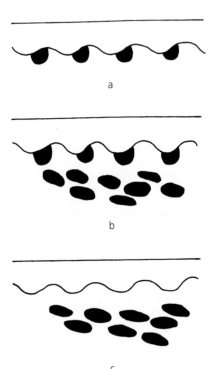

Figure 17.2 Schematic representation of the three main types of naevus.
a = junctional; *b* = compound; *c* = intradermal (see text)

COMPOUND NAEVUS

- slightly older age group than junctional naevus
- microscopy shows junctional component and nests of cells within the dermis
- rarely become malignant

INTRADERMAL NAEVUS

- usually in adults
- flat, raised, nodular or pedunculated
- pigmented or non-pigmented
- microscopically no junctional activity with naevus cells only in the dermis
- marked neural differentiation
- virtually never become malignant

SPITZ NAEVUS

- also known as benign juvenile melanoma
- occurs in adults and children
- benign behaviour

- usually solitary lesion
- most common in lower extremities and face
- grossly usually pink in colour because of sparsity of melanin pigment
- microscopically usually compound or intradermal naevus with spindle-shaped and epithelioid melanocytes
- nuclear pleomorphism and mitotic figures are common resulting in simulation of a malignant melanoma
- other histological features include oedema, colloid bodies, vascular ectasia and artefactual clefts above naevus cells at dermal–epidermal junction

HALO NAEVUS

- pigmented naevus surrounded by an area of skin depigmentation or halo
- lesion usually undergoes spontaneous evolution
- benign
- microscopy shows compound or intradermal naevus with marked surrounding lymphocytic infiltrate

BLUE NAEVUS

- dome-shaped nodule which is blue or blue-black in colour
- occurs most commonly on hands, feet, neck and arms
- microscopically lesion is present in dermis or subcutaneous fat with little or no junctional component
- lesion is composed of long slender spindle-shaped melanocytes with abundant melanin
- many pigmented melanophages are also present
- rarely get malignant forms

CONGENITAL NAEVUS

- found in approximately 1% of newborn infants
- variable in size but may be large
- if greater than 20 cm in diameter, referred to as giant melanocytic naevus
- melanotic or amelanotic
- may be covered with hair
- grossly may have the distribution of a garment
- giant naevi should be excised as soon as possible because of risk of malignant transformation
- lesser risk of malignancy in smaller naevi
- microscopically compound or intradermal naevus
- melanocytes extend deeply into subcutaneous fat and are aggregated around skin appendage structures

DYSPLASTIC NAEVUS

- may be sporadic or familial
- increased risk of malignant melanoma
- in familial type have family history of atypical moles and melanomas
- usually multiple naevi but may get solitary lesions
- most commonly found on trunk
- clinically often have irregular border and irregular pigmentation and are often large in size

- microscopy shows proliferation of atypical melanocytes at dermal–epidermal junction
- melanocytes are organised in a lentiginous pattern
- inflammatory response and fusion of adjacent rete ridges

Cutaneous malignant melanoma

- increasing incidence in developed countries
- highest incidence in Queensland (40/100 000)
- more common in fair-skinned persons
- average age is 50 years
- occasionally multiple, especially with dysplastic naevus syndrome
- in women the commonest site is the legs
- in men the commonest site is the back

AETIOLOGY

UV sunlight

- exposure to sunlight, especially when fair-skinned

Pre-existing naevus

- found in approximately 20% of melanomas
- junctional and compound naevi are more likely to become malignant, especially giant congenital naevi
- dysplastic naevi, especially the familial type, are more likely to become malignant

Xeroderma pigmentosa

- in this condition there is an increased risk of cutaneous malignant melanoma, squamous carcinoma and basal cell carcinoma

CHANGES SUGGESTIVE OF MALIGNANT TRANSFORMATION

Table 17.2 Changes in a mole which suggest malignant transformation (adapted from Davis 1982)

Parameter	Change
Size	Enlargement. Malignant melanoma tends to enlarge gradually over several months
Outline	Becomes irregular (indented and notched)
Colour	Becomes darker, then there is irregularity of colour with various shades of brown, black, pink, etc
Elevation	Becomes thicker and nodular
Surface	Normal skin markings are lost
Surroundings	Lumps in surrounding tissue may be satellite tumours
Symptoms	Tingling, itch, serous discharge, recurrent minor bleeding

TYPES OF CUTANEOUS MALIGNANT MELANOMA

- there are four main types of cutaneous malignant melanoma

Lentigo maligna melanoma

- develops from lentigo maligna (malignant melanoma *in situ*)
- usually blue/black in colour
- occurs on face and sun-exposed skin
- elderly patients
- usually good prognosis as tend to be superficial lesions
- 5-year survival is approximately 90%
- microscopy shows diffuse replacement of basal cell layer of epidermis by atypical melanocytes
- in lentigo maligna atypical melanocytes are confined to dermal–epidermal junction
- in lentigo maligna melanoma there is dermal invasion by atypical melanocytes
- overlying epidermis is atrophic

Superficial spreading malignant melanoma

- most common type of cutaneous malignant melanoma
- may develop from superficial spreading melanoma *in situ*
- grossly pigmented lesion, often with irregular edge
- may rarely bleed or ulcerate
- microscopy shows proliferation of atypical melanocytes at dermal epidermal junction with pronounced pagetoid spread into epidermis
- penetration into dermis is present in invasive melanoma
- with *in situ* superficial spreading melanoma, only radial (horizontal) growth phase is present with no evidence of dermal infiltration (vertical growth phase)
- prognosis depends on Breslow depth of invasion (see p. 263)

Nodular malignant melanoma

- second commonest type of cutaneous melanoma
- nodular lump in skin
- melanotic or amelanotic
- may present with itch and bleeding due to surface ulceration
- microscopy shows vertical growth pattern with little or no radial growth
- prognosis depends on Breslow depth of invasion
- prognosis is poor because of pronounced vertical growth

Acral lentiginous malignant melanoma

- occurs on soles and palms and in ungal and subungal regions
- occurs in areas where the epidermis is thick
- poor prognosis

Rare varieties of cutaneous malignant melanoma

- desmoplastic melanoma. There is a marked fibroblastic reaction. Prognosis is poor
- neurotrophic melanoma. This shows a tendency to infiltrate cutaneous and subcutaneous nerves. Prognosis is poor

SPREAD OF CUTANEOUS MALIGNANT MELANOMA

- to regional lymph nodes
- locally within skin and subcutaneous tissue
- later blood spread to liver, bones, lungs and brain

CLINICAL STAGES

Table 17.3   Staging of malignant melanoma (adapted from Adam and Efron 1983)

Stage I
Localized melanoma, without metastasis to distant or regional nodes
Multiple primary melanomas
Locally recurrent melanoma within 4 cm of the primary site

Stage II
Metastasis limited to regional lymph nodes
Primary melanoma present or removed with simultaneous metastasis
Primary melanoma controlled with subsequent metastasis
Locally recurrent melanoma with metastasis
In-transit metastasis beyond 4 cm from the primary site

Stage III
Disseminated melanoma
Visceral and/or multiple lymphatic metastases
Multiple cutaneous and/or subcutaneous metastases

PROGNOSIS

- depends largely on Breslow depth of invasion (Table 17.4) (measured from granular cell layer of epidermis to deepest tumour cell). Melanomas less than 0.76 mm thick have a good prognosis, 0.76–1.5 mm have an intermediate prognosis and greater than 1.5 mm have a poor prognosis
- Clark classification (Figure 17.3)
- prognosis also depends on stage

Table 17.4   Prognosis of stage I malignant melanoma according to tumour thickness (Koh 1991)

Tumour thickness (mm)	5-year survival (%)
<0.75	96
0.76–1.49	87
1.5–2.49	75
2.5–3.99	66
>4.0	47

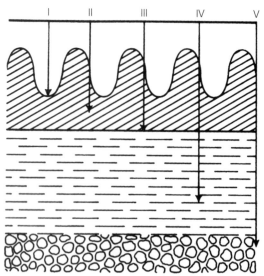

Figure 17.3 The Clark level of invasion of malignant melanoma.
I = Intraepidermal; II = papillary dermis; III = interface between papillary and reticular dermis; IV = reticular dermis; V = subcutaneous fat

- women have a better prognosis than men
- age under 50 years have a better prognosis
- tumour on back, neck, arms, palms, soles have a worse prognosis
- very rarely spontaneous regression of malignant melanoma

VASCULAR LESIONS OF SKIN

Naevus flammeus

- common birth mark, occurring in as many as 50% of infants
- includes salmon patch and port-wine stain
- salmon patch tends to involute with time, whereas port-wine stain shows no tendency to regress
- microscopy shows dilatation of dermal vessels
- port-wine stain may be associated with vascular malformations of the meninges, brain or retina in the Sturge-Weber syndrome

Spider naevus

- common acquired lesions
- microscopy shows central arteriole with radiating capillaries
- common in pregnancy, liver failure and hyperthyroidism

Capillary haemangioma

- common
- also known as strawberry naevus or juvenile haemangioma
- presents at birth or shortly afterwards
- elevated purple, red macule
- occurs most commonly in head and neck region
- tend to regress over period of months to years
- microscopy shows multilobulated tumour composed of closely packed capillary channels

Cavernous haemangioma

- occurs in children and may be present at birth
- occurs most commonly in head and neck region
- larger, deeper and less well circumscribed than capillary haemangioma
- little tendency to regress
- may be associated with Mafucci's syndrome
- microscopy shows dilated thin walled vessels lined by flat endothelial cells
- may get combined capillary and cavernous haemangioma

Pyogenic granuloma (lobular capillary haemangioma)

- common
- variant of capillary haemangioma
- can occur at any age
- predilection for fingers and head and neck area
- solitary, rapidly growing, ulcerated, polypoid blue-red nodule
- may have a history of trauma
- microscopically comprises a capillary haemangioma with a marked inflammatory response
- resembles granulation tissue

Angiolymphoid hyperplasia with eosinophilia (histiocytoid haemangioma, epithelioid haemangioma)

- usually occurs in head and neck region
- often multiple
- usually middle-aged adults
- microscopy shows proliferation of blood vessels lined by plump endothelial cells with surrounding lymphoid aggregates and eosinophils

KAPOSI'S SARCOMA

(See Chapter 22)

ANGIOSARCOMA

- occurs in the head and neck area of elderly patients
- aggressive with recurrence and metastases
- may occur following mastectomy, in area of lymphoedema
- may occur after radiation therapy
- poor prognosis
- microscopy shows vascular channels lined by atypical endothelial cells

GLOMUS TUMOUR

- arises from glomus body (structure involved in temperature regulation)
- usually young adults
- haemorrhagic spot beneath finger or toe nail
- may be painful
- multiple lesions may occur in children with an autosomal dominant pattern of inheritance
- microscopy shows sheets of glomus cells (round cells with central pale nucleus) and blood vessels
- rarely there are malignant forms (glomangiosarcoma)

SKIN APPENDAGE TUMOURS

Benign

HAIR FOLLICLE ORIGIN

Pilomatrixoma

- also known as calcifying epithelioma of Malherbe
- dermal and subcutaneous calcified nodule
- occurs most commonly on face, scalp, neck or upper limbs
- usually young adults
- microscopy shows mass of dark small cells with ghost outlines of necrotic cells
- later calcify
- rarely undergo malignant transformation

Trichoepithelioma

- usually solitary nodule in head and neck region
- rarely multiple and may be familial
- microscopy shows epithelial elements with central keratin-filled horn cysts
- may calcify
- may get a foreign body reaction

ECCRINE SWEAT GLAND ORIGIN

Syringoma

- usually occur in head and neck of adults
- may be multiple
- microscopy shows gland-like structures in dermis lined by two cell layers
- a fibrous stroma is present
- benign

Eccrine poroma

- occurs as a solitary lesion, often on soles of foot
- connected to epidermis
- consists of broad bands of cells with eosinophilic cytoplasm
- rarely becomes malignant

APOCRINE SWEAT GLAND ORIGIN

Hidradenoma papilliferum (papillary hidradenoma)

- occurs on the vulva and perianal area in females
- microscopy shows papillary formations lined by apocrine type cells

Cylindroma

- occurs most commonly on scalp and is often multiple
- turban tumour
- usually occurs in adults
- females more often than males
- microscopy shows nests of dark-staining cells surrounded by thick basement membrane type material

SEBACEOUS GLAND ORIGIN

Sebaceous hyperplasia

- occurs most commonly on the face or forehead
- grossly comprises yellow papules
- microscopy shows increased numbers of normal appearing sebaceous glands

Sebaceous adenoma

- may be associated with visceral malignancy, especially of the colon (Muir-Torre syndrome)
- usually solitary lesions on head of adults
- microscopy shows well circumscribed collection of sebaceous cells

MALIGNANT SKIN APPENDAGE TUMOURS

- may arise *de novo* or may develop from pre-existing benign skin appendage tumours
- malignant hair follicle tumours and apocrine carcinomas are very rare
- malignant tumours of eccrine origin include microcystic adnexal carcinoma, mucinous carcinoma and adenoid cystic carcinoma
- sebaceous carcinomas occur around the eyelids
- sebaceous carcinomas have the potential for recurrence and metastasis
- microscopically they are comprised of malignant sebaceous type cells

MERKEL CELL CARCINOMA (NEUROENDOCRINE CARCINOMA, TRABECULAR CARCINOMA)

- neuroendocrine carcinoma
- normal Merkel cells are found in skin and are part of APUD system

- Merkel cell carcinomas are rare tumours, occurring most commonly in the upper body of the elderly
- presents with red/blue nodules
- microscopy shows sheets of tumour cells with a high mitotic rate
- aggressive tumours which spread widely and locally recur
- must be differentiated from metastatic small cell carcinoma of lung
- immunohistochemically get 'dot-like' paranuclear positivity with anti-cytokeratin antibodies
- on electron microscopy get dense-core neuroendocrine granules and paranuclear arrays of filaments

DERMATOFIBROMA (BENIGN FIBROUS HISTIOCYTOMA)

- common tumour of dermis
- grossly there is a small elevated nodule covered by intact squamous epithelium
- microscopy shows proliferation of spindle shaped cells and blood vessels with dermis
- surface epithelium shows hyperplastic changes
- benign lesion with little tendency to recur

The soft tissues

18

TUMOUR-LIKE LESIONS OF SOFT TISSUES

Fibromatoses

- broad group of benign fibrous tissue proliferations of similar histology
- behaviour is intermediate between benign fibrous lesions and fibrosarcomas in that they have a propensity for recurrence but do not metastasise

Palmar fibromatosis (Dupytren's contracture)

- common
- involves superficial fascia of palm
- clinically there are firm nodules or cord in the palm
- difficulty in flexing joints
- males affected more commonly than females
- may be associated with epilepsy and alcohol abuse
- microscopy shows poorly circumscribed proliferation of fibrous tissue

Plantar fibromatosis (Ledderhose's disease)

- affects the fascia of the sole of the foot
- usually do not get contraction deformity
- microscopically similar to palmar fibromatosis

Peyronie's disease

- penile fibromatosis
- fibrous plaques develop in the corpora cavernosa of the penis
- get pain and curvature on erection
- microscopically similar to other types of fibromatosis

Desmoid fibromatosis

- divided into extra-abdominal, abdominal wall and intra-abdominal
- may be sporadic, familial or associated with familial adenomatous polyposis (FAP)
- more common in females
- peak incidence is second to fourth decades
- may arise during pregnancy
- may develop in a pre-existing scar

- marked tendency to recur
- may be treated with anti-oestrogens, e.g. tamoxifen
- extra-abdominal desmoid fibromatosis most commonly arises in fascia of shoulder girdle, chest, back and thigh
- microscopy shows proliferation of spindle-shaped fibroblasts
- lesion infiltrates widely
- there is little nuclear pleomorphism and a low mitotic rate

Nodular fasciitis

- common
- occurs as painful, rapidly growing nodule in young adults
- common sites are forearm, chest wall, back
- cause is unknown
- benign lesions which rarely recur
- recurrence is usually the result of incomplete excision
- microscopy shows interlacing bundles of mature fibroblasts in myxoid stroma
- mitotic figures may be numerous

Proliferative myositis and proliferative fasciitis

- subcutaneous or intramuscular nodules
- essentially variants of nodular fasciitis
- usually occur in arms and legs of elderly patients
- rapid growth but benign and rarely recurs
- microscopy shows proliferation of cells with prominent nucleoli and abundant cytoplasm
- mitotic figures are common
- infiltrates fat and muscle

Keloid

- overgrowth of scar tissue beyond original wound. Similar to hypertrophic scar but in this the scar tissue is confined to the wound
- occurs in young adults, especially of negroid race
- occurs spontaneously or following trauma or vaccination
- microscopy shows thick glassy eosinophilic bands of collagen in hyalinised scar tissue
- does not regress and may recur after surgical removal

Retroperitoneal fibrosis

- rare
- fibrous tissue in retroperitoneal space
- may be associated with scleroderma, mediastinal fibrosis, Riedel's thyroiditis, sclerosing cholangitis, orbital pseudotumour and drugs such as methysergide and methyldopa
- more common in males
- often presents with ureteric obstruction
- may get oedema of legs due to IVC obstruction

- may also get pyrexia and malaise
- an abdominal mass may be palpable
- microscopy shows dense fibrous tissue with inflammatory cell infiltration

BENIGN TUMOURS OF SOFT TISSUE

Lipoma

- benign fatty lesion
- composed of mature fat cells
- usually solitary but may be multiple
- common
- usually subcutaneous but occasionally deep-seated
- occasionally causes pressure symptoms
- grossly well circumscribed fatty mass
- microscopically composed of mature fat cells

Angiolipoma

- often multiple
- usually painful nodule
- male predominance
- upper limbs and trunk are most commonly affected sites
- microscopy shows mature adipose tissue with small vascular channels containing fibrin thrombi

Spindle-cell and pleomorphic lipoma

- more common in males
- most arise on upper back, shoulders or back of neck
- microscopy shows mature fat cells admixed with spindle cells (spindle-cell lipoma) or floret type giant cells (pleomorphic lipoma)
- often mixture of spindle-cell lipoma and pleomorphic lipoma and considered to share overlapping clinical and morphological features
- benign lesions with little or no tendency to recur

Intramuscular lipoma

- deep seated lipoma within skeletal muscle
- often poorly circumscribed and infiltrating
- may recur
- thigh and trunk are commonest locations

Synovial lipoma

- also known as lipoma arborescens
- collections of mature fat cells within synovium

Intraneural lipoma (fibrolipomatous hamartoma of nerve)

- slowly growing swelling, most often on median nerve
- symptoms of compression neuropathy
- microscopically affected nerve is expanded by adipose tissue

Leiomyoma

- benign tumour of smooth muscle
- occur in uterus, gastrointestinal tract, testis, skin, soft tissues
- in skin arises from arrector pili muscle
- may be multiple
- commonly found in scrotum
- may arise in deep soft tissue but uncommon
- microscopy shows bundles of regular spindle cells with eosinophilic cytoplasm
- positive immunohistochemical staining for desmin aids diagnosis
- angioleiomyoma or vascular leiomyoma is variant
- this is often painful and the most common site is the lower leg
- microscopically angioleiomyoma is composed of thick walled vascular channels and smooth muscle cells

Rhabdomyoma

- benign tumour of skeletal muscle
- rare
- may be divided into adult and fetal forms
- adult form almost always occurs in head and neck region
- more common in males
- fetal type is also most common in head and neck region
- microscopically adult type is composed of mature skeletal muscle fibres
- fetal type is composed of more immature skeletal muscle
- mature skeletal muscle fibres consist of deeply eosinophilic cells with visible cross-striations
- fetal rhabdomyoma may be difficult to distinguish from rhabdomyosarcoma

Lymphangioma

- usually presents in childhood and may be present at birth
- common in axilla and head and neck area (cystic hygroma)
- presents as soft fluctuant mass
- grossly multicystic lesions
- microscopy shows cystic spaces lined by flattened cells
- cystic spaces are filled with proteinaceous fluid
- aggregates of lymphocytes may be present between cystic spaces

Giant cell tumour of tendon sheath

- common
- virtually confined to digits, especially fingers
- lobulated lesions

- more common in females
- tendency to recur locally
- microscopy shows sheets of regular polygonal cells with multinucleate giant cells
- rarely get malignant transformation

Solitary fibrous tumour

- most common in pleura and peritoneum but may occur at any site
- usually presents with mass
- may be systemic symptoms
- rarely malignant forms
- microscopy shows spindle-shaped cells with areas of hyalinisation
- immunohistochemically stain positively with antibodies against CD34

Intramuscular myxoma

- usually adults
- most common site is muscles of thigh or lower limb
- occasionally multiple
- microscopy shows bland spindle-shaped cells in abundant myxoid stroma

SOFT TISSUE TUMOURS OF INTERMEDIATE MALIGNANT POTENTIAL

Dermatofibrosarcoma protuberans

- nodular mass involving dermis and subcutaneous tissue
- locally aggressive with propensity for recurrence, but rarely metastasise
- usually age 20–50 years
- most common on trunk, groin and lower extremities
- microscopy shows monomorphic population of spindle-shaped cells arranged in a storiform pattern
- infiltrates subcutaneous tissue and dermis
- immunohistochemically positive for CD34

Atypical fibroxanthoma

- uncommon
- occurs in the skin of the head and neck area of elderly patients
- ulceration is common
- microscopy shows pleomorphic spindle-shaped cells with high mitotic rate
- immunohistochemistry is useful to distinguish from spindle cell squamous carcinoma, malignant melanoma and angiosarcoma
- good prognosis
- amost never metastasise, but may rarely recur

Haemangiopericytoma

- tumour of pericytes
- occur in adults

- benign and malignant forms occur
- presents as slow-growing painless mass
- may pulsate
- may be associated with hypoglycaemia, especially if arising in retroperitoneum
- most common sites include thigh, pelvis and retroperitoneum
- grossly comprises vascular, haemorrhagic mass
- microscopy shows spindle-shaped cells with intervening vascular channels lined by endothelial cells
- signs of possible malignancy include marked nuclear pleomorphism, a high mitotic rate and the presence of necrosis
- haemangiopericytoma-like areas may occur in a variety of other soft tissue lesions and these should be excluded before making a diagnosis of haemangiopericytoma

MALIGNANT TUMOURS OF SOFT TISSUES (SARCOMAS)

- rare
- aetiology is unkown
- previous irradiation may predispose to some sarcomas
- Kaposi's sarcoma is associated with immune deficiency
- characteristic chromosomal abnormalities occur in some sarcomas, e.g. myxoid liposarcoma, extraskeletal mesenchymal chondrosarcoma, synovial sarcoma (see below)
- usually metastasise via blood-stream

STAGING AND HISTOLOGICAL GRADING

(Table 18.1)

PROGNOSIS

- depends on:
  - type of sarcoma
  - degree of nuclear pleomorphism
  - mitotic count
  - presence or absence of necrosis
  - low grade sarcomas have a better 5-year survival than high grade

DIAGNOSIS

- FNA may be of value
- trucut or incisional biopsy may also be used

Malignant fibrous histiocytoma

- commonest sarcoma in elderly
- cell of origin is fibroblast
- diagnosis of exclusion, when alternative differentiation cannot be demonstrated
- in many cases, if extensive immunohistochemical and ultrastructural studies are performed, an alternative diagnosis can be reached
- most commonly occurs in lower limb musculature or in retroperitoneum
- microscopic variants include pleomorphic, myxoid, giant cell, inflammatory and angiomatoid

Table 18.1 Staging and histological grading of soft tissue sarcomas

Stage	Extent of disease
*TNM classification**	
T0	No evidence of primary tumour
T1	Tumour of 5 cm or less in its greatest dimension and without extension to bone, major blood vessel or major nerve
T2	Tumour more than 5 cm in greatest dimension but without extension to bone, major blood vessel or major nerve
T3	Tumour with extension to bone, major vessel and nerve
Tx	Not assessed
N0	Regional nodes not involved
N1	Regional nodes involved
Nx	Not assessed
M0	No distant metastases
M1	Distant metastases
Mx	Not assessed
Histopathological grading	
G1	High degree of differentiation
G2	Medium degree of differentiation
G3	Low degree of differentiation (undifferentiated)
Gx	Not assessed

*TNM system does not apply to Kaposi's sarcoma, dermatofibrosarcoma, desmoid tumour and sarcomas arising from dura, brain or hollow viscera.

- pleomorphic variant is most common
- in this variant get pleomorphic cells, often with giant cells, arranged in a storiform (cartwheel) pattern
- usually get high mitotic rate and presence of necrosis
- local recurrence is common
- metastases commonly occur to lung, liver and bone
- deep seated tumours are very aggressive
- very large tumours have a worse prognosis

Fibrosarcoma

- malignant tumour of fibroblasts
- now very uncommon histological diagnosis
- may get adult and infantile types
- most frequent sites are thigh and trunk
- male predominance in both adult and infantile forms
- microscopy shows spindle-shaped cells with no specific differentiation
- a herring-bone pattern is often apparent

- diagnosis of exclusion with no specific differentiation demonstrable by immuno-histochemistry or electron microscopy
- metastases to lungs, bones, liver
- prognosis depends on histological grade, site and adequacy of surgery
- infantile types have a better prognosis than adult types

Liposarcoma

- male predominance
- tumour of adulthood
- rare in children
- principal subtypes include well differentiated, myxoid, round cell and pleomorphic
- common sites are thigh, trunk, retroperitoneum and upper limbs
- myxoid liposarcoma has a characteristic chromosomal translocation (t12/16)
- microscopically characterised by presence of lipoblasts
- lipoblasts have indented scalloped hyperchromatic nuclei and vacuolated cytoplasm
- well differentiated liposarcoma is composed largely of mature fat
- myxoid liposarcoma has a myxoid stroma and a characteristic vascular pattern
- pleomorphic liposarcoma is composed of pleomorphic cells
- metastases occur to liver and lung
- rarely spreads to lymph nodes

PROGNOSIS

- limb tumours have a better prognosis than retroperitoneal
- pleomorphic and round cell sarcomas have a worse prognosis
- approximate 5-year survivals are well differentiated (90%), myxoid (90%), round cell (25%) and pleomorphic (20%)

Leiomyosarcoma

- malignant tumour showing smooth muscle differentiation
- occurs in retroperitoneum, subcutaneous tissue and skin
- occasionally arises from walls of blood vessels, especially inferior vena cava or large veins of lower limbs
- microscopically composed of spindle-shaped cells
- nuclei are cigar-shaped
- smooth muscle differentiation may be demonstrated by immunohistochemistry (desmin positive) or by electron microscopy
- cutaneous leiomyosarcomas have a good prognosis and rarely metastasise
- retroperitoneal tumours often reach a large size, commonly metastasise and have a poor prognosis

Rhabdomyosarcoma

- malignant tumour showing skeletal muscle differentiation (may be demonstrated by immunohistochemistry or electron microscopy)
- commonest sarcoma of children and young adults

- commonest sites include head and neck region, orbit, sinuses, palate, ear and mastoid, retroperitoneum, limbs, bladder, prostate and vagina
- three main histological subtypes occur:

EMBRYONAL TYPE

- occurs in head and neck region and in genitourinary tract
- occurs in children usually before age 10 years with an average age of 4 years
- microscopically composed of small round hyperchromatic cells
- deletions of long arm of chromosome 11
- occasional cells with pink cytoplasm and with demonstrable cross-striations
- botryoid type of embryonal rhabdomyosarcoma occurs when tumour arises beneath a mucosal surface and grows in an exophytic 'grape-like' manner
- microscopy shows abundant myxoid stroma in botryoid type

ALVEOLAR TYPE

- occurs in young adults
- most common in limbs
- characteristic chromosomal translocation (t2/13)
- microscopically tumour grows in alveolar pattern with tumour cells lining fibrous septae

PLEOMORPHIC TYPE

- occurs in adults
- microscopically composed of bizzare pleomorphic cells
- usually occurs on limbs

PROGNOSIS

- embryonal rhabdomyosarcomas have a better prognosis than alveolar or pleomorphic subtypes
- prognosis depends on site

Kaposi's sarcoma

- occurs in three forms:
  - endemic tumour in parts of Africa
  - sporadic tumour outside Africa
  - in association with immunodeficiency, especially AIDS (see Chapter 22)
- microscopically composed of interconnecting vascular channels

Synovial sarcoma

- peak incidence is age 10–35 years
- slight male predominance
- most occur around the knee
- may also arise in the trunk and head and neck region and mediastinum
- no longer believed that lesions arise from synovium
- may present with pain or mass
- characteristic chromosomal translocation (tX/18)

- microscopy shows biphasic or monophasic types
- in biphasic type, epithelial and spindle cells are present
- epithelial cells may form cords or nests
- immunohistochemically epithelial areas stain positively for cytokeratins and epithelial membrane antigen. Spindle cell component stains positively for vimentin
- may get radiological and microscopic evidence of calcification
- local recurrences and metastases are common
- overall 5-year survival is approximately 50%

Epithelioid sarcoma

- most cases occur in distal extremities, especially around hand and wrist
- occurs in young adults with a male predominance
- presents with ulcerated mass or skin nodules
- marked capacity for local spread
- spreads along fascial or neurovascular structures
- microscopy shows epithelioid cells with central necrosis
- tumour cells stain positively with cytokeratin markers
- high recurrence rate
- tendency to metastasise to lymph nodes and lungs
- poor prognosis

Extraskeletal myxoid chondrosarcoma

- rare
- occurs principally in fourth to sixth decades with a slight male predominance
- more common in lower limbs
- characteristic chromosomal translocation (t9/22)
- microscopy shows lobulated appearance
- lacy pattern of tumour cells in myxoid stroma
- slowly growing tumours which are prone to local recurrence
- may rarely metastasise

Alveolar soft part sarcoma

- uncommon
- usually adolescents or young adults with a slight female predominance
- most common site is lower limbs
- poor prognosis with eventual metastases to lungs
- microscopy shows large tumours cells with eosinophilic cytoplasm, exhibiting alveolar growth pattern
- characteristically there is PAS positive crystalline material within tumour cells
- these can also be demonstrated by electron microscopy
- commonly there is vascular invasion at periphery of tumour
- controversy over pattern of differentiation but now believed to show skeletal muscle differentiation

Bones and joints

19

NORMAL STRUCTURE

- two main groups of bones:
  1. Long bones of the appendicular skeleton and of the hands and feet
     - under portion at each end (epiphysis)
     - cylindrical portion in the middle (diaphysis)
     - transition zone between (metaphysis)
     - in long bones which are growing the epiphysis and metaphysis are separated by the epiphyseal cartilage (growth plate)
  2. Flat bones of the axial skeleton, e.g. skull, scapula, clavicle, vertebrae and pelvic bones
- there are two morphologically different types of bone:
  - compact (cortical) bone – provides structural stability
  - trabecular (cancellous or medullary) bone – provides intramedullary network
- three types of specialised bone cells exist:
  1. Osteoblasts
     - arise from pluripotential fetal mesenchymal cells
     - give rise to collagen of the bony matrix
     - contain abundant alkaline phosphatase which plays a role in mineralisation of the bone
  2. Osteocytes
     - osteoblasts embedded in osseous matrix
  3. Osteoclasts
     - large multinucleated cells
     - exhibit features of monocytes or macrophages and are derived from these cells
     - lie in Howship's lacunae and reabsorb adjacent bone
- osteoid is the bony matrix and is composed of type I collagen. This becomes mineralised. Bone also has a ground substance of glycoproteins and proteoglycans
- cortex of bone is surrounded by periosteum which is composed of fibrous tissue

Blood supply

- principal nutrient artery from major axial artery enters shaft to divide into ascending and descending branches
- periarticular plexus supplies the metaphysis
- epiphysis supplied by vessels from non-articular cortex
- prior to the development of the growth plate there are frequent anastomoses between epiphyseal and metaphyseal circulations in infants
- mature growth plate acts as a barrier between the two systems which helps to localise infection
- periosteal vessels supply the outer one-third of the cortex

BONE AND JOINT INFECTIONS

Acute pyogenic osteomyelitis

- usually caused by bacterial organisms
- most commonly involves metaphysis of long bones, especially lower femur, upper tibia, upper humerus, lower radius and vertebral bodies
- most commonly reaches bone by haematogenous spread
- may also reach bone by extension from a contiguous site or by direct implantation
- origin of bacteraemia may be skin infection, dental sepsis or nasopharyngeal sepsis
- predisposing factors include diabetes, IV drug abuse, systemic steroids, rheumatoid arthritis, sickle cell anaemia, surgery and fractures
- the most commonly isolated organism is *Staphylococcus aureus*
- *Haemophilus influenzae, Escherichia coli, Proteus*, streptococci and *Klebsiella* may also be found
- *Salmonella* osteomyelitis may complicate sickle cell anaemia
- in some cases, no organisms are isolated, especially if antibiotics have already been given

PATHOLOGY

- depends on stage (acute, subacute, chronic)
- initially an acute inflammatory response consisting of neutrophils and later monocytes
- increased intraosseous pressure causes venous obstruction and thrombosis and cell death
- later arterial thrombosis and infarction of medullary contents
- may be spontaneous decompression, if exudate passes through cortex into subperiosteal space
- segmental necrosis of bone occurs, the dead piece of the bone being known as the sequestrum
- small sequestra removed by osteoclasts
- large sequestra may cause chronic infection
- in infants, and uncommonly in adults, epiphyseal infection may spread into the joint to produce septic arthritis
- involucrum is reactive bone formed by the periosteum around the sequestra
- may get formation of intraosseous Brodie's abscesses
- sclerosing osteomyelitis of Garré typically involves the jaw and is associated with extensive new bone formation

CLINICAL FEATURES, TREATMENT AND COMPLICATIONS

- often presents with fever, malaise, bone pain
- metaphyseal tenderness
- radiologically there is lytic focus of bone destruction surrounded by zone of sclerosis
- increased ESR, anaemia, leucocytosis, positive blood cultures
- treatment is early intravenous antibiotics with or without surgical drainage
- role of early surgery is controversial
- chronic infection causes fibrosis, ischaemia, sequestra formation
- damage to growth plate in children may cause limb shortening
- damage to joint surface may cause later degenerative arthritis
- other complications include pathological fracture, amyloidosis, endocarditis and development of squamous carcinoma

Chronic osteomyelitis

- may follow incomplete resolution of acute osteomyelitis
- may be due to delay in diagnosis, extensive bone necrosis, inadequate antibiotic therapy, inadequate surgical debridement or weakened host defence
- may be characterised by acute flare-ups

PATHOLOGY

- dense avascular scar tissue and bone
- chronic inflammatory cells
- pus discharges through sinuses which connect to skin
- radical surgery to excise sequestra may be required
- late complications include amyloidosis and development of squamous carcinoma in sinus tract

Septic (infectious) arthritis

- most common organisms are *Gonococcus, Staphylococcus, Streptococcus, Haemophilus influenzae*
- in infants less than 2 years, *Haemophilus influenzae* is common
- may be secondary to osteomyelitis or to adjacent soft tissue abscess
- knee and hip joints commonly affected
- in adults there is often a predisposing joint condition, e.g. rheumatoid arthritis
- classical presentation is sudden development of acutely painful, swollen joint
- systemic findings of fever, leucocytosis and increased ESR common
- if severe infection or if not treated then may get permanent joint damage with stiffness and ankylosis
- late complications include infarction of bone epiphysis, dislocation of joint, osteomyelitis or perforation of capsule to form periarticular soft tissue abscess

Tuberculosis

- common in Third World
- becoming more common in industrialised nations, because of influx of immigrants and immunosuppression, e.g. AIDS
- primary focus of infection is usually lung
- blood spread to bone or joint
- microscopy shows caseating granulomatous inflammation consisting of histiocytes and Langhan's type giant cells
- organisms can be identified by Ziehl-Neelson staining
- tuberculous osteomyelitis usually affects metaphyseal region of bones
- tuberculous arthritis causes affected synovium to grow as a pannus over articular cartilage and erode into bone
- chronic disease results in fibrous ankylosis and obliteration of joint space
- joints most commonly affected are hips, knees and ankles

Tuberculosis of vertebrae (Pott's disease)

- usually presents with fever, pain, weight loss
- often occurs in thoracic vertebrae

- occasionally lumbar vertebrae
- rarely cervical vertebrae
- infection may spread through intervertebral disc to involve multiple vertebrae
- may also extend into surrounding soft tissues, e.g. psoas muscle to form psoas abscess
- may get compression fractures resulting in scoliosis, kyphosis and neurological deficits
- other complications include tuberculous arthritis, sinus tract formation and amyloidosis

Syphilis

- due to spirochaete *Treponema pallidum*

CONGENITAL
Parrot's syphilitic osteochondritis

- spirochaete lodges near growth plate during fifth month *in utero* causing osteochondritis and periostitis

Clutton's joints

- symmetrical painless effusion, especially in the knees
- usually age 8–16 years

ACQUIRED
Gummatous inflammation

- a gumma is composed of central necrosis surrounded by lymphocytes and histiocytes
- spirochaetes may be demonstrated by silver stains
- causes arthritis and synovitis
- usually early in tertiary stage of syphilis

Charcot's joints

- tertiary syphilis
- end stage painless destruction of weight-bearing joints
- associated with tabes dorsalis

Periostitis

- any age
- especially older children
- occurs in tibia, resulting in sabre shin
- subperiosteal inflammation causes new bone formation in cortex

Brucellosis

- direct contact with infected farm animals or products
- entry via skin, eyes, gastrointestinal tract, respiratory tract
- causes fever and systemic symptoms

- may have bone or joint involvement
- in children may get acute arthritis
- in adults, vertebrae may be affected with granulomatous inflammation

Lyme arthritis

- caused by infection with spirochaete *Borrelia burgdorferi*
- initial site of infection is skin
- dissemination to joints occurs in days to weeks
- remitting, migrating arthritis involving large joints, especially knees, shoulders, elbows and ankles
- microscopy shows a chronic papillary synovitis, resembling that seen in rheumatoid arthritis
- organisms may be revealed by silver staining

TUMOURS

- primary bone tumours are rare and are often in younger patients
- secondary bone tumours are more common, especially in elderly patients

DIAGNOSIS

- clinical, including age of patient, bone involved and site within bone
- radiology
  - plain x-ray
  - tomograms
  - CT
  - MRI
- pathology – FNA and open biopsy may be used for preoperative confirmation of diagnosis
- in diagnosing all bone tumours, close correlation should be made between clinical, radiological and pathological findings

CLASSIFICATION

(Table 19.1)

BENIGN BONE FORMING TUMOURS

Osteoma

- occurs almost exclusively in skull, paranasal sinuses and facial bones
- in head and neck region may present with symptoms of nasal and paranasal obstruction
- most occur in fourth to fifth decades
- radiography shows a sharply circumscribed, radio-opaque mass protruding from the bone surface
- multiple osteomas may be found in Gardner's syndrome (osteomas, epidermal cysts, fibromatoses, adenomatous colonic polyposis)
- microscopically composed of mature bone

Table 19.1 Primary bone tumours (modified from the 1972 WHO classification)

1. *Bone forming tumours*

Benign	Malignant
1. Osteoma	1. Osteosarcoma
2. Osteoid osteoma	2. Parosteal osteosarcoma
3. Osteoblastoma	

2. *Cartilage forming tumours*

Benign	Malignant
1. Chondroma	1. Chondrosarcoma
2. Osteochondroma	
3. Chondroblastoma	
4. Chondromyxoid fibroma	

3. *Giant cell tumours*

Wide spectrum of behaviour, benign–malignant

4. *Marrow tumours*

Malignant
1. Ewing's sarcoma
2. Myeloma
3. Malignant lymphoma

5. *Vascular tumours*

Benign	Intermediate	Malignant
1. Haemangioma	1. Haemangioendothelioma	1. Angiosarcoma
2. Lymphangioma	2. Haemangiopericytoma	
3. Glomus tumour		

6. *Other connective tissue tumours*

Benign	Malignant
1. Desmoplastic fibroma	1. Fibrosarcoma
2. Lipoma	2. Liposarcoma
	3. Undifferentiated sarcoma

7. *Other tumours*

Benign
1. Chordoma
2. Adamantinoma

8. *Unclassified tumours*

9. *Tumour-like lesions*

1. Solitary bone cyst
2. Aneurysmal bone cyst
3. Metaphyseal fibrous defect
4. Fibrous dysplasia
5. Eosinophilic granuloma
6. Brown tumour of hyperparathyroidism

- totally benign
- recurrence is rare
- asymptomatic lesions require no treatment

Osteoid osteoma

- common
- usually less than 1 cm in diameter
- usually in second decade of life
- more common in males
- most common sites are femur and tibia
- often chronic pain which is worse at night and which is relieved by aspirin
- radiologically has a highly characteristic appearance. Typically get a zone of marked sclerosis surrounding a well-demarcated area of radiolucency
- microscopy shows central highly vascular nidus with spicules of immature bone lined by osteoblasts and osteoclasts
- surrounding this nidus sclerotic bone is present
- treatment is excision
- recurrence is rare but is greater if nidus is not completely removed

Osteoblastoma

- microscopically similar to osteoid osteoma but of greater size (>1 cm)
- less common than osteoid osteoma
- peak incidence is second decade
- more common in males
- most common sites are spine, femur, skull, tibia
- presents with pain and swelling
- radiology shows well circumscribed radiolucent area
- microscopically similar to osteoid osteoma
- treatment is curettage or surgical resection
- local recurrence rare
- very occasionally malignant change occurs, especially after radiotherapy

MALIGNANT BONE FORMING TUMOURS

Osteosarcoma

- WHO definition: 'Malignant bone tumour characterised by the direct formation of bone or osteoid by the tumour cells'
- may arise *de novo* or secondary to lesions such as Paget's disease, osteogenesis imperfecta, bone infarct, chronic osteomyelitis and fibrous dysplasia
- some cases are familial and may coexist with retinoblastoma
- may occur following irradiation for benign bone lesions
- most cases with *de novo* osteosarcoma are age 10–20 years
- more common in males
- cases associated with Paget's disease are usually in elderly patients
- marked predilection for metaphyseal regions of long bones, especially distal femur, proximal tibia and proximal humerus
- presents with bone pain and swelling

- raised serum alkaline phosphatase
- radiography usually shows a mixed lytic and sclerotic appearance
- soft tissue mass with new bone formation
- other radiological features include Codman's triangle (periosteal new bone formation), sun-ray spiculation and onion skinning
- grossly usually large, metaphyseal lesion which invades medulla, penetrates cortex and produces periosteal elevation
- may extend into surrounding soft tissues
- microscopy shows malignant stromal cells associated with osteoid
- cartilaginous, myxoid and fibrous areas may also be present
- often bizarre nuclei and numerous mitotic figures
- metastatic spread occurs via blood stream to the lungs
- surgical resection of pulmonary metastases may improve prognosis
- treatment is surgery and chemotherapy
- prior to chemotherapy, 5-year survival was 10–20%
- prognosis now dramatically improved with new chemotherapy
- lesions of flat bones have poorer prognosis than those in the extremities

Parosteal osteosarcoma

- highly differentiated osteosarcoma
- arises from juxtacortical region of long bones
- peak incidence is in the second decade
- females more commonly affected than males
- most common sites are lower femur and upper tibia
- presents as painless mass
- radiologically has characteristic frequently diagnostic appearance
- dense mushroom-shaped mass attached to the outer metaphyseal cortex by a broad base
- microscopy shows islands of bone separated by a fibrous stroma
- long-term survival is 80–90%
- may recur locally

Osteosarcoma arising in Paget's disease

- usually elderly patients
- usually long-standing Paget's disease
- all are high grade anaplastic tumours
- may be multicentric tumours
- poor prognosis
- other sarcomas, e.g. malignant fibrous histiocytoma and fibrosarcoma may arise in Paget's disease
- most common sites are large tubular bones and flat bones of the axial skeleton

BENIGN CARTILAGINOUS TUMOURS

Chondroma

- common
- most commonly involves small bones of hand and feet
- if grows within medullary cavity of bone, then called enchondroma

- if projects outwards from bone then called ecchondroma
- presents with swelling or pathological fracture
- most common in second to fourth decades
- radiology shows lucent area with spicules of calcification
- multiple enchondromas occur in Ollier's disease
- get multiple enchondromas combined with haemangiomas in Maffucci's syndrome
- microscopically chondromas are composed of lobules of cartilage separated by a fibrous stroma
- areas of endochondral calcification may occur
- cartilage can be quite cellular but this does not indicate malignancy
- solitary lesions rarely become malignant
- with multiple lesions (especially in Ollier's disease or Maffucci's syndrome) there is a risk of malignant transformation
- treatment is curettage with or without bone grafting
- rarely recur

Osteochondroma (osteocartilaginous exostosis)

- common benign tumour
- many are asymptomatic
- cartilage capped bony projection which projects from cortical surface of bone
- most common sites are lower end of femur and upper end of humerus
- usually young patients
- usually presents with painless swelling
- radiology shows bony outgrowth with narrow to broad stalk
- multiple osteochondromas may occur in a familial disorder
- grossly there is bony protuberance covered by cartilage
- microscopy shows cartilage cap covering underlying bone
- malignant transformation occurs rarely in solitary lesions and is more common with multiple lesions

Chondroblastoma

- benign neoplasm
- affects epiphysis of long bones, especially femur, tibia and humerus
- 95% of cases occur between ages 5 and 25 years
- males are affected more commonly than females
- most common symptom is pain
- radiology shows well defined lytic lesion with a thin margin of increased bone density
- microscopically composed of small round cells (chrondroblasts) with multinucleate giant cells
- other microscopic features are a chondroid matrix and characteristic calcification with a chicken wire pattern
- treatment is curettage with bone grafting
- curettage may be followed by recurrence
- occasionally behave aggressively with the development of metastases, even when typical histology
- rarely undergo sarcomatous transformation, especially following radiation

Chondromyxoid fibroma

- rare
- usually age 10–30 years
- most common sites are lower femur and upper tibia
- presents with pain and swelling
- radiology shows eccentrically located lytic metaphyseal lesion
- lobules of myxoid matrix
- microscopy shows spindle-shaped cells embedded in a chrondromyxoid stroma
- characteristically lobulated architecture
- treatment is curettage or resection
- may recur
- rarely malignant change occurs

MALIGNANT CARTILAGINOUS TUMOURS

Chondrosarcoma

- primary chondrosarcoma arises *de novo*
- secondary chrondrosarcoma arises from benign cartilaginous lesions such as an enchondroma or osteochondroma
- occasionally occur after radiation or in Paget's disease
- peak incidence for primary chondrosarcoma is fifth to seventh decades
- secondary chondrosarcomas occur at a younger age
- males are more commonly affected than females
- most common site is bones of pelvis followed by femur, humerus and ribs
- presents with pain and swelling
- radiology shows mottled partially calcified areas
- microscopy shows cellular lobulated cartilage
- may be graded 1 to 3 depending on degree of pleomorphism and other features
- in high grade tumours anaplastic cells occur
- rapidly spreads within medullary cavity of bone
- may also extend into surrounding soft tissues
- distant metastases are most often to the lungs
- treatment is *en bloc* excision
- prognosis depends on stage, site and histological grade

MISCELLANEOUS BONE TUMOURS

Giant cell tumour (osteoclastoma)

- generally benign but often locally aggressive neoplasms
- usually age 20–40 years
- males more common than females
- involves epiphyseal region of bones
- most common sites are lower femur, upper tibia and lower radius
- presents with pain and swelling
- may arise in Paget's disease

- radiology shows lytic lesion with fine to coarse trabeculations
- microscopy shows vascular stroma with mononuclear tumour cells and diffusely distributed osteoclast-like giant cells
- treatment is curettage or *en bloc* excision
- recurrence is common following curettage
- may get malignant transformation, especially following radiotherapy

Ewing's sarcoma

- highly malignant
- belongs to group of neuroectodermal tumours
- occurs in young people, with median age of approximately 30 years
- one of small blue cell tumours of childhood (also includes lymphoma, neuroblastoma, rhabdomyosarcoma)
- characteristic chromosomal translocation (t11/22)
- males more commonly affected than females
- any bone may be affected but predilection for long tubular bones, especially femur
- presents with pain and swelling
- may be constitutional symptoms of high ESR, high white cell count, pyrexia and anaemia
- radiology shows ill-defined, lytic lesion with an 'onion skin' or 'sunburst' periosteal reaction
- grossly there is friable necrotic tumour
- microscopically composed of dense small round cells with uniform dark nuclei
- cells contain glycogen
- abundant necrosis is often present
- immunohistochemical staining with antibody against MIC2 gene product is useful in diagnosis
- with advent of multiagent chemotherapy, treatment has undergone considerable evolution in recent years

Multiple myeloma

- neoplasm of plasma cells
- usually multiple bones affected, especially vertebrae, ribs, skull and pelvis
- occasionally solitary lesions occur (plasmacytoma)
- secretes monoclonal immunoglobulins
- usual age is 50–70 years
- males more commonly affected than females
- presents with bone pain, pathological fractures, anaemia, high serum calcium, weight loss and renal failure
- ESR is often markedly elevated
- Bence-Jones proteins are detected in the urine
- serum electrophoresis is useful in diagnosis
- diagnosis usually confirmed by bone marrow biopsy
- radiology shows multiple punched out lytic lesions
- microscopy shows sheets of plasma cells of varying differentiation
- complications include renal failure, amyloidosis, hypercalcaemia, anaemia and infections
- prognosis depends on stage of disease and degree of differentiation of plasma cells

- usual treatment is alkylating agents
- median survival is 2–3 years
- most die of infections or renal failure

VASCULAR TUMOURS OF BONE

- these are rare

Benign

HAEMANGIOMA

- most common site is vertebral bodies
- most common in fifth decade
- rarely may be multiple and associated with extraosseous haemangiomas
- usually presents with pain
- may be asymptomatic
- biopsy may cause severe haemorrhage
- microscopy shows dilated vascular spaces lined by endothelial cells
- radiology shows lytic intramedullary lesions

LYMPHANGIOMA

- rare
- may be multiple
- microscopically consist of dilated lymphatic channels

GLOMUS TUMOUR

- benign
- most common site is terminal phalynx
- causes severe pain
- derived from specialised smooth muscle cells of glomus body
- microscopically composed of regular round cells with vascular stroma

Intermediate

- rare
- include epithelioid haemangioendothelioma and haemangiopericytoma
- unpredictable behaviour

Malignant

ANGIOSARCOMA

- rare
- highly malignant
- femur, tibia and humerus are most commonly affected
- rapid growth occurs destroying bone
- metastases to lung

- microscopy shows atypical endothelial cells lining vascular spaces
- diagnosis may be aided by positive staining with anti-endothelial antibodies
- treatment is *en bloc* excision or amputation
- prognosis is poor

OTHER TUMOURS OF BONE

Desmoplastic fibroma

- rare
- non-metastasising but locally aggressive and infiltrative
- similar to soft tissue desmoid and represents skeletal counterpart
- usually presents with swelling and pain
- most common site is mandible
- microscopy shows spindle-shaped cells resembling fibroblasts
- high recurrence rate following curettage

Lipoma

- rare
- similar to soft tissue lipoma and composed of mature adipose tissue
- benign

Fibrosarcoma

- malignant spindle cell neoplasm exhibiting fibroblastic differentiation
- usually presents with pain and swelling
- may be secondary to Paget's disease, giant cell tumour, chronic osteomyelitis, bone infarct or fibrous dysplasia
- may occur after bone irradiation
- most common sites are femur and tibia
- radiology shows lytic destructive lesion
- microscopy shows malignant spindle cell neoplasm often arranged in a herring-bone pattern
- differentiated from osteosarcoma by lack of osteoid
- may be graded 1 to 3
- prognosis depends on grade

Malignant fibrous histiocytoma

- usually present with pain or swelling
- sarcoma with large tumour cells often arranged in storiform pattern
- may arise in Paget's disease
- most common sites are femur and tibia
- microscopy shows anaplastic spindle-shaped tumour cells, often with giant cells
- differentiated from osteosarcoma by lack of osteoid
- aggressive tumours with poor prognosis

Chordoma

- rare
- malignant slowly growing neoplasms which occur along the axial skeleton
- origin is embryonic notochord remnants
- most common in fifth to seventh decades
- more common in males
- most common site is sacrococcygeal area
- locally invasive
- rarely metastasise
- often present with nerve root compression
- grossly lobulated appearance
- microscopy shows vacuolated (physaliphorous) cells lying in a myxoid matrix
- may get cartilaginous variant
- wide surgical excision is treatment of choice
- may recur
- may dedifferentiate into a high grade sarcoma

Adamantinoma

- rare
- marked predilection for tibia
- epithelial origin
- may be associated with osteofibrous dysplasia
- most common in second and third decades
- presents with pain and swelling
- radiology shows sharply defined lytic defect (soap bubble appearance)
- microscopy shows epithelioid cells of varying patterns set in fibrous stroma
- may metastasise to lymph nodes or lung
- metastasis may occur late

TUMOUR-LIKE LESIONS OF BONE

Solitary bone cyst (simple or unicameral bone cyst)

- male predilection
- most common in second and third decades
- most common sites are humerus and femur
- presents as an incidental finding on x-ray or with a fracture
- radiology shows lucent areas in metaphysis with expanded cortex
- curettage may be followed by recurrence
- extremely rarely sarcomatous transformation
- microscopically wall is composed of fibrous tissue, often with granulation tissue and haemosiderin pigment

Aneurysmal bone cyst

- benign but expansile multicystic lesion
- may be rapidly growing and destructive

- may get aneurysmal bone cyst-like areas in neoplasms such as giant cell tumour and chrondroblastoma
- usually age 20 years or younger
- most common sites are metaphyseal region of long bones or vertebral body
- presents with painful swelling
- may spread to involve adjacent bones, especially in vertebrae
- radiology shows multiloculated lytic lesion
- grossly get blood-filled cavity with fibrous and bony septa
- microscopy shows blood-filled spaces with fibrous septa containing giant cells and osteoid
- prognosis is good but may recur locally following curettage

Metaphyseal fibrous defect and non-ossifying fibroma

- common
- two conditions are histologically similar
- metaphyseal fibrous defect involves the cortex of the bone whereas non-ossifying fibroma is larger and involves the medullary cavity
- most common sites are tibia and femur
- presents as an incidental finding on x-ray, with pain or with a fracture
- may be multiple and associated with neurofibromatosis
- most common in children
- radiology shows sharply circumscribed lytic lesion
- microscopy shows fibrous tissue, often with inflammatory cells and new bone formation
- prognosis is good
- frequently disappear spontaneously

Fibrous dysplasia

- probably hamartomatous
- developmental in nature
- presents with incidental finding on x-ray with pain or with fracture
- usually one bone affected (monostotic)
- usually between ages 5 and 20 years
- rarely polyostotic with skin pigmentation and precocious puberty in females (Albright's syndrome)
- polyostotic form usually presents earlier in life
- most common sites are craniofacial bones, femur and tibia
- radiology usually shows lucent area
- very rarely malignant change occurs with development of sarcoma
- microscopy shows irregularly shaped trabeculae of woven bone in a cellular fibrous stroma
- treatment is curettage or excision of affected bone
- may get recurrence following curettage

Eosinophilic granuloma

- derived from Langerhan's cells
- part of spectrum of histiocytosis X (also includes Hand-Schuller-Christian disease and Letterer-Siwe disease)

- solitary or multiple bone lesions
- may not be true neoplasm but may be reactive or disorder of immune system
- most common in first three decades of life
- more common in males
- most common sites are skull and long bones
- radiography shows punched out lytic lesion
- clinically presents with pain or may be incidental x-ray finding
- microscopy shows Langerhan's cells with reactive eosinophils, plasma cells and multinucleated giant cells
- Langerhan's cells may be identified by positive staining with S–100 protein or by ultrastructural demonstration of Birbeck granules
- solitary lesions usually cured by curettage
- may develop additional lesions

Brown tumour of hyperparathyroidism

- rare nowadays
- associated with hyperparathyroidism
- increased serum calcium
- in severe hyperparathyroidism there is osteitis fibrosa cystica
- subperiosteal lesions, especially involving middle phalanges, symphysis pubis, sacroiliac joints and distal clavicle
- microscopy shows osteoblasts with fibrous tissue and multinucleate giant cells
- characteristically get multiple fractures
- control of hyperparathyroidism allows bone lesions to regress or disappear

HIP DISORDERS IN CHILDREN

Congenital dislocation of hip (CDH)

- genetic and environmental factors important in aetiology
- first born child most commonly affected
- more common in females

GENETIC

- affected children may have a familial history

ENVIRONMENTAL

- more common with breech presentation
- more common with Caesarian section
- position of infant after birth may be important

PATHOLOGY

- fibrocartilaginous labrum is inverted
- ligamentum teres and pulvinar fat pad are enlarged
- acetabulum is shallow
- capsule stretches and infolds between the head and acetabulum
- femoral neck is anteverted
- nucleus of capital epiphysis is small and delayed

COMPLICATIONS

- ischaemia of epiphysis
- avascular necrosis and deformity of femoral head

Perthes' disease

- avascular necrosis of femoral head
- predisposing factors include low social class, elderly parents, low birth weight and trauma to hips
- more common in males
- 12% bilateral
- usually age 3–10 years
- presents with painful irritable hip and limp

PATHOLOGY

- inflammation of epiphysis
- death of marrow cells, osteoclasts and osteoblasts
- increased joint space
- repair phase with ingrowth of vascular granulation tissue
- new bone laid down in dead trabeculae
- collapse and fragmentation of necrotic trabeculae
- later flattening and irregularity of femoral head with premature degenerative osteoarthritis
- treatment is initially conservative with good results
- may require surgery

Slipped upper femoral epiphysis

- usually young (teens)
- separation of upper femoral epiphysis with trivial trauma
- presents with pain in hip and limp
- often have a history of minor trauma
- males more common than females
- children may be obese with delayed sexual development
- occasionally there is an overt metabolic abnormality
- diagnosis is by lateral x-ray
- capital epiphysis slips posteriorly
- tears anterior periosteum off neck
- elevates posterior periosteum off neck to form new bone
- anterior part of the neck undergoes partial reabsorption

COMPLICATIONS

- avascular necrosis of femoral head
- bony collapse
- secondary osteoarthritis
- cartilage necrosis (acute chondrolysis)

TREATMENT

- surgical pinning

OSTEOARTHRITIS (OA)

- degenerative joint disease
- most common in elderly patients
- characterised by progressive erosion of articular cartilage
- may be primary or secondary to a variety of causes (secondary osteoarthritis)
- joints most commonly affected include hips, knees and vertebrae
- symptoms include pain, morning stiffness and limitation of movement
- radiology shows subchondral bone sclerosis, cyst formation and osteophytes

Aetiology

ABNORMAL STRESS FACTORS

- Perthes' disease
- intra-articular fracture
- slipped upper femoral epiphysis
- congenital dislocation of the hip
- varus knee deformity
- ligament abnormalities
- obesity

ABNORMAL CARTILAGE

- increased cross-linking of collagen resulting in decreased tensile strength
- pannus formation, e.g. in rheumatoid arthritis inhibits cartilage nutrition
- pyogenic infection may release toxins which attack the cartilage
- crystal disease, e.g. gout results in depolymerisation of proteoglycans
- abnormal synovium affects cartilage nutrition
- minor changes in cartilage composition may occur on a genetic basis

Pathology

- fibrillation of cartilage surface
- fissures occur into basal layers of cartilage
- shearing forces result in loss of flakes of cartilage which expose subchondral bone
- sloughed flakes of cartilage and subchondral bone float in joint (joint mice)
- osteophytes (bony outgrowths) develop at margin of articular surface
- sclerosis of subchondral bone secondary to microfractures
- cysts occur in subchondral bone
- synovitis occurs
- in women, Heberden's nodes in the fingers represent prominent osteophytes at the distal interphalangeal joints

RHEUMATOID ARTHRITIS (RA)

- chronic systemic inflammatory disorder
- symmetrical chronic polyarthritis
- other organs affected include heart, blood vessels, lungs, skin and eyes
- occurs in 2–3% of the population

- most common age 40–50 years
- females more common than males
- cause unknown but may be autoimmune disease
- often familial association
- association with HLA-DR4

Clinical

- symmetrical polyarthritis of small joints of hands and feet
- ankles, wrists, knees and elbows may also be affected
- systemic symptoms of weight loss, fever, muscle pain and malaise
- may occur in monoarticular form in large weight-bearing joint
- affected joints are swollen, warm, painful and stiff
- usually chronic relapsing disease
- rheumatoid factor positive in 80%

Pathology

- initially synovium becomes oedematous, thickened and hyperplastic
- synovial inflammatory infiltrate, composed of lymphoid follicles, plasma cells and macrophages
- synovial fluid is turbid and increased in volume
- inflamed and hyperplastic synovium creeps over the articular surface, forming a pannus
- pannus causes erosion of underlying cartilage
- pannus also penetrates bone forming subchrondral cysts, resulting in osteoporosis
- eventually fibrous and then bony ankylosis
- skin rheumatoid nodules occur in 25% of patients. Arise in forearm, elbows, occiput and lumbosacral areas
- may also occur in lungs, spleen, heart and aorta
- microscopy shows fibrinoid necrosis surrounded by lymphocytes and histiocytes
- may also get vasculitis

ANKYLOSING SPONDYLITIS

- one of seronegative arthritides
- rheumatoid factor negative
- 95% are positive for HLA-B27 antigen
- more common in males
- aetiology is unknown
- may be abnormal immune response in genetically predisposed individuals
- most commonly affected joint is sacroiliac
- usually presents with backache and stiffness
- peripheral joints may also be involved
- microscopy shows chronic synovitis resulting in destruction of articular cartilage
- later fibrous and bony ankylosis
- uveitis, aortitis and amyloidosis may also occur

OTHER SERONEGATIVE ARTHRITIDES

- Reiter's syndrome (arthritis, non-gonococcal urethritis, conjunctivitis). Usually male patients and probably autoimmune reaction to previous infection
- psoriatic arthritis
- enteropathic arthritis, associated with ulcerative colitis or Crohn's disease

METABOLIC BONE DISEASE

Hyperparathyroidism

(See p. 243)

Osteoporosis

- decreased bone mass
- may be localised to a single bone or may involve entire skeleton
- sedentary life style is associated with faster bone loss
- faster bone loss in older population
- osteoporosis may be primary or secondary
- primary osteoporosis is most common in females after the menopause

PATHOLOGICAL CAUSES

(Table 19.2)

CLINICAL

- bone pain
- collapse fractures of vertebrae with loss of height, lumbar lordosis or kyphoscoliosis
- pathological fractures of long bones, e.g. neck of femur
- blood biochemistry normal
- do not get x-ray changes until significant bone loss
- photon absorption densitometry allows more accurate assessment
- axial skeleton is most commonly affected, especially lumbar spine
- increased incidence of radial and femoral neck fractures
- microscopy shows thinning of bony trabeculae

Osteomalacia

- defect in mineralisation of bone matrix
- causes include calcium deficiency, low phosphate or deficiency of vitamin D or some disturbance in its metabolism
- causes of deficient vitamin D include dietary inadequacy, decreased sunlight, malabsorption, hepatic disease and renal disease
- usually present with back pain or pathological fracture
- may also get proximal myopathy

Table 19.2 Classification of osteoporosis

Primary Postmenopausal or senile osteoporosis Juvenile idiopathic osteoporosis	

Secondary
Endocrine
  Cushing's disease
  Hyperparathyroidism
  Hyperthyroidism
  Acromegaly
  Hypogonadism
	Malignant disease
	  Carcinomatosis
	  Myelomatosis
	  Lymphoma

Mechanical
  Immobilisation
  Disuse
  Weightlessness
	Chronic disease
	  Rheumatoid arthritis
	  Tuberculosis
	  Renal disease
	  Ankylosing spondylitis

Drugs
  Corticosteroids
  Alcohol
  Heparin
	Inherited disorders
	  Osteogenesis imperfecta
	  Vitamin D-resistant rickets
	  Marfan's syndrome
	  Down's syndrome

Nutritional Generalised malnutrition or scurvy	

- serum calcium is low or normal
- microscopy shows increased ratio of unmineralised osteoid to mineralised bone
- Looser's zones or Milkman's fractures may be seen radiologically

Rickets

- childhood manifestation of defective bone mineralisation
- aetiology is similar to osteomalacia, but renal causes are more common
- in infants, head and chest are most commonly affected
- may get frontal bossing and squared appearance to head
- deformation of chest produces 'rachitic rosary' (swelling of costochondral junctions of ribs)
- may get pigeon-breast deformity

Paget's disease (osteitis deformans)

- unknown cause
- possibly due to a slow virus, e.g. measles
- increase in bone turnover with increased reabsorption and also increased formation of new disorganised bone
- may be divided into initial osteolytic stage, a mixed osteolytic and osteosclerotic stage and a burnt out quiescent osteosclerotic stage

CLINICAL

- common over 60 years
- slight male predominance
- occasionally one bone affected (monostotic Paget's disease), but usually multiple bones (polyostotic)
- may be incidental finding or may present with bone pain
- may get cranial nerve palsy due to base of skull entrapment by sclerotic bone
- may get bowing of tibia
- kyphosis of spine
- spinal stenosis
- new bone is vascular and rarely high output cardiac failure occurs
- serum calcium and phosphate are normal but increased calcium may occur if patient is immobilised
- high serum alkaline phosphatase is found with high urinary hydroxyproline
- radiology shows enlarged bones with thick coarsened cortex

PATHOLOGY

- histological hallmark is mosaic pattern of lamellar bone
- in initial lytic phase there is osteoclastic activity with resorptive pits
- see abnormally large osteoclasts
- in mixed phase there is prominent osteoblastic activity
- intervening fibrous stroma is very vascular

COMPLICATIONS

- nerve entrapment
- high output cardiac failure
- spinal stenosis
- fractures especially of the femur
- sarcomatous transformation may occur in 5–10% of patients with severe polyostotic disease
- may get osteosarcoma, fibrosarcoma, chondrosarcoma or malignant fibrous histiocytoma
- most commonly arise in long bones, pelvis, skull and spine
- Paget's sarcomas have a poor prognosis

FAT EMBOLISM SYNDROME

- syndrome of acute respiratory insufficiency associated with embolisation of bone marrow fat to lungs after musculoskeletal trauma
- many patients have some evidence of fat embolism after fractures of long bone but may not be clinically important
- may also occur after soft tissue trauma and burns

CLINICALLY

- respiratory distress
- petechial rash
- neurological symptoms, e.g. irritability, restlessness, delirium, coma
- tachycardia
- jaundice

- anaemia, low platelets and DIC may occur
- fatal in approximately 10% of cases
- diagnosis is by clinical suspicion and low PO_2 in absence of other causes of hypoxia

PATHOGENESIS

- mechanical obstruction of pulmonary and cerebral microvasculature by fat
- chemical injury due to free fatty acids released from fat globules resulting in toxic injury to vascular endothelium

PATHOLOGY

- globules of fat within alveolar and other capillaries
- may require frozen section and fat stains to demonstrate fat because this is dissolved out by routine pathological processing
- small vessels blocked with fat, fibrin, platelets and white blood cells
- loss of surfactant with small areas of atelectasis
- alveolar collapse results in segmental consolidation
- hyaline membranes form with fibroblastic proliferation
- later fibrous tissue formation occurs
- fat emboli in systemic circulation cause microinfarcts in viscera
- petechiae in skin and conjunctiva occur
- in central nervous system petechial haemorrhages occur in white matter and small vessels become blocked by fat with secondary haemorrhagic necrosis

AVASCULAR BONE NECROSIS

- usually present with bone pain and tenderness

CAUSES

- many cases are idiopathic
- trauma
- infection
- radiation therapy
- connective tissue disorders
- pregnancy
- alcohol abuse
- chronic pancreatitis
- Gaucher's disease

PATHOLOGY

- necrosis of bone and bone marrow with ingrowth of vascular granulation tissue
- later new bone forms by creeping substitution

The nervous system

20

NORMAL STRUCTURE

- brain is divided into forebrain, midbrain and hindbrain
- forebrain includes cerebral cortex, basal ganglia, lateral ventricles, thalamus, hypothalamus and third ventricle
- the cerebral cortex, basal ganglia and lateral ventricles form the cerebral hemispheres
- four basal ganglia are situated deep in the cerebral hemispheres
- the thalamus acts as a relay station for sensory pathways to the cerebral cortex
- the hypothalamus forms the floor of the third ventricle and is involved with autonomic nervous system control, cardiovascular regulation, temperature regulation, food intake and water balance, gastrointestinal activity and emotional responses
- the midbrain (mesencephalon) connects with the pons and the cerebrum
- the midbrain contains the nuclei of the third and fourth cranial nerves
- the hindbrain includes the cerebellum, pons, medulla and fourth ventricle
- the cerebellum lies in the posterior cranial fossa and consists of two hemispheres and a midline vermis
- the cerebellum receives input from all the sensory organs and via the motor centres it regulates equilibrium, muscle tone and posture
- the pons forms part of the floor of the fourth ventricle and is connected to the cerebellum via the middle cerebellar peduncle
- the pons plays a role in the regulation of respiration and contains nuclei of the Vth, VIth, VIIth and VIIIth cranial nerves
- the medulla is continuous with the spinal cord through the foramen magnum
- the nuclei of the IXth, Xth, XIth and XIIth cranial nerves reside in the medulla
- all spinal cord tracts are represented
- centres for control of cardiac and respiratory function lie in the medulla
- the pituitary gland consists of a vascular and cellular anterior lobe (adenohypophysis) and a less vascular posterior lobe (neurohypophysis). The latter is connected with the tuber cinereum via the pituitary stalk
- the pituitary fossa is roofed by a fold of dura, the diaphragma sellae
- the spinal cord extends from the foramen magnum to the lumbar area
- the tapering lower end of the spinal cord is termed the conus medullaris from which the filum terminale extends down to the coccyx

Circulation of cerebrospinal fluid (CSF)

- CSF is formed by the choroid plexus of the lateral, third and fourth ventricles. The two large lateral ventricles produce most of the CSF which flows into the third ventricle via the interventricular foramina of Monro

- from the third ventricle, CSF passes through the aqueduct of Sylvius into the fourth ventricle and from there into the subarachnoid space via the median and lateral openings of the foramina of Magendie and Luschka
- CSF is resorbed by the arachnoid villi which lie mainly in the superior sagittal sinus

Blood supply of the brain

- the brain is supplied by the internal carotid and vertebral arteries. These form an anastomosis around the optic chiasma and pituitary gland. This is termed the circle of Willis (Figure 20.1)

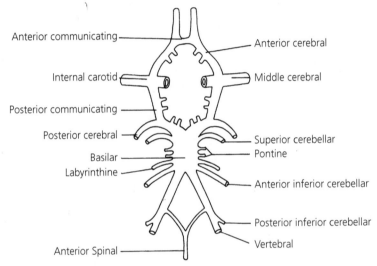

Anterior communicating
Anterior cerebral
Internal carotid
Middle cerebral
Posterior communicating
Posterior cerebral
Superior cerebellar
Basilar
Pontine
Labyrinthine
Anterior inferior cerebellar
Posterior inferior cerebellar
Anterior Spinal
Vertebral

Figure 20.1 Schematic diagram of the vascular supply to the brain

Meninges

- there are three meningeal layers, the dura mater, arachnoid mater and pia mater
- the dura mater lines the cranial vault and cranial fossae and extends down the spinal cord to the second sacral vertebra
- all venous sinuses except the inferior sagittal and straight sinuses lie between the periosteum and the dura mater
- arachnoid mater is applied to the inner surface of the dura
- the spinal subarachnoid space is large and communicates through the foramen magnum with the subarachnoid space of the posterior cranial fossa
- the pia mater invests the brain and spinal cord closely and contains small blood vessels

Histology

- central nervous system (CNS) contains neurons and neuroglial cells
- the cell bodies of the neurons reside in the grey matter or in the basal ganglia. Leaving each cell body is a single axon or nerve fibre which forms a synapse with other neurons or with the motor end-plates of striated muscles
- the non-neuronal cells of the CNS are termed neuroglia and are of four types:
  - *astrocytes* have numerous star-like processes and provide structural support
  - *oligodendrocytes* are responsible for myelination of axons and are the predominant cell in the white matter
  - *microglia* are small cells which become phagocytic in response to injury. They are related to macrophages
  - *ependymal* cells form the lining of the ventricular system and spinal canal
- the cerebrum has an outer layer of grey matter arranged in a variable number of layers
- the deep hemisphere consists mainly of white matter
- the spinal cord has an inner butterfly-shaped region of grey matter and an outer layer of white matter

CONGENITAL ABNORMALITIES

Craniosynostosis

- an abnormality of one or more of skull sutures leading to premature fusion and resultant deformity
- incidence is 1 in 20 000 births in the UK
- common form of the disease affects the sagittal suture and causes narrowing of the skull with elongation to compensate for brain growth
- produces a rise in intracranial pressure with neurological deficit if no corrective measures are undertaken

Encephalocoele

- herniation of meninges and brain tissue through a skull defect
- usually occur in occipital region of skull
- usually occipital lobes of brain and cerebellum herniate
- may occasionally occur in parietal and frontal regions of skull
- vary greatly in size and prognosis. Large lesions with an incomplete skin covering are frequently fatal

Anencephaly

- type of neural tube defect
- affected infants rarely survive more than a few hours
- head is flattened and the vault of skull and brain are replaced by a dark red soft mass of tissue
- histology shows vascular structures, glial tissue and choroid plexus
- may be associated with spina bifida
- associated with polyhydramnios
- may be detected by ultrasound from 12 weeks' gestation

Spina bifida, meningomyelocoele and meningocoele

- variants of neural tube defect
- abnormalities of neural tube in caudal region give rise to these conditions
- prenatal diagnosis may be made by high serum levels of α-fetoprotein
- incidence of neural tube defects varies throughout the world and is especially high in Northern Ireland
- spina bifida cystica affects 4.5 per 1000 live births
- mothers with a previously affected pregnancy may obtain a degree of protection from further abnormalities by folic acid and vitamin supplements
- twice as common in females as males
- in spina bifida occulta failure of fusion of the posterior vertebral arches occurs, most commonly in the lumbosacral region
- may have associated abnormalities of the overlying skin such as dimpling, pigmentation or patch of hair
- frequently asymptomatic, although neurological symptoms affecting the bladder and lower legs may develop in adult life
- spina bifida cystica is a more severe defect where both meningeal and neural tissue may be involved
- in a meningomyelocele, herniation of both meninges and neural tissue occurs through a bony defect in the vertebrae. The lesion usually consists of a sac of dura and arachnoid covered by skin and with spinal cord elements
- meningomyelocoeles most commonly occur in the lumbar region
- affected infants usually have denervation of leg musculature and sphincter problems in the bladder and rectum
- may get meningitis
- in a meningocoele, herniation of meninges occurs through a bony defect
- spinal cord may be in the correct position in a meningocoele
- may also have Arnold-Chiari malformation and develop hydrocephalus

Arnold-Chiari malformation

- consists of a series of abnormalities affecting mainly the medulla and cerebellum in children. A rare adult form is also recognised. In one type there is herniation of the cerebellar tonsils through the foramen magnum
- some forms may be associated with a meningomyelocoele
- more severe cases are associated with hydrocephalus

Hydrocephalus

- the majority of cases are caused by obstruction to the flow of CSF
- more rarely may be caused by excess production of CSF by a choroid plexus papilloma
- can be classified as *non-communicating* where the obstruction is within the ventricular system and CSF cannot pass into the subarachnoid space, or *communicating* where the obstruction is outside the ventricular system and there is communication between the subarachnoid space and the ventricular system
- hydrocephalus in the newborn or early in life may be due to stenosis or forking of the aqueduct of Sylvius, the Arnold-Chiari malformation (see above) or the Dandy-Walker malformation (occlusion of the foramina of the fourth ventricle)
- other causes of hydrocephalus are fibrosis of the subarachnoid space following meningitis and subarachnoid haemorrhage

- clinical features in children include enlarging head, bulging fontanelle, epilepsy, headache and mental retardation
- after infancy obstructive hydrocephalus is frequently due to a tumour in the posterior fossa, midbrain or third ventricle. Subarachnoid haemorrhage and meningitis may cause adhesions with resultant hydrocephalus
- occasionally no cause is found
- if hydrocephalus develops slowly, the inner skull table becomes eroded and diverticula of the ventricles form

INFECTION OF CNS

Meningitis

- may be due to bacterial, viral or fungal organisms
- infection is usually haematogenous, but direct spread may occur from the paranasal sinuses or may be secondary to penetrating injury
- can occur at any age
- predominant bacterial organisms are *Escherichia coli* in neonates, *Haemophilus influenzae* in infants and children, *Neisseria meningitidis* in teenagers and young adults and *Streptococcus pneumoniae* in elderly patients
- *N. meningitidis*, a Gram-negative diplococcus, is the commonest cause of bacterial meningitis in the UK
- the organism is found in the nasopharynx in 10% of the population
- *N. meningitidis* is frequently responsible for epidemics of meningitis, often associated with a skin rash
- septicaemia may lead to adrenal haemorrhage and circulatory collapse (Waterhouse-Friderichsen syndrome)
- patients who have had prior splenectomy are susceptible to pneumococcal meningitis
- clinical features of meningitis include pyrexia, headache, vomiting, coma, neck rigidity, photophobia and nuchal rigidity
- diagnosis is by lumbar puncture and CSF analysis.
- The CSF appears cloudy. In bacterial meningitis, polymorphs are present, the protein level is raised and the sugar level is decreased
- viral meningitis differs from bacterial in having a CSF lymphocytosis, a normal or only slightly raised protein concentration and a normal or slightly increased sugar content
- tuberculous meningitis and fungal meningitis are also associated with a CSF lymphocytosis
- tuberculous and fungal meningitis (e.g. *Cryptococcus*) are rare, but may be seen in immunosuppressed patients, e.g. AIDS
- macroscopic examination of bacterial meningitis shows fibrinous exudate and pus formation on the surface of the brain
- microscopic examination shows an acute inflammatory exudate consisting mainly of polymorphs
- in viral meningitis, the predominant inflammatory cells are lymphocytes
- in tuberculous meningitis, granulomas are seen histologically
- complications of meningitis include cerebral infarction due to thrombosis of a vessel, hydrocephalus due to fibrous adhesions and cranial nerve palsy
- bacterial meningitis requires prompt antibiotic therapy whereas viral meningitis is usually self-limiting

Brain abscess

- infection of the paranasal sinuses, the middle ear or the mastoid may spread directly to the brain causing frontal lobe, temporal lobe and cerebellar abscesses respectively
- incidence of brain abscess has fallen with effective antibiotic treatment for sinusitis, middle ear infections and mastoid infections
- a generalised systemic infection with haematogenous spread may cause metastatic abscesses in the brain
- metastatic brain abscesses most commonly develop in the area of brain supplied by the middle cerebral artery
- cyanotic congenital heart disease, e.g. Fallot's tetralogy may be associated with cerebral abscess
- cranial trauma (surgical or accidental) and chronic lung disease predispose to brain abscess
- brain abscesses may complicate bacterial endocarditis
- clinically there is usually initial evidence of a meningeal reaction followed by focal neurological signs
- abscess acts as a space-occupying lesion causing a rise in intracranial pressure (ICP) and may result in uncal and tonsillar herniation
- microscopically abscess contains cell debris and polymorphs with a surrounding zone of fibrous tissue
- surgery with drainage of abscess may be necessary
- epilepsy may occur after treatment of abscess

Spinal abscesses

- spinal abscesses are most commonly extradural
- haematogenous spread of infection to a vertebral body may result in a focus of osteomyelitis and accumulation of extradural pus
- may also occur secondary to spinal injuries or surgical trauma
- patients usually present with backache and nerve root pain with systemic upset
- cord compression eventually develops
- commonest causative organisms are staphylococci
- infection usually starts in adjacent vertebrae and destroys the intervertebral disc with collapse and kyphoscoliosis

AIDS and the central nervous system

- the CNS is frequently affected in AIDS patients (see Chapter 22)

CEREBROVASCULAR DISEASE

Transient ischaemic attacks

- a transient ischaemic attack (TIA) is an episode of focal neurological disturbance lasting for less than 24 hours and which is followed by total recovery
- TIAs are usually caused by atheroma of the carotid arteries. This may result in decreased blood flow or in peripheral embolism

- symptoms include contralateral weakness and numbness together with ipsilateral monocular blindness
- atheromatous plaques affecting the vertebral arteries cause vertigo, ataxia and diplopia
- rare causes of TIA include polycythaemia rubra vera, cardiac arrhythmias and hypotension
- TIAs may go on to complete stroke in the same anatomical territory
- benefits of surgery (endarterectomy) are most clearly seen in patients with severe carotid artery stenosis

Stroke

- a stroke is a focal neurological defect of sudden onset which lasts greater than 24 hours and which is due to vascular disease
- 85% of strokes are due to cerebral infarction and 15% due to intracerebral haemorrhage
- hypertension is the most important risk factor associated with stroke. Hypertension promotes the development of atheroma in the extra- and intracranial arteries. Microaneurysms of Charcot-Bouchard may be secondary to hypertension
- these aneurysms develop in the intracerebral branches of the major arteries, especially in branches of the middle cerebral artery. They may rupture and cause intracerebral haemorrhage
- smoking is also a major risk factor for stroke

Cerebral infarction

- most cases occur as a result of extracranial vascular disease
- cause may be occlusion of carotid or vertebral arteries by atheroma, embolism or hypotension which may occur secondary to myocardial infarction or cardiac arrhythmia
- emboli may arise in the heart, e.g. from the left atrium in patients with atrial fibrillation, from a mural thrombus following myocardial infarction or from infective endocarditis
- emboli may also arise from atheromatous plaques in aorta, carotid or vertebral arteries
- clinically cerebral infarction causes a reduction in the level of consciousness and neurological defect
- in cases of generalised cerebral hypoperfusion, the watershed areas of the cerebral circulation, e.g. between the anterior and middle cerebral arteries become infarcted (boundary zone infarction)
- other causes of cerebral infarction include cortical vein thrombosis due to infection or dehydration, cyanotic congenital heart disease producing septic emboli, congenital vascular malformations, traumatic injury to vessels of neck and arteritis involving the vertebral, carotid or intracerebral arteries
- macroscopic appearance of cerebral infarction depends on size of lesion and time of survival
- recent infarcts are soft and swollen. They may be anaemic or haemorrhagic depending upon whether some blood flow through the infarct has been restored
- the initial swelling and oedema may cause an increase in ICP and brain shift
- breakdown of the infarcted area occurs after some time and a fluid-filled cyst surrounded by gliosis remains

Intracerebral haemorrhage

- hypertension is most important risk factor
- clinical syndrome is of various neurological deficits, depending on the anatomical site
- hypertensive patients have a tendency to develop microaneurysms (Charcot-Bouchard aneurysms) in the intracerebral branches of the major arteries, especially the lenticulostriate branch of the middle cerebral artery. These microaneurysms rupture, resulting in intracerebral haemorrhage
- other lesions which may result in intracerebral haemorrhage include berry aneurysms (see below), vascular malformations, septic emboli resulting in mycotic aneurysms, amyloidosis, vasculitis, haemorrhage into an area of infarction, bleeding into intracranial tumours, trauma and bleeding diatheses
- grossly intracerebral haemorrhage tracks through the white matter and often ruptures into ventricles
- a rise in ICP may cause tentorial herniation and secondary midbrain haemorrhage
- an area of intracerebral haemorrhage may be difficult to distinguish from a haemorrhagic infarct

Subarachnoid haemorrhage (SAH)

- SAH is due to rupture of a berry aneurysm in approximately 65% of cases
- in up to 25% of cases no cause is found
- arteriovenous malformations account for approximately 5% of cases as do blood dyscrasias
- other causes of SAH include extension of an intracerebral haemorrhage into the subarachnoid space
- affected patients develop sudden headache and neck stiffness with or without neurological deficit. The level of consciousness may be lowered
- patients may progress rapidly to coma and death
- late complications if patient survives include cerebral infarction after an interval of 3–7 days. This is due to vasospasm in the artery distal to the aneurysm. Communicating hydrocephalus may develop due to presence of blood in the subarachnoid space causing arachnoiditis and impairing the resorption of CSF. Non-communicating hydrocephalus may also occur due to organisation and fibrosis

Berry aneuryms

- berry aneurysms (also known as saccular or congenital aneurysms) may occur *de novo* or in association with conditions such as the Ehlers-Danlos syndrome, coarctation of the aorta and polycystic kidneys. The incidence at various sites is given in Table 20.1
- occur in between 1 and 2% of the adult population
- more common in women
- may be multiple
- berry aneurysms vary in size and shape
- rupture of a berry aneurysm is the most common cause of SAH
- most often develop at bifurcation of arteries
- following SAH from a berry aneurysm, the greatest incidence of rebleeding occurs between the 5th and 9th days
- giant berry aneurysms may act as a space occupying lesion and patients may present with raised intracranial pressure, epilepsy or cranial nerve palsies

Table 20.1 Sites of berry aneurysms

Site	Percentage
Middle cerebral artery	19
Anterior cerebral and anterior communicating arteries	41
Internal carotid and posterior communicating arteries	37
Basilar artery circulation	3
Total	100

Other intracerebral aneurysms

- mycotic aneurysms are uncommon aneurysms in which an inflammatory reaction causes destruction of the internal elastic lamina and media with resultant weakness and dilatation of the wall. These may be due to septic emboli. Complications include intracerebral infarction or haemorrhage
- true traumatic aneurysms are rare. They most commonly involve vessels such as the anterior cerebral artery in relation to the falx or the carotid artery near the tentorium

HEAD INJURIES

- consequences of head injury include primary damage occurring at the time of the injury (cerebral contusions, lacerations of scalp, fracture of skull, diffuse axonal damage, intracranial haemorrhage) or secondary damage occurring as a complication of the injury (raised intracranial pressure, hypoxia, swelling, infection)

Primary brain damage

LOCALISED BRAIN DAMAGE

- when the brain moves within the skull as in a deceleration injury it does so about a fixed axis between the fixed parts (the brainstem) and the unfixed parts (cerebral hemispheres)
- localised brain damage is commonest in the frontal and temporal lobes which may become contused or lacerated
- localised brain damage may be at the site of impact (coup injury) or on the side of the brain diametrically opposite to the site of injury (contracoup injury)

DIFFUSE AXONAL INJURY

- the rotational forces between the relatively fixed brainstem and the unfixed cerebral hemispheres causes shearing forces which tear the axons of the white matter
- seen on cut section of the brain as small areas of haemorrhage, especially in the brainstem and corpus callosum

- usually bilateral, asymmetrical and associated with intraventricular bleeding
- usually get immediate prolonged unconsciousness
- the deeper the coma the more widespread the diffuse axonal damage
- microscopy shows evidence of widespread damage to axons in form of axonal retraction bodies

Secondary brain damage

- further clinical deterioration after primary brain damage is likely to be due to secondary damage

HAEMATOMA

- *extradural* haematoma is associated with a skull fracture and tearing of the middle meningeal artery or vein
- with extradural haematoma the patient often does not lose consciousness immediately, but has a lucid interval before the onset of symptoms
- with acute *subdural* haematoma the patient is less likely to have a lucid interval
- acute *intracerebral haematoma* produces focal signs and patients often fail to recover consciousness
- chronic subdural haematoma presents days or months after original trauma with confusion, fluctuating level of consciousness and focal neurological signs
- *subarachnoid haemorrhage* may occur in severe head injuries
- blood in the subarachnoid space produces vasospasm and further ischaemic damage

BRAIN SWELLING

- increase in brain volume may be due either to an increase in cerebral blood volume (congestive brain swelling) or to cerebral oedema
- cerebral oedema may occur adjacent to contusions
- brain swelling causes compression of cerebral capillaries and further ischaemic damage to the brain
- raised intracranial pressure causes brain shifts and herniations and eventually cerebral perfusion ceases and death ensues

INFECTION

- usually secondary to a compound skull fracture or to fracture of the skull resulting in portal of entry for organisms. Meningitis or brain abscess may ensue

HYPOXIA

- may occur as a consequence of brainstem damage, chest injury or aspiration
- hypoxia worsens cerebral ischaemia

HYPOTENSION

- may be due to blood loss, cardiac tamponade or spinal injury
- low systemic blood pressure, especially when associated with elevated intra-cranial pressure, decreases cerebral perfusion and worsens cerebral ischaemia

RAISED INTRACRANIAL PRESSURE AND BRAIN SHIFTS

- the various forms of secondary brain damage tend to cause serious complications via a final common pathway of raised intracranial pressure and brain shift
- when pressure increases above the tentorium, a shift of the cingulate gyrus occurs under the falx
- trans-tentorial herniation compresses the ipsilateral third cranial nerve causing dilatation of the pupil and ptosis
- brainstem distortion and ischaemia produce decerebrate rigidity
- compression of the posterior cerebral artery causes infarction of the medial occipital cortex
- displacement of the cerebellar tonsils from the posterior fossa through the foramen magnum into the spinal canal (tonsillar herniation) is associated with decrease in level of consciousness
- in tonsillar herniation death may occur due to compression of the medulla and the respiratory centre
- late sequelae of head injuries include epilepsy and hydrocephalus

PERIPHERAL NERVE INJURIES

- three types of nerve injury have been described:

NEUROPRAXIA

- a physiological block in conduction without anatomical axonal interruption
- caused by blunt injuries, high velocity missile injuries adjacent to the nerve, compression and ischaemia or excessive stretching of the nerve
- grossly the nerve appears intact and normal
- segmental demyelination is seen on microscopic examination
- complete return of motor and sensory function usually occurs

AXONOTEMESIS

- anatomical disruption of the axon without serious disruption of the endoneurial or perineurial framework
- results in motor and sensory loss distal to the injury secondary to axonal degeneration
- usually good return of function

NEUROTEMESIS

- partial or complete division of nerve with disruption of axons, myelin sheath and connective tissue support
- if the nerve is transected completely a proximal stump neuroma develops composed of disorganised and proliferating axons with connective tissue and Schwann cells (traumatic neuroma)
- recovery is poor

Chronic injuries of peripheral nerves

- compression by narrowing of the compartment through which nerve passes, e.g. carpal tunnel syndrome

- repetitive stretching as nerve passes over a structure such as a cervical rib
- impingement by narrowing of the normal boundaries of a compartment, e.g. thoracic outlet syndromes
- repeated dislocations, e.g. in ulnar paralysis

PRIMARY INTRACRANIAL TUMOURS

General

- sixth commonest malignant tumour in adults and second commonest in children
- meningiomas and neurilemmomas are more common in females, but other primary brain tumours are more common in males
- predisposing factors include the administration of ionising radiation in childhood. This results in an increased risk of meningioma and astrocytoma
- genetic associations include tuberous sclerosis (astrocytoma) and Turcot's syndrome (glioblastoma, medulloblastoma)
- prolonged immunosuppression is a risk factor for development of astrocytomas and malignant lymphomas
- neurilemmomas may develop in von Recklinghausen's disease
- primary intracranial tumours may arise from the brain or from other intracranial structures including the meninges, cranial nerves and pituitary gland
- tumours of the brain may arise from neurons, neuroglial cells or from blood vessels
- tumours of neurons or of neuroglial cells are termed neuroepithelial tumours. The majority of these are derived from neuroglial cells, e.g. astrocytomas, oligodendrogliomas and ependymomas
- neuronal tumours are very rare
- diagnosis is usually by CT or MRI combined with frozen section examination

Location

- in children two-thirds of brain tumours are infratentorial
- in adults two-thirds of tumours are supratentorial
- 60% of tumours in childhood are astrocytomas, arising in the cerebellum or brainstem
- medulloblastoma usually arises in the midline of the cerebellum
- ependymomas arise from the ventricular system of the brain
- craniopharyngiomas arise in the suprasellar region
- glioblastomas and astrocytomas are common in the frontal and temporal lobes, are less frequent in the parietal lobes and are uncommon in the occipital lobes
- haemangioblastomas are most common in the cerebellum, although they also occur in the medulla and spinal cord
- oligodendrogliomas occur in the cerebral hemispheres and rarely in the posterior fossa
- meningiomas occur at any site on the brain surface

Clinical features

- local effects include focal neurological deficits and epilepsy and are due to destruction of brain tissue and surrounding oedema

- epilepsy is especially associated with slowly growing oligodendrogliomas
- in silent areas such as the non-dominant temporal lobe, the corpus callosum, the frontal lobe and the thalamus, neurological signs occur late in the disease process
- increased ICP may result in headache, nausea or papilloedema and is due to either the mass of the tumour with surrounding oedema or to obstruction of the ventricular system. Eventually the rise in ICP may produce brain shifts
- tumours of the CNS in general do not metastasise

Tumours of neuroepithelial tissue

ASTROCYTOMAS

- occur as well differentiated cerebral tumours in children, especially in brainstem and cerebellum
- in adults, occur mainly in cerebral hemispheres
- tumour is ill-defined and merges into normal brain
- infiltration of the brain causes enlargement and distortion of the involved hemisphere
- tumour may spread across the corpus callosum
- clinical presentation depends upon site at which tumour arises
- usually slow-growing
- microscopically, although mixed cell types occur, most are predominantly of one cell type
- *fibrillary astrocytomas* consist of tumour cells containing abundant intracytoplasmic glial filaments
- *protoplasmic astrocytomas* are composed of stellate cells with fine processes
- *gemistocytic astrocytomas* are composed of plump cells with abundant eosinophilic cytoplasm
- *subependymal giant cell astrocytomas* arise in the thalamus in patients with tuberous sclerosis
- all these tumours are well differentiated (low grade) and contain regularly shaped cells with few mitotic figures
- astrocytomas frequently undergo progressive loss of differentiation and transform into *anaplastic astrocytomas*
- *pleomorphic xanthoastrocytomas* contain cells with abundant foamy cytoplasm. They have a good prognosis
- *pilocytic astrocytomas are well differentiated and have a better prognosis than other astrocytomas*
- they are composed of fusiform cells with wavy fibrillary processes which are hair-like (pilocytic)
- intracytoplasmic Rosenthal fibres may be found in pilocytic astrocytomas
- *anaplastic astrocytoma* contains areas of well differentiated astrocytoma together with anaplastic areas
- behaviour is intermediate between well differentiated astrocytoma and glioblastoma multiforme
- prognosis of astrocytoma depends upon grade and site of tumour
- brainstem astrocytomas are often inoperable due to involvement of vital structures
- cerebellar astrocytomas are resectable in children in the vast majority of cases
- prognosis of cerebral astrocytomas is more favourable in children
- brainstem astrocytomas are usually high grade tumours
- positive immunohistochemical staining for glial fibrillary acidic protein (GFAP) may aid in diagnosis

OLIGODENDROGLIOMAS

- account for approximately 3% of primary intracranial tumours
- occur at any age, but uncommon in children
- slowly growing tumours of the cerebral hemispheres, especially the frontal lobes
- rare in posterior fossa and spinal cord
- rarely, aggressive anaplastic form occurs
- typically present with epilepsy or slowly progressive focal neurological signs
- intracranial calcification is often seen on x-ray
- grossly oligodendrogliomas have a distinctive plum colour
- microscopically cells have small rounded nuclei with clear cytoplasm and distinct cell borders. Cells have a box-like appearance
- fine branched blood vessels are characteristic
- may stain positively with GFAP
- younger patients have a better prognosis than older patients

EPENDYMOMAS

- more common in children than in adults
- bimodal age distribution with a peak at 5 years and a smaller broader peak in adult life
- account for approximately 3% of primary intracranial tumours
- arise from the ependymal lining of the lateral, third and fourth ventricles and in the spinal cord
- most commonly arise from the fourth ventricle
- most in children are intracranial, whereas in adults they are equally distributed between the cranial cavity and the spine
- may spread throughout the subarachnoid space and rarely metastasise outside the CNS
- tend to be slow growing
- may present with hydrocephalus due to blockage of ventricular system
- microscopy shows small cells with rosette or pseudorosette formation
- when situated in the fourth ventricle, total removal is often impossible
- treatment has improved in recent years with surgical resection and postoperative radiotherapy
- myxopapillary ependymomas occur at the lower end of the spinal cord and arise from the filum terminale

CHOROID PLEXUS TUMOURS

- occur in the ventricular system of the brain
- may arise at any age
- often present with raised ICP due to obstruction of ventricular system
- uncommon, accounting for less than 1% of all primary intracranial tumours
- grossly papillary tumours attached to the ventricular wall
- most are well differentiated choroid plexus papillomas, but malignant choroid plexus carcinomas rarely occur
- microscopically papillomas are composed of fibrovascular cores covered by epithelium

GLIOBLASTOMA MULTIFORME

- commonest primary neuroepithelial tumour
- usually middle-aged and elderly patients

- clinical presentation depends on site of tumour but usually history is short
- account for approximately 30% of all primary intracranial tumours
- majority occur in the cerebral hemispheres, especially the frontal and temporal lobes
- on gross examination brain is usually heavy and swollen and tumour is irregular in shape, often with satellite nodules
- areas of haemorrhage and necrosis are common
- microscopically high grade tumours with marked nuclear pleomorphism
- get necrotic areas with surrounding palisading of tumour cells and proliferation of vascular endothelial cells
- treatment is usually palliative
- long-term survival is very poor
- glioblastomas may spread throughout the ventricular system of the brain and over the spinal cord and rarely metastasise outside the CNS
- may stain positively with GFAP

MEDULLOBLASTOMAS

- most common primitive neuroectodermal tumour (PNET) of brain
- occur predominantly in children and adolescents
- approximately 30% of intracranial tumours in childhood are medulloblastomas
- in young children usually arise in vermis in midline of cerebellum, but in young adults arise more laterally in cerebellum
- highly malignant tumours
- clinically present with ataxia, brainstem signs and vomiting
- hydrocephalus may result from obstruction of the fourth ventricle
- microscopically highly cellular and composed of small hyperchromatic cells with scanty cytoplasm
- may get rosette formation
- may get desmoplastic variant
- distant metastases outside the CNS occur rarely
- at operation as much tumour as possible is removed, and radiation is given to cover the entire CNS and spinal cord because of the seeding propensity of the tumour

Tumours of nerve sheath origin

SCHWANNOMAS

- synonyms include neurilemmoma and neurinoma
- neoplasm of Schwann cells
- tumours arise most commonly from the sensory cranial nerves, especially the vestibular division of the VIIIth nerve (acoustic neuroma)
- presentation of acoustic neuroma is deafness, tinnitus and enlargement of the internal auditory meatus
- also arise from dorsal spinal nerve roots
- most common in middle-aged adults
- more common in females
- if multiple, may be associated with von Recklinghausen's disease (neurofibromatosis)
- grossly encapsulated neoplasms
- microscopically composed of spindle-shaped cells with wavy nuclei arranged in Antoni A areas (nuclei are arranged in parallel bundles) and Antoni B areas (hypocellular myxoid areas)

- may get degenerative changes
- immunohistochemically stain diffusely positive with S-100 protein
- Schwannomas are extremely slow growing
- malignant Schwannomas are rare in the cranium or spine but are more common in peripheral nerves

NEUROFIBROMAS

- composed of Schwann cells, fibroblasts and other cellular elements
- often multiple and occasionally malignant
- rarely occur intracranially
- may be associated with von Recklinghausen's disease
- immunohistochemically stain focally positive with S-100 protein

Tumours of meninges

MENINGIOMAS

- rare in children and most common in older adults
- originate from the arachnoid layer of the meninges
- more common in females
- account for approximately 15% of all primary intracranial tumours
- increased incidence in von Recklinghausen's disease
- increased incidence of carcinoma of breast with meningiomas
- clinically usually present as slowly growing space-occupying lesion
- may result in neurological defects if present at base of skull
- may arise from spinal cord
- typical feature is the presence of thickening of the adjacent skull bone which may be either internal (endostosis) or external (exostosis)
- 90% of meningiomas are supratentorial
- grossly encapsulated firm tumours which indent the underlying brain
- rarely forms a flat sheet of tumour on the inner aspect of the dura (meningioma en plaque)
- several microscopic subtypes occur, including *meningothelial, fibroblastic, transitional* and *psammomatous*
- vast majority are benign, but malignant forms occur
- vascularity and frequent inaccessible site may make surgery difficult
- recurrence depends on the completeness of removal

Primary malignant lymphomas

- very rare tumours in immunocompetent patients
- primary cerebral lymphomas increasing in incidence because of association with AIDS and renal transplant patients
- usually high grade non-Hodgkin's lymphomas of B-cell lineage
- usually present with focal neurological signs, epilepsy or raised intracranial pressure
- often have multiple deposits in the brain and the usual treatment is irradiation of the entire brain
- tumour cells characteristically aggregate around blood vessels
- positive immunohistochemical staining for lymphoid markers aids in diagnosis
- prognosis is very poor
- must exclude distant spread from lymphoma elsewhere

Tumours of vascular origin

HAEMANGIOBLASTOMAS

- occur mainly in adults
- most common in the cerebellum, but also occur in the spinal cord
- supratentorial haemangioblastomas are rare
- relatively benign course
- clinically present with cerebellar signs, e.g. ataxia and raised ICP
- in some cases there is polycythaemia due to erythropoietin production by the tumour
- occur in von Hippel-Lindau syndrome where they are often multiple (includes renal and pancreatic cysts, renal cell carcinoma and phaeochromocytoma)
- this syndrome is associated with a mutation on the short arm of chromosome 13
- microscopically composed of numerous vascular channels lined by plump endothelial cells and surrounded by lipid-laden vacuolated cells

Other malformative tumours and tumour-like conditions

CRANIOPHARYNGIOMAS

- occur in both children and adults but with a peak incidence in the second decade
- cystic or solid mass at base of brain
- arise from remnants of Rathke's pouch
- commonly suprasellar (94%)
- presents as space-occupying lesion with headache or with visual disturbance or with endocrine dysfunction due to pituitary or hypothalamic damage
- radiological calcification is seen in many cases
- grossly many are cystic and are filled with fluid containing cholesterol crystals
- cyst lining is commonly squamous epithelium
- solid areas of the tumour consist of squamous and columnar epithelium embedded in fibrous stroma
- craniopharyngiomas are slow growing
- may invade the surrounding brain making complete excision difficult
- rupture with release of keratin or cholesterol crystals may cause sterile fibrosing meningitis

EPIDERMOID CYSTS

- may occur at any age
- most common site is cerebellopontine angle
- may present with raised ICP or with sterile meningitis due to release of contents
- microscopically lined by squamous epithelium without skin appendage structures

DERMOID CYSTS

- much less common than epidermoid cysts
- microscopically lining is squamous epithelium with skin appendages in wall
- most commonly occur in posterior fossa, in ventricles, at base of brain or in spinal cord

COLLOID CYSTS

- benign cysts at the anterior end of the third ventricle near the foramina of Monro
- may cause acute hydrocephalus and sudden death
- macroscopically thin-walled cysts containing soft colloid material
- microscopically lined by columnar or cuboidal epithelium, often containing cilia
- transventricular surgery and complete resection is the treatment of choice

VASCULAR MALFORMATIONS

- cavernous angiomas are often multiple and may result in focal neurological signs, epilepsy and subarachnoid haemorrhage
- cerebral hemispheres and pons are most commonly affected areas
- grossly consist of a tangled mass of blood vessels
- microscopically composed of thick and thin-walled blood vessels
- arteriovenous malformations consist of mixture of arteries and veins
- commonly present in second to fourth decades with neurological signs, epilepsy, subarachnoid or intracerebral haemorrhage or headaches
- most common site is supratentorial region, especially in distribution of middle cerebral arteries
- microscopically composed of tangle of arteries and veins, surrounded by areas of gliosis with haemorrhage
- Sturge-Weber-Dimitri syndrome is characterised by a port wine stain on the face, localised to the region supplied by the trigeminal nerve and a vascular malformation of the ipsilateral cerebral hemispheres. There is atrophy and calcification in the surrounding brain

Tumours of the anterior pituitary gland

PITUITARY ADENOMAS

- majority occur in adults
- may be hormone secreting (approximately 75%) or non-functioning (approximately 25%)
- x-ray may reveal enlargement of the pituitary fossa
- hormone-secreting tumours usually present with symptoms related to the production of a single hormone, e.g. acromegaly or Cushing's disease
- non-functioning tumours usually present as a space-occupying lesion or with pan-hypopituitarism
- many pituitary adenomas are small (microadenoma)
- adenomas which secrete growth hormone cause gigantism in prepubertal children and acromegaly in adults
- adenomas which secrete prolactin (prolactinomas) are the most common functioning adenomas of the pituitary
- females with prolactinomas present with amenorrhoea, galactorrhoea and infertility
- in males the adenoma may be clinically silent but may cause infertility and decreased libido
- prolactinomas may be treated medically with bromocriptine
- adrenocorticotrophic hormone (ACTH)-secreting adenomas cause Cushing's disease
- hyperthyroidism may result from TSH-secreting adenomas
- rarely more than one hormone may be secreted by an adenoma

- pituitary adenomas may also secrete follicle stimulating hormone and luteinising hormone
- non-functioning pituitary adenomas produce symptoms at a late stage when they are large. Clinical symptoms may be caused by compression of the optic chiasma or thalamus
- progressive destruction of the pituitary gland may eventually result in pan-hypopituitarism
- adenomas 10 mm in diameter or less are termed microadenomas
- microscopically pituitary adenomas are composed of regular cells growing in sheets or nests or a variety of other patterns
- immunohistochemistry may be used to demonstate hormone produced by tumour cells
- electron microscopy may reveal secretory granules of characteristic size and density

PITUITARY CARCINOMA

- primary carcinoma of the anterior pituitary is very rare

METASTATIC TUMOURS IN THE CENTRAL NERVOUS SYSTEM

- blood-borne either via the arterial supply or via the vertebral veins which do not contain valves and which allow retrograde flow
- deposits are usually discrete and often occur in the cerebral hemispheres
- secondary deposits are often multiple
- frequently occur in the distribution of the middle cerebral artery or in the cerebellar hemispheres
- commonest primary sites of tumour are lung, skin (malignant melanoma), kidney, colon, soft tissue and breast

SPINAL TUMOURS

- extradural tumours arise in the space between the dura and the vertebral column
- extradural tumours may be secondary or rarely neurofibromas or meningiomas may occur
- commonest intradural tumours are meningiomas, which are usually situated outside the spinal cord (extramedullary)
- other extramedullary intradural tumours include Schwannomas which arise from the spinal nerves
- intramedullary, intradural tumours include ependymomas, astrocytomas and vascular tumours
- myxopapillary ependymomas characteristically arise at the lower end of the spinal cord
- clinically symptoms are related to the spinal cord or to spinal nerve roots
- cord symptoms include spastic weakness below the lesion followed by sensory loss and sphincter disturbance
- involvement of anterior nerve roots causes lower motor neuron-type of weakness
- involvement of the posterior root causes pain
- diagnosis is aided by myelography, CT and MRI scanning

TUMOURS OF PERIPHERAL NERVES

Schwannomas

- neoplasm of Schwann cells
- see p. 316

NEUROFIBROMAS

- see p. 317
- consist of mixture of Schwann cells with other cell types
- more commonly arise from peripheral nerves
- grossly presents with skin nodule
- microscopically composed of fibroblasts, Schwann cells and other cell types
- rarely get malignant change

Neurofibromatosis (von Recklinghausen's disease)

- inherited as autosomal dominant disorder
- in type I neurofibromatosis these are multiple neurofibromas, café-au-lait spots, megacolon, vascular lesions, gastrointestinal stromal tumours and various brain tumours
- the responsible gene (NFI) is located on chromosome 17
- may get development of malignant peripheral nerve sheath tumours
- type II (central) neurofibromatosis is due to an abnormality of a gene located on chromosome 22
- characterised by a variety of CNS tumours, especially bilateral acoustic schwannnomas
- meningiomas, astrocytomas and tumours of other types also occur

Organ transplantation 21

NOMENCLATURE

Allograft

- donor and recipient are not immunologically identical

Isograft

- donor and recipient are identical twins

Xenograft

- transplant between different species

Matching

- ABO blood group
- HLA (human leucocyte antigens) on chromosome 6
- HLA peptide matching

Contraindications for donors

- extracranial malignancy
- infection (donors are screened for CMV, AIDS, hepatitis viruses)
- generalised disease

PATHOLOGY OF ALLOGRAFT REJECTION

Classification

- hyperacute rejection – occurs with minutes
- acute rejection – occurs in first few weeks
  - cellular
  - humeral/vascular
- chronic rejection – occurs after a few weeks

HYPERACUTE REJECTION

- this rarely occurs and is caused by preformed circulating antibodies to antigens on graft
- rejection is rapid (within minutes) and caused by damage to endothelium. Platelet aggregation and DIC occurs
- organ becomes swollen and cyanotic
- hyperacute rejection is irreversible and organ infarcts often occur
- occasionally occurs in kidney and liver

ACUTE REJECTION

- occurs in first few weeks after transplantation
- patient is often unwell with a temperature
- manifested by decreased function of donor organ
- cellular and humeral (vascular) types occur

Acute cellular rejection

- microscopy shows interstitial mononuclear cell infiltration (T lymphocytes, activated macrophages, plasma cells). Cells also infiltrate epithelial structures, e.g. renal tubules, biliary or bronchial epithelium
- damage occurs due to production of lymphokines and due to direct cytotoxicity
- lymphocytes of recipient interact with endothelial cells in transplant which function as antigen presenting cells
- acute cellular rejection is reversible with increased immunosuppression

Acute humeral or vascular rejection

- occurs when antibodies to donor antigens develop following transplantation
- microscopically medium and small arteries are usually affected, e.g. interlobular arteries in kidneys
- the arterial intima becomes oedematous with infiltration by mononuclear cells
- disruption of elastic fibres and fibrinoid necrosis
- in kidney glomeruli may become necrotic
- arterial thrombosis occurs which may result in infarcts
- interstitial haemorrhage and microinfarcts are common
- grossly surface of kidney showing humeral rejection is flea bitten

CHRONIC REJECTION

- occurs after weeks or months or later
- microscopy shows thickening of arteries or arterioles
- ischaemic damage occurs to organ

DIFFERENTIAL DIAGNOSIS OF TRANSPLANT REJECTION

Recurrence of original disease

CYCLOSPORIN A TOXICITY

- cyclosporin A is used as part of immunosuppressive regimen in renal transplant patients
- may result in nephrotoxicity

- tubulo-interstitial or glomerular scarring
- vacuolation of tubular cells and giant mitochondria occur
- hyaline change in arterioles

INFECTION

- opportunistic infections occur due to immunosuppression
- may be due to reactivation of latent infection, especially CMV

MALIGNANCY DEVELOPING IN TRANSPLANT PATIENTS

- most common malignancy is non-Hodgkin's B-cell lymphoma (post-transplant lymphoproliferative disorder)
- most of these lymphomas are EBV driven
- Kaposi's sarcoma may also occur
- skin and anogenital squamous lesions may also occur due to infection by HPV
- there is an increased risk of CNS tumours

SIDE EFFECTS OF IMMUNOSUPPRESSION

- infection
- malignancy
- bone marrow toxicity
- Cushing's syndrome (due to steroids)
- hirsutism and diabetes and other side-effects of steroids

RENAL TRANSPLANTATION

- rejection, recurrence of original disease, cyclosporin A toxicity and infections may all occur
- may be monitored by renal biopsy
- malignancy and some infections are contraindications to renal transplant
- other complications include:

Acute tubular necrosis (ATN)

- common especially if donor ischaemia
- get slow return of renal function postoperatively with decreased urine output
- may be confirmed on renal biopsy with flattening of tubular epithelium and casts within lumina of tubules. Mitotic figures in tubular epithelium suggest regenerative activity
- FNA can be useful in diagnosing ATN and distinguishing this from rejection

Obstruction

- Bowman's spaces surrounding glomeruli may be dilated and contain casts of Tamm-Horsfall protein
- tubular dilatation may be seen and tubules may contain casts
- presence of neutrophils in tubules indicates superimposed infection

Glomerulonephritis (GN)

- may be due to *de novo* or recurrent GN
- membranoproliferative GN (dense deposit type II) is most likely type of GN to recur
- IgA nephropathy and focal segmental glomerulosclerosis may also recur
- membranous GN may occur *de novo* or may be secondary to infection, e.g. hepatitis B

Renal vein thrombosis

- characterised by rapid deterioration of renal function

CARDIAC TRANSPLANTATION

- rejection is more common in heart than in other organs
- rejection is usually monitored by biopsy
- transvenous endomyocardial biopsy is most commonly utilised
- contraindications to cardiac transplantation include malignancy, HIV infection and some other infections
- in acute rejection microscopy shows interstitial oedema, lymphocytic infiltration and myocyte necrosis
- myocyte necrosis usually implies severe rejection
- as changes may be patchy in myocardium, several biopsies (usually four) should be taken
- in chronic rejection there is narrowing of coronary arteries due to fibromuscular thickening

LUNG TRANSPLANTATION

- risk of infection with CMV, pneumocystis and fungi
- infections are usually diagnosed by sputum culture and bronchiolo-aolveolar lavage
- rejection is usually diagnosed by transbronchial biopsies
- microscopy shows a perivascular mononuclear cell infiltrate
- get fibrointimal thickening of blood vessels
- bronchiolitis obliterans may occur
- graft versus host disease may occur from peribronchial lymphoid tissue within the transplant
- graft versus host disease is manifested by diarrhoea, skin rash and bone marrow failure
- combined heart and lung transplant may be performed and is monitored by endomyocardial and transbronchial biopsy

LIVER TRANSPLANTATION

- HLA matching is less important than in other organs
- usually monitored by liver biopsy
- hyperacute rejection rarely occurs

- acute cellular rejection is characterised by infiltration of portal tracts by T lymphocytes and other lymphoid cells
- microscopy shows swollen endothelial cells
- get infiltration of biliary epithelium by lymphoid cells
- changes may be focal and may be missed on biopsy
- in chronic rejection there is arterial narrowing due to fibro-intimal hyperplasia and infiltration by foamy histiocytes
- bile ductules are also damaged. They become fibrosed and destroyed
- infection may also occur
- ascending cholangitis may develop
- CMV or EBV infection may occur
- recurrent disease in the liver may also be a problem, e.g. viral hepatitis and autoimmune diseases such as primary biliary cirrhosis

PANCREATIC TRANSPLANTATION

- difficult to biopsy pancreas after transplantion
- pancreas is susceptible to ischaemic changes
- vascular thrombosis is quite common
- in acute rejection mononuclear cell infiltration and endovasculitis occur
- duct obstruction may occur resulting in pancreatitis

SMALL BOWEL TRANSPLANTATION

- ischaemic injury to mucosa may result in bacterial invasion and sepsis
- more prone to rejection than other solid organs
- graft versus host disease may occur due to abundant lymphoid tissue within graft
- cyclosporin A is toxic to the gut vasculature

Acquired immune deficiency syndrome (AIDS)

FEATURES

- definition includes patients with laboratory evidence of HIV infection and with a number of specified diseases. Such diseases include oesophageal, tracheal or pulmonary candidiasis, cryptosporidosis, herpes simplex or cytomegalovirus (CMV) infection, *Pneumocystis carinii* pneumonia, atypical mycobacterial infection, Kaposi's sarcoma or cerebral lymphoma
- causative virus is human immunodeficiency virus (HIV-1)
- a related virus HIV-II, which also causes AIDS, has been identified in West Africa
- HIV belongs to the Lentivirinae subfamily of retroviruses
- virus produces cytopathic effects in the CD4 subset of human T lymphocytes
- this deficiency of CD4 lymphocytes (helper/inducer lymphocytes) causes a state of profound immunodeficiency
- remarkable heterogeneity of the envelope protein around the virus
- the CD4 molecule, as well as being present on T lymphocytes, is found in lower density in other cells such as macrophages and some B lymphocytes. The CD4+ T lymphocyte has a central role in the immune response interacting with macrophages, other T lymphocytes, B lymphocytes and natural killer cells

SPREAD

- principal mode of spread of HIV virus is sexual intercourse
- may spread by intravenous drug abusers sharing contaminated needles
- transfusion of infected blood or blood products
- donated organs or semen
- may also spread from mother to fetus
- needlestick injury and mucosal exposure to infected blood or body fluids are potentially dangerous, but risk of infection is small
- virus is widespread and is found throughout body fluids of infected patients, but semen and blood are especially infectious
- homosexual men remain at greatest risk of HIV infection
- intravenous drug abusers constitute a high risk group
- haemophiliacs were infected before the introduction of screening of blood and blood products. Spread via transfusion of infected blood has been eradicated in western countries since screening was introduced. The risk of infection by this route remains high in countries with inadequate screening of blood
- in central Africa the male:female ratio of HIV positivity is almost equal and heterosexual intercourse appears to be the principal mode of spread. Perinatal transmission is also important

CLINICAL FEATURES

- following infection seroconversion takes place within 6 weeks
- this process of seroconversion may be asymptomatic, but some patients develop fever, sore throat, arthralgia, lymphadenopathy and a rash
- patients then move into an asymptomatic phase with the development of antibodies to core and surface proteins
- viraemia is detected by the presence of the core protein (p24) and this precedes the appearance of IgG and IgM antibodies to the entire virus
- progression of disease is marked by a fall in CD4 helper/inducer lymphocytes
- following the acute phase many patients have persistent generalised lymphadenopathy (PGL) involving chiefly cervical, axillary and submandibular lymph nodes
- most individuals develop progressive disease after a median time of 7–10 years
- non-specific constitutional symptoms such as night sweats, diarrhoea, weight loss and fever develop
- opportunistic infections such as oral candidiasis, oral hairy leukoplakia, herpes zoster, oral or genital herpes simplex and other infective skin conditions occur
- the final phase is characterised by further constitutional symptoms of fever, weight loss, diarrhoea, neurological disease, dementia, myelopathy and peripheral neuropathy together with other secondary infections such as candidiasis, tuberculosis, salmonella, herpes zoster, cytomegalovirus and *Pneumocystis carinii* pneumonia
- malignancies such as Kaposi's sarcoma and non-Hodgkin's lymphoma may also develop

MANIFESTATIONS OF AIDS IN ORGAN SYSTEMS

Lymph nodes

- persistent generalised lymphadenopathy (PGL) is common prior to the onset of fully developed AIDS
- microscopically in the early stages the enlarged lymph nodes exhibit an increase in the size and number of lymphoid follicles. The follicles contain prominent germinal centres and outside the follicles there is a proliferation of immunoblasts and plasma cells
- with increasing immunodeficiency and decrease in CD4 count, lymph nodes later show follicular involution and lymphocyte depletion
- within extrafollicular areas there is marked depletion of lymphocytes and increased vascularity
- other conditions which may involve lymph nodes in AIDS include Kaposi's sarcoma, malignant lymphoma and mycobacterial infection (especially atypical mycobacteria). Malignant lymphomas are usually high grade, non-Hodgkin's and of B-cell lineage

Lungs

- *Pneumocystis carinii* pneumonia is the commonest manifestation of AIDS in the lung
- the organism is pathogenic only in the presence of immunodeficiency

- usually present with protracted cough, dyspnoea and fever
- chest x-ray shows bilateral prehilar shadowing, mainly involving the middle and lower zones of the lungs
- diagnosis is by broncho-alveolar lavage or transbronchial biopsy
- microscopy shows pink foamy exudate within alveolar spaces
- organism exhibits positivity with silver stains and Grocott's methanamine silver stain is useful in diagnosis
- cytomegalovirus (CMV) infection is also common in AIDS
- often occurs in association with *P. carinii* pneumonia – microscopy shows interstitial pneumonitis with thickening of alveolar walls, lymphocytic infiltration and proliferation of pneumocytes
- the pathognomonic microscopic feature is characteristic large intranuclear inclusions surrounded by a clear halo (owl's eye appearance)
- immunohistochemical staining with antibodies against CMV may assist in diagnosis
- atypical mycobacterial infection with organisms such as *Mycobacteria avium intracellulare* and *Mycobacterium kansasii* is also frequent
- the incidence of *Mycobacterium tuberculosis* infection is also increased
- unusual inflammatory reactions occur in immunodeficient AIDS patients and classical necrotising granulomatous inflammation may not be seen in tuberculosis
- atypical mycobacteria elicits a histiocytic reaction and the histiocytes contain abundant intracytoplasmic organisms
- Ziehl-Neelsen stain is useful in demonstrating acid-fast bacilli in mycobacterial infection
- bacterial pneumonia with the usual organisms is also common
- candidal infection may occur secondary to oral candidiasis
- invasive aspergillosis may occur
- pulmonary *Cryptococcus* infection produces focal, miliary or pneumonic lesions. Lung involvement may be part of generalised cryptococcosis involving meninges, liver, kidneys and other organs
- *Toxoplasmosis* and *Histoplasmosis* infection may also occur
- Kaposi's sarcoma may involve the lungs and may produce multiple haemorrhagic lesions
- malignant lymphoma may involve the lungs

Mouth and gastrointestinal tract

- the mouth and gastrointestinal tract are affected in many AIDS cases
- AIDS enteropathy is the generic term which includes all the non-neoplastic disorders which may occur in the intestine in AIDS patients
- gingivitis and dental abscesses are common
- oral candidiasis is common
- oral hairy leukoplakia is almost pathognomonic of AIDS and consists of white shaggy patches on the lateral margins or undersurface of tongue
- microscopically hairy leukoplakia shows hyperkeratosis and acanthosis with balloon degeneration of keratinocytes
- reactivation of Epstein-Barr virus (EBV) infection is thought to be causative in the development of hairy leukoplakia
- retrosternal pain and dysphagia are common due to oesophageal ulceration. Ulceration is usually due to candidal infection (secondary to oral candidiasis) or to CMV or herpes simplex virus (HSV) infection

- histological diagnosis is difficult in small biopsies. Therefore special stains for fungi (PAS) or immunohistochemistry for CMV or HSV are useful
- intestinal infection with diarrhoea, malabsorption and weight loss is common in AIDS
- the commonest infecting organism causing diarrhoea is the protozoan *Cryptosporidium*. The organism infects both the large and small intestine
- in histological sections the organism appears as a small basophilic spherule attached to the luminal surface of the gut
- cytomegalovirus (CMV) is a common cause of gastrointestinal infection in AIDS
- ulceration occurs in colon and also in small intestine
- diarrhoea is the most common symptom, but occasionally intestinal perforation or severe haemorrhage occur
- microscopic diagnosis depends on recognition of the characteristic inclusions or identification of infected cells by immunohistochemistry
- microsporidosis causes diarrhoea in a significant number of AIDS patients. The organism (an intracellular protozoan, *Enterocytozoon bieneusi*) is best identified in a small intestinal biopsy. Giemsa stains may be useful in diagnosis as well as electron microscopy
- *Giardia lamblia* is a common protozoon with a worldwide distribution. It infects the upper small intestine and may cause diarrhoea and malabsorption. Infection may occur in healthy patients but is increased in patients with AIDS
- the organism may be identified in a duodenal aspirate or in a duodenal or jejunal biopsy. Cyst detection in faeces may also be diagnostic
- *Isospora belli* is a protozoan organism which may cause infection in AIDS patients
- organisms can be seen on the surface of enterocytes in small bowel or on rectal biopsy
- *Salmonella* infection is also common in AIDS and may be a cause of diarrhoea
- *Mycobacterium avium intracellulare* infection may occur in AIDS. Organisms may be identified on Ziehl-Neelsen staining
- anorectal ulceration and proctitis are common, especially in homosexual males. Infection by *Neisseria gonorrhoeae, Treponema pallidum, Entamoeba histolytica* and herpes simplex virus may occur
- anal intraepithelial neoplasia (AIN) and anal squamous carcinomas may occur, especially in homosexuals
- acalculous cholecystitis may occur in AIDS patients
- Kaposi's sarcoma and malignant lymphomas may develop in the gastrointestinal tract in AIDS patients

Skin

- dermatological problems are very common in patients with AIDS
- seborrhoeic dermatitis is common in AIDS
- herpes simplex infection may result in severe prolonged, painful ulceration
- herpes zoster infection is also common
- molluscum contagiosum occurs in many patients. Lesions may be multiple and are often unusually large
- anal and genital condylomata caused by human papilloma virus (HPV) infection are common
- anal intraepithelial neoplasia (AIN) and invasive anal squamous carcinomas may occur
- other cutaneous squamous carcinomas caused by HPV infection may occur

- HIV infection and syphilis may coexist
- bacterial infections such as impetigo and folliculitis may occur
- fungal infection may occur
- the skin may be involved by tumours such as Kaposi's sarcoma and malignant lymphoma
- bacillary angiomatosis presents as a cutaneous lesion and is caused by a rickettsia-like organism (*Rochalimaea quintana*). Microscopically it consists of vascular tissue containing clusters of organisms which may be demonstrated using the Warthin Starre stain

Nervous system

- the central and peripheral nervous system are commonly affected in AIDS
- over 50% of HIV-infected patients eventually develop cerebral abnormalities which include dementia, meningoencephalitis, encephalopathy involving the white matter, peripheral neuropathy and myositis
- opportunistic infections of the central nervous system are common, including cryptococcal meningitis, toxoplasmosis and CMV
- may also get retinitis and progressive multifocal leukoencephalopathy (PML)
- neurosyphilis may occur
- some develop cerebral lymphomas. These are usually high grade B-cell lymphomas
- Kaposi's sarcoma has not been described in the brain
- the AIDS dementia complex is characterised by motor, cognitive and behavioural abnormalities. This is seldom seen in the early asymptomatic phase of HIV infection and is associated with increasing immunosuppression as the disease progresses. Symptoms range from loss of concentration and forgetfulness to slowing of speech and mental responses. In late stages severe dementia may occur

AIDS-RELATED NEOPLASMS

- these include Kaposi's sarcoma, malignant lymphoma, oral, cutaneous and cervical squamous carcinoma and cloacogenic anorectal carcinoma
- Kaposi's sarcoma is common in central and southern Africa. In these countries it has a chronic indolent course, occurring mainly on the lower legs of elderly men. Kaposi's sarcoma is the commonest AIDS-related neoplasm and in patients with AIDS it behaves in an aggressive fashion
- multiple lesions affecting skin, gastrointestinal tract, mouth, lymph nodes, lungs and other organs may occur
- in skin the early stages appear as flat purple or dark red lesions usually on the trunk, arms, legs or face. This is known as the patch stage. Later plaque and nodular stages develop
- microscopy of the well-established lesion shows a cellular tumour composed of interlacing fascicles of spindle cells forming vascular channels
- complications of Kaposi's sarcoma include ulceration and infection with bleeding and anaemia
- radiotherapy may be effective for early skin lesions but recurrence is common
- malignant lymphoma is common in AIDS patients, usually high grade non-Hodgkin's of B-cell lineage
- these lymphomas behave aggressively and are often extranodal

- primary cerebral lymphoma is usually rare, but there is a markedly increased incidence in AIDS
- cerebral lymphoma in AIDS has a poor prognosis
- other sites frequently involved are the gastrointestinal tract, mucocutaneous junctions and bone marrow
- cutaneous and anogenital squamous carcinomas may occur in AIDS secondary to HPV infection

Index

Page numbers in *italics* refer to figures and tables.